Hearing Disorders

HEARING DISORDERS

SECOND EDITION

Edited by

Jerry L. Northern, Ph.D.

Professor of Otolaryngology,
University of Colorado School of Medicine;
Head, Division of Audiology,
University Hospital, Denver

Allyn and Bacon
Boston • London • Toronto • Sydney • Tokyo • Singapore

ISBN 0-205-13539-0

Printed in the United States of America

98 97 96 95 94 93   10 9 8 7 6 5 4 3 2

In memory of my deaf grandparents, T. Y. and Edna,
who provided the spark of my interest in hearing disorders,
and who were always there when I needed help.

Contents

Preface

Although hearing impairment is a communicative disorder about which much is known, significant gaps in our knowledge preclude total success in treatment of patients with hearing handicaps. The management of persons with hearing disorders is the responsibility of numerous professionals, many of whom view the handicap from different perspectives. Information about hearing loss is published in a broad variety of professional journals, textbooks, popular magazines, and trade publications. These materials are not always easily available to persons interested in learning more about hearing disorders.

The purpose of this book is to provide general information about the medical aspects of hearing impairment in easily understood chapters written by some of the nation's foremost authorities on hearing problems. My goal is to provide a comprehensive review of the clinical implications of hearing disorders and an overview of the techniques currently in use to evaluate hearing problems, including contemporary approaches to the treatment and management of persons with hearing impairment, tinnitus, and dizziness.

Hearing-impaired persons represent the major concern of specialists in a wide variety of professional areas, and they are also of peripheral interest for many service-oriented and allied health personnel. Although each group of specialists may focus its attention on different aspects of the hearing problem, a common core of background knowledge is essential. Unfortunately, little cross-disciplinary teaching is used in most training programs. Audiologists train audiologists; educators educate educators; and physicians teach physicians. As a result, training has been specialized to the utmost —possibly to the detriment of the person with the hearing loss.

This book brings together in a single text specialists in a wide variety of fields. Each has written here about the current status of basic auditory science and the clinical arts in their area of expertise. This book provides medical background information for nonmedical readers as well as basic reference material for physicians. Among specialists to whom *Hearing Disorders* will be of interest are audiologists and otolaryngologists, allied health professionals, and health agency personnel who deal with the hearing impaired. Persons with hearing loss, parents of hearing-handicapped children, teachers of the hearing impaired, and hearing-aid dispensers will find information in the book that will be of value. Students preparing for comprehensive examinations will find these chapters to be stimulating review material, but not as encumbered with details as a reference book.

The second edition of *Hearing Disorders* is more medically oriented than the first edition. Seven chapters are totally new to this edition and cover such topics as auditory evoked potentials, laboratory and radiology techniques used in otologic diagnosis, the treatment of tinnitus, and the evaluation and management of vestibular disorders. The remaining chapters have been revised and updated through the efforts of thirty-four contributors. The chapters are divided into four sections: Part I describes the clinical evaluation of patients with hearing problems; Part II describes the manifestations, diagnosis, treatment, and management of patients with nine common hearing disorders; Part III contains four chapters dealing with vestibular disorders; and Part IV discusses various other aspects of hearing, including physiology of the auditory mechanism, medical management of the hearing-handicapped child, direct stimulation of the auditory nerve (the cochlear implant), and tinnitus.

The range of information presented in this text is the result of a cooperative endeavor by a group of dedicated people who recognize the need for multidisciplinary efforts to explore unknown areas of hearing loss. Credit for any value derived from this book belongs equally to all contributing authors.

J.L.N.

Contributing Authors

David L. Asher, Ph.D.
*Assistant Professor of Otolaryngology,
University of Colorado School of Medicine,
Denver*

Dennis V. Barcz, M.D.
*Assistant Professor, Department of
Otolaryngology, University of Colorado School
of Medicine; Attending Physician, Department
of Otolaryngology, Children's Hospital, Denver*

LaVonne Bergstrom, M.D.
*Professor of Surgery, Division of Head and Neck
Surgery, University of California, Los Angeles,
School of Medicine*

Charles I. Berlin, Ph.D.
*Professor of Otorhinolaryngology and
Biocommunication, and Director, Kresge
Hearing Research Laboratory of the South,
Louisiana State University School of Medicine
in New Orleans*

Derald E. Brackmann, M.D.
*Clinical Professor of Otology, University of
Southern California School of Medicine;
Chief of Otology, St. Vincent Medical Center,
Los Angeles*

Peter Dallos, Ph.D.
*Professor and Chairman, Department of
Neurobiology and Physiology, Northwestern
University Medical School, Chicago*

Eugene L. Derlacki, M.D.
*Professor Emeritus of Otolaryngology and Head
and Neck Surgery, Northwestern University
Medical School; Senior Staff Member,
Department of Otolaryngology, Northwestern
Memorial Hospital, Chicago*

Marion P. Downs, M.A., D.H.S.
*Professor Emerita of Otolaryngology, University
of Colorado School of Medicine, Denver*

John Gilroy, M.D., F.R.C.P.(C.)
*Professor and Chairman, Department of
Neurology, Wayne State University School
of Medicine; Chief, Department of Neurology,
Harper-Grace Hospital, Detroit*

Donald W. Goin, M.D.
*Associate Clinical Professor, Department of
Otolaryngology, University of Colorado School
of Medicine, Denver*

Kurt Hecox, M.D., Ph.D.
Professor, Department of Neurology, University of Wisconsin Medical School, Madison

William F. House, M.D.
Clinical Professor of Otolaryngology, University of Southern California School of Medicine; Physician, Section of Otolaryngology, St. Vincent Medical Center, Los Angeles

John T. Jacobson, Ph.D.
Associate Professor and Acting Director, School of Human Communication Disorders, Dalhousie University; Assistant Professor, Department of Otolaryngology, Dalhousie University Faculty of Medicine, Halifax, Nova Scotia

Bruce W. Jafek, M.D.
Professor and Chairman, Department of Otolaryngology, University of Colorado School of Medicine, Denver

Robert W. Keith, Ph.D.
Professor and Director, Division of Audiology and Speech Pathology, University of Cincinnati College of Medicine, Cincinnati

David M. Lipscomb, Ph.D.
Professor of Audiology and Speech Pathology, The University of Tennessee, Knoxville

George E. Lynn, Ph.D.
Professor of Audiology and Associate in Neurology, Wayne State University School of Medicine, Detroit

Charles A. Mangham, M.D., M.S.
Assistant Clinical Professor, Department of Otolaryngology, University of Washington School of Medicine; Physician, Section of Otolaryngology and Facial Plastic Surgery, The Mason Clinic, Seattle

Robert E. Mischke, M.D.
Associate Clinical Professor, Department of Otolaryngology, University of Colorado School of Medicine; Staff Physician, Mercy and St. Joseph's Hospitals, Denver

Thomas W. Norris, Ph.D.
Professor and Director, Division of Audiology and Speech Pathology, University of Nebraska College of Medicine, Omaha

Jerry L. Northern, Ph.D.
Professor of Otolaryngology, University of Colorado School of Medicine; Head, Division of Audiology, University Hospital, Denver

Nigel R. T. Pashley, M.B., B.S., F.R.C.S.(C.)
Associate Professor of Pediatrics and Otolaryngology, University of Colorado School of Medicine; Chairman, Department of Pediatric Otolaryngology, Head and Neck Surgery, The Children's Hospital, Denver

Jack L. Pulec, M.D.
Associate Clinical Professor of Otolaryngology, University of Southern California School of Medicine; Physician, Department of Otolaryngology, Hospital of the Good Samaritan, Los Angeles

Jeffrey S. Rose, M.D.
Chief Resident, Department of Radiology, University of Colorado Health Sciences Center, Denver

Allen F. Ryan, Ph.D.
Associate Professor of Otolaryngology, University of California, San Diego, School of Medicine, La Jolla

Jay W. Sanders, Ph.D.
Professor of Audiology, Division of Hearing and Speech Sciences, Vanderbilt University, Nashville

Steven J. Staller, Ph.D.
Clinical Instructor in Otolaryngology, University of Colorado School of Medicine; Research Director, Denver Ear Institute, Denver

Janet M. Stewart, M.D.
Associate Professor, Department of Pediatrics, University of Colorado School of Medicine; Director of Birth Defects Clinic, University Hospital, Denver

Patricia L. Thompson, M.A.
Research Associate in Otolaryngology, University of Colorado Health Sciences Center, Denver

Jack A. Vernon, Ph.D.
Professor of Otolaryngology, University of Oregon Health Sciences Center School of Medicine, Portland

W. Dixon Ward, Ph.D.
Professor of Communication Disorders,
University of Minnesota Medical School—
Minneapolis

Marlin Weaver, M.D.
Clinical Professor of Otolaryngology,
University of Colorado School of Medicine;
Physician, Department of Otolaryngology,
University Hospital, Denver

Joseph D. White, Jr., D.M.D., M.D.
Chief Resident, Department of Otolaryngology,
University of Colorado Health Sciences Center,
Denver; Major, United States Army Medical
Corps

C. Thomas Yarington, Jr., M.D.
Clinical Professor of Otolaryngology,
University of Washington School of Medicine;
Head, Section of Otolaryngology and Plastic
Surgery, The Mason Clinic, Seattle

I

The Clinical Evaluation

1

The Otologic Evaluation

Bruce W. Jafek
Dennis V. Barcz

In evaluating otologic function, a close working relationship between the physician and audiologist is essential. Each contributes relatively unique expertise, but the observations should be complementary; the best results are obtained if each understands the working diagnosis and hypothesis of the other. Immediate consultation should take place, possibly followed by re-examination or joint examination in complex cases or in those in which the results are unclear or not in agreement. Neither professional can function in a vacuum, yet both the audiologist and physician should have a knowledge of the others' techniques and findings. The audiologist should be able to perform a quick otoscopic examination to evaluate the possibility of obstruction in the external auditory canal, whereas the physician should be able to use tuning forks to confirm the audiologic evaluation and to arrive at the proper diagnosis.

The otologic evaluation includes a complete otologic and related medical history; an otologic and pertinent general examination; and detailed specialized testing as indicated, including the audiologic assessment.

THE OTOLOGIC HISTORY

Throughout the evaluation, keep the patient's chief complaint clearly in mind, as this is central to both establishing the diagnosis as well as achieving patient satisfaction: *Why* did the patient come to see you? What can you *do* to relieve this symptom?

The otologic history must include inquiring into the five "cardinal signs" of ear pathology: (1) hearing loss, (2) ear pain (otalgia), (3) ear discharge (otorrhea), (4) head noise (tinnitus), and (5) dizziness (vertigo). If any of these symptoms are found, detailed characterization helps lead to the diagnosis.

The following outline provides a preliminary "skeleton" on which to organize the history:

1. Hearing loss
   a. Is it unilateral or bilateral? Which side?
   b. Is it continuous or intermittent?

1

c. Is it acute or chronic? Is the onset associated with other symptoms (e.g., noise exposure or illness)?

d. Is the loss in volume of sound or in the ability to understand (discrimination)?

e. Is there a family history of hearing loss?

f. Is there a history of ear surgery? What were the results?

g. What is the patient's occupation? Is there occupational or recreational noise exposure?

h. Is there a history of specific ototoxic exposure to meningitis, measles, mumps, syphilis, high fever, diuretics, aminoglycoside antibiotics (e.g., streptomycin, gentamicin, or tobramycin), or unconsciousness?

i. Does the patient use a hearing aid?

2. Pain or earache (otalgia)
   a. Is it unilateral or bilateral? Which side?
   b. Is it continuous or intermittent? Is it recurrent?
   c. Is it acute or chronic?
   d. Is it associated with recent upper respiratory infection?

3. Discharge (otorrhea)
   a. Is it unilateral or bilateral? Which side?
   b. Is it continuous or intermittent?
   c. Is it acute or chronic?
   d. What is the character: clear, purulent, or bloody?
   e. Is it associated with previous upper respiratory infection or water in the ear?

4. Head noise (tinnitus)
   a. Is it unilateral or bilateral? Which side?
   b. Is it continuous or intermittent?
   c. Is it acute or insidious in onset?
   d. What is the character of the noise? High-pitched ("like a steam pipe"), low-pitched ("like the ocean"), or pulsating? (It should be noted that otologic noises are nonspecific. "Voices" are not of otologic origin and psychiatric consultation may be appropriate.)
   e. Is the patient taking any drugs (e.g., aspirin or quinine)?

5. Dizziness (vertigo). Dizziness is the general term for many forms of unsteadiness.

Dizziness may have multiple etiologies, some of which are otologic in origin. It should therefore be carefully characterized by the examiner. Vertigo (of otologic origin) implies motion, is usually accompanied by rhythmic eye movements known as nystagmus, and may be due to peripheral or central vestibular disorders. Disequilibrium, on the other hand, implies the illusion of spatial disorientation or uncoordination, is not accompanied by nystagmus, and is usually due to a systemic disorder or nonvestibular neurologic disease. "Subjective" vertigo implies that the patient senses motion of his or her body, whereas "objective" vertigo means that the environment seems to move around the patient. These final terms are of descriptive value, however, and not of differential diagnostic value.

a. What is the chronology: continuous or intermittent? What is the interval between episodes? Is it acute or gradual in onset?

b. Are there coexisting constitutional symptoms such as nausea, vomiting, or both? Is there falling? Which direction?

c. Are there temporally associated otologic symptoms such as pressure in the ear, and hearing loss?

d. Are there ocular symptoms such as double vision, blurred vision, problems in darkness, or spots before the eyes (scotomata)?

e. Is there central nervous system/ataxia, such as numbness in extremities or speech problems (dysarthria)?

f. Is there disequilibrium: light-headedness, headache, or blackouts?

g. Is there a history of contributing conditions such as diabetes, thyroid disorder, allergy, syphilis, neurologic disorder, cardiac disorder, or arteriosclerosis?

Because of the proximity of the vestibule to the cochlea, the presence (or absence) of vestibular symptoms is extremely important in the otologic evaluation and deserves additional comment.

The history is the single most important tool in the differential diagnosis of vestibular disorders. A common technique is to ask the patient to describe a typical attack in as great a detail as possible, *without using the word "dizzy."*

In sorting out the various etiologies of dizziness, it is important to remember the four systems that serve to orient the body in space and to maintain balance and posture: (1) ocular (vision), (2) otologic and vestibular (hearing), (3) musculoskeletal (proprioceptive), and (4) nervous (the central nervous system integrates input via peripheral nerves). Dysfunction in any one system may produce dizziness, but this dizziness is often compensated for by the other systems. When two systems are incapacitated or lost, the patient experiences major problems in orientation. Thus, a person who has absent vestibular responses does well until he is in the dark and loses visual orientation. A blind person becomes severely disabled with impairment of the vestibular apparatus.

In addition to the detailed otologic history, a careful medical history must be obtained. Of special interest are neurologic, cardiac, ophthalmologic, hematologic, and allergic symptoms. Medications should also be recorded.

Obviously no symptom alone is diagnostic, so correlation of a constellation of symptoms is necessary for accurate diagnosis. For example, acute hearing loss may suggest many diagnoses (e.g., otitis media or sud-

den hearing loss), whereas an associated vertigo and "fullness of the ear" focus the clinician's attention on Meniere's disease. Similarly, ear pain, hearing loss, and ear drainage may have several etiologies, whereas associated pain on movement of the pinna suggests otitis externa, which can then be confirmed by the physical examination.

EXAMINATION OF THE EAR

Examination of the ear begins with inspection and palpation of the external ear (pinna) and periauricular (surrounding) structures, including the mastoid bone (posterior and inferior) and parotid lymph nodes (auricular lymphatic drainage). The presence of any drainage from the ear canal is noted, and the pinna is retracted posteriorly and superiorly to evaluate pain on motion as well as to get a preliminary idea of the course and state of the external auditory canal. The appearance and anatomy of the normal external ear is shown in Figure 1-1.

Additional detailed examination of the ear requires light and magnification. Light can be provided directly with an otoscope or microscope, or indirectly with a head mirror. The neophyte generally uses the lighted otoscope, which provides excellent illumination and magnification as shown in Figure 1-2. Removal of impacted ceru-

Figure 1-1. Lateral view of right ear (pinna) illustrates external landmarks.

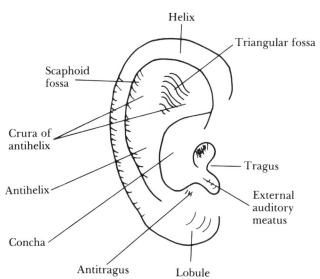

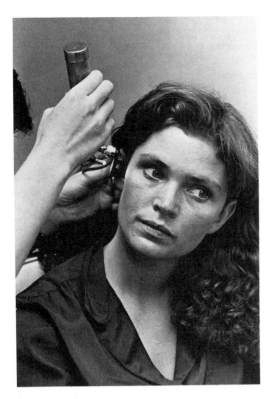

Figure 1-2. Examination of ear canal using lighted otoscope. Pinna is pulled posterior and superior to straighten the cartilaginous portion of the external auditory canal.

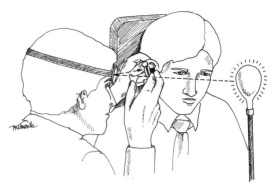

Figure 1-3. Head mirror examination of ear canal and tympanic membrane. The light is reflected (arrow) off examiner's head mirror into the ear speculum.

men or a foreign body from the ear canal, however, may require the use of either the operating microscope or ear speculum and head mirror.

The most important step in preparing to examine the eardrum is to make sure the ear canal and surface of the tympanic membrane are clean. Wax, pus, and particulate matter must be meticulously removed.

There are three methods of cleaning the ear canal: (1) a cerumen spoon or cotton applicator can be used to remove matter under direct vision, (2) the ear canal can be irrigated with tap water at body temperature (inadvisable if a perforation is seen or suspected), or (3) a small angulated suction tip can be used to aspirate pus or other liquid material from the ear canal.

The examination of the tympanic membrane is usually performed with the patient positioned as follows: sitting, leaning forward slightly, and turning the head to

one side. The examiner may be either standing or sitting, but should be comfortable. A good rule is to bring the patient to the examiner.

For a right-handed examiner using the head mirror, the external light is positioned over the patient's shoulder and the reflecting head mirror over the examiner's left eye, as shown in Figure 1-3. The head mirror has a hole in the center, through which the area to be examined is visualized while shading the examiner's eye from the direct glare of the light source. The examiner's other eye remains open.

The external ear is pulled posteriorly and superiorly to straighten the external auditory canal, and the ear speculum is advanced just beyond the last ear canal hair that marks the junction between the lateral, hairy, cartilaginous canal and the medial, hairless, bony canal. The examiner should select the largest ear speculum that comfortably fits the external canal.

A closed speculum is used with the pneumatic otoscope; this gives a lighted, magnified view of the tympanic membrane and allows assessment of tympanic membrane mobility by gently applying positive and negative pressure. Some experience is required to interpret mobility, but this is rapidly acquired as the results are correlated with patterns obtained with tympanometry.

When the tympanic membrane is examined with the operating microscope, the patient is generally positioned supine, although the examination may be done with a wall-mounted scope and the patient seated in the examining chair as shown in

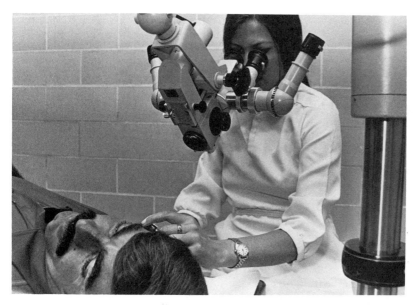

Figure 1-4. Microscopic examination of external ear canal and tympanic membrane.

Figure 1-4. Again, an appropriately sized ear speculum is positioned at the junction of the bony and cartilaginous ear canal as the pinna is retracted posteriorly and superiorly to straighten the canal. The microscope is illuminated and greater degrees of magnification (6–40 power) are used to view various aspects of the tympanic membrane. Additional advantages for using the microscope are that the examiner's hands are free to manipulate instruments and more detailed pneumatic otoscopy can be accomplished. Operative manipulation, such as myringotomy with pressure-equalizing tube placement, is also possible. Finally, newer microscopes allow rapid magnified examination of the tympanic membrane and are excellent for photographic documentation.

Regardless of the method of examination selected, the goal is to visualize the tympanic membrane and such middle ear structures as might be visible through a perforation, as well as to assess tympanic membrane mobility.

The normal tympanic membrane landmarks are shown in Figure 1-5. It is sometimes difficult to see the more anterior portion of the tympanic membrane because of overhang of the external auditory canal caused by the temporal mandibular joint.

The normal tympanic membrane is pearly gray in color, and is often thin enough so that the incus can be visualized through it in the posterior, superior quadrant of the membrane. The chorda tympani nerve may also be seen, coursing anterosuperiorly between the incus and malleus to exit the middle ear anteriorly. (The chorda tympani provides taste sensation to the anterior two thirds of the tongue.) The most obvious landmark is the handle of the malleus, with its distal umbo centered in the tympanic membrane and more proximal short process. The light reflex ("cone of light") is generally triangular with its apex on the umbo and base directed anteriorly and inferiorly. The anulus is a white thickening of the periphery of the tympanic membrane, except superiorly in the region of the pars flaccida (Shrapnell's membrane). Inferior to the short process of the malleus, the tympanic membrane is thicker owing to the middle fibrous layer; this area is termed the *pars tensa*. Externally on the lateral surface the tympanic membrane is covered by thin squamous epithelium, whereas the internal or medial surface is lined by a flattened endothelium.

For simplicity, the ear is divided into the external, middle, and inner ear as shown in Figure 1-6. The external ear focuses sound waves toward the tympanic membrane, and the middle ear conducts and

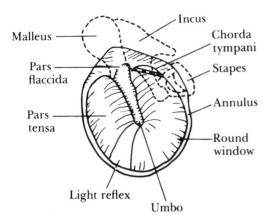

Figure 1-5. Lateral view of the tympanic membrane with landmarks labeled.

amplifies vibrations to the inner ear. The inner ear transduces sound pressure (waves) energy to neural impulses, carrying these on to the interpretative centers in the brain. This is discussed in greater detail in Chapters 21 and 22.

TUNING FORK TESTS

Audiologic testing is discussed in detail in Chapters 2 and 3. A basic, screening assessment of audiologic function can be undertaken with tuning forks. These results *must correlate* with the results of the otologic assessment, audiogram, and acoustic impedance measurements. When disagreement exists, either the patient is not fully cooperating with the behavioral tests or error exists within the other testing procedures. In any event, the disagreement must be resolved.

Audiometric assessment by the otolaryngologist usually includes basic tuning fork testing supplemented, when appropriate, by the Mueller speaking tube and Bárány Noise Box.

Much has been said about which tuning fork to use, of what material it should be made, and how to activate it. Historic aspects of these tests are interesting; the article by Johnson (1970) is a good starting point.

It is important for each clinician to become familiar with the normal and abnormal responses with tuning forks the way he uses them. We use aluminum tuning forks and usually test with a 512 Hz fork.

The 1024 Hz fork is used to supplement this information, to determine if there is a sufficient air-bone gap at that frequency. We do not recommend use of the 256 Hz fork because of the tactile sensation it produces by bone conduction. The tactile vibrations may be mistaken by the patient for sound. In addition, because more sound intensity is required at 256 Hz to reach the normal hearing threshold, the tuning fork must be hit sufficiently so the patient will perceive the sound. Finally, the pitch of the 256 Hz tuning fork is so low that the tone is easily masked by environmental and clinical noise. Striking the tuning fork too hard may create overtones that may confuse the patient. The fork can be activated by hitting it on your knee or your heel.

The Weber Test

Place the stem of a vibrating tuning fork on the skull in the midline, usually firmly in the middle of the forehead, as shown in Figure 1-7. The patient is asked to indicate in which ear the sound is heard loudest, and the test is recorded as "Weber midline 512" (indicating that the sound did not lateralize with the 512 Hz tuning fork) or "Weber right 512" (indicating lateralization to the right ear with the 512 Hz tuning fork).

With unilateral hearing impairment, lateralization of the sound to the poorer hearing ear indicates an element of conductive hearing loss in that ear, whereas lateralization to the better hearing ear suggests that the problem in the involved ear is sensorineural.

Alternatively, the stem of the tuning fork for the Weber test may be placed on the nasal bones or the teeth when a louder bone-conduction stimulus is required.

The Rinne Test

The Rinne test is a comparison of bone-conduction and air-conduction transmission of sound. The stem of the vibrating tuning fork is placed initially on the *lamina perforata* of the mastoid (the flat surface of the mastoid just behind the upper portion of the pinna), as near to the posterosuperior edge of the ear canal as possible without touching the pinna. This placement avoids the variable factor of

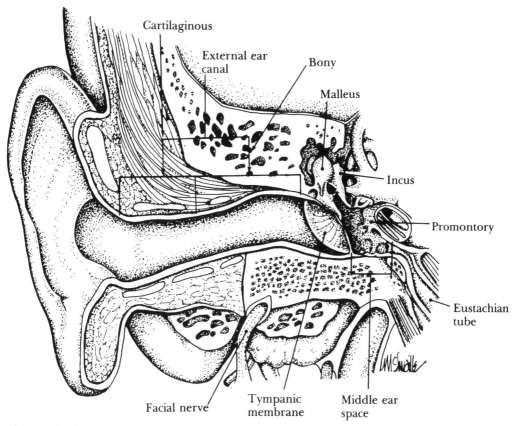

Cartilaginous

External ear canal

Bony

Malleus

Incus

Promontory

Eustachian tube

Facial nerve

Tympanic membrane

Middle ear space

Figure 1-6. Diagrammatic representation of limits of external, middle, and inner ear.

soft tissue thickness. The body of the tuning fork is directed laterally as shown in Figure 1-8.

The ear is next tested "by air" by holding the same vibrating tuning fork vertically, approximately 2 inches lateral to the opening of the external canal with the tuning fork tines held superiorly in the coronal plane of the skull.

The patient is asked whether the sound is louder with the fork "behind" the ear or "in front of" the ear, and the results are recorded for each ear separately as "Rinne AC > BC-R-512" (meaning air conduction was perceived as louder than bone conduction when testing the right ear with the 512 Hz fork). Some otologists use the terminology "Rinne negative" for BC > AC and "Rinne positive" for AC > BC.

When testing the contralateral ear for a conductive hearing loss, it is necessary to use a Bárány noisemaker in the nontest ear to prohibit lateralization of the sound to the conductive loss ear owing to the Weber phenomenon.

The Rinne test is also described by testing bone conduction until the patient no longer perceives the sound, and then quickly testing air conduction by asking if the patient "now hears the sound" as the tuning fork is placed in front of the ear. This method is slower than the technique previously described without providing additional accuracy.

Modified Schwabach Test

The Schwabach test, as originally described, is a comparison of tuning fork sound duration as heard by the patient and examiner. The modification involves a comparison of both the patient's and examiner's bone- and air-conduction levels.

The fork is rapped softly and moved back and forth between the examiner's and patient's ear (in front of the ear to test air conduction, and behind the ear with the stem on the mastoid to test bone conduction). The patient is asked to let the exam-

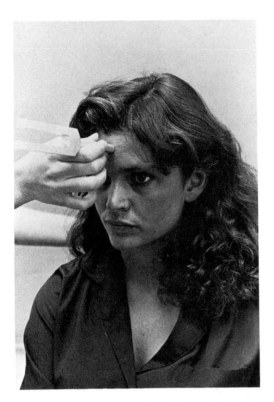

Figure 1-7. Placement of vibrating tuning fork in middle of forehead to administer Weber test.

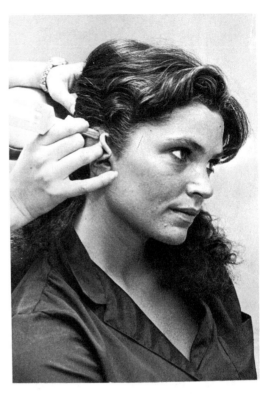

Figure 1-8. Placement of vibrating tuning fork postauricularly to administer bone-conduction portion of Rinne test.

iner know when the sound is no longer heard, and the examiner then listens to the tuning fork and records whether he or she still perceives the sound. The information is recorded as "patient R = AC examiner R = AC 512," meaning that the patient perceived the sound in his right ear by air conduction longer than the examiner with the 512 Hz fork. The other ear is tested similarly.

Interpretation of the test results depends on a knowledge of the examiner's hearing thresholds at each test frequency and is quite reproducible. Several tuning forks of different frequencies may be used to rapidly map the patient's audiogram relative to the audiogram of the examiner.

The Mueller speaking tube, with Bárány noisemaker masking the opposite ear, may be used to supplement tuning fork tests in the otologic examination. The speaking tube is used for loud speech and provides from 120 to 154 dB sound pressure level (SPL), depending on how loudly the examiner speaks into the tube. The Bárány noisemaker is an effective masking device because its frequency response is from 500 to 6000 Hz, with maximum power output of 130 dB SPL at 1000 Hz. With this frequency response, the noisemaker is very good for masking the opposite ear when testing the patient's ability to hear and understand speech. The output of both of these elementary devices is often in excess of signal generated by conventional audiometers. The technique can be used to verify audiometric findings in patients with severe losses.

VESTIBULAR FUNCTION TESTS

Vestibular anatomy and physiology is discussed in detail in Chapter 17.

Briefly summarized, the vestibular system consists of six semicircular canals, arranged in three pairs with one set of three to a side; the utricle and saccule; and the central nervous connections. The three semicircular canals on one side are in

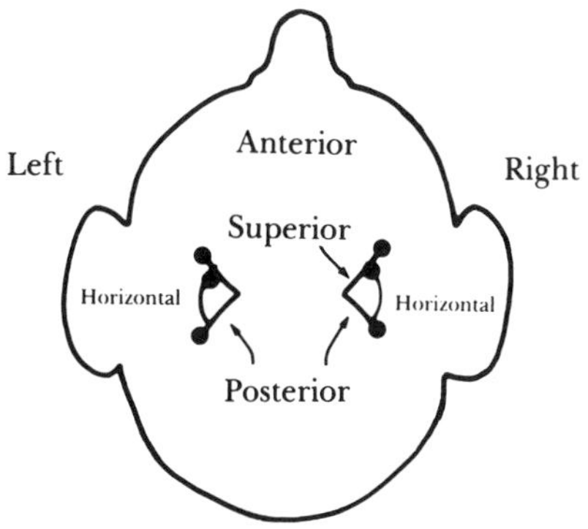

Figure 1-9. Schematized representation of superior, posterior, and lateral semicircular canals with ampullae. Left superior canal is parallel to right posterior, etc., to give bilateral representation of motion.

planes at right angles to one another and each is paired with one on the opposite side, lying in a parallel plane. The two horizontal canals make one pair, and the left superior canal is paired with the right posterior, and so on (Fig. 1-9). The dilated or ampullated ends of the two paired canals are oriented in opposite directions about the axis of rotation of their planes, so that movement of the head (and endolymph fluid) in the plane of the canals results in motion of the fluid toward the ampulla (ampullopetal) in one and away from the ampulla (ampullofugal) in the other. Thus, the semicircular canals respond to angular acceleration and deceleration by displacement of the hair cells of the crista of the ampulla by the cupula as it is acted on by the inertially moved endolymph.

The utricle and saccule, on the other hand, respond to linear acceleration and deceleration and gravity, again through the inertial activity of the endolymph, but this time acting on the otoliths, which rest in a gelatinous mass on the hair cells of the maculae of the utricle and saccule (Fig. 1-10).

Deflection of the hair cells produces an increase (or decrease) over the resting state of the number of impulses in the vestibular division of the eighth cranial nerve. This information is carried centrally and subsequently back peripherally over the vestibulospinal and vestibulo-ocular tracts,

producing increased (or decreased) muscle tone in the extraocular and skeletal muscles to compensate for the acceleration and deceleration to maintain balance and spatial orientation. Dysfunction of the system may produce nystagmus, past-pointing, and falling, as well as the symptom of vertigo.

Clinically, the vestibular system can be tested by (1) observation of the resting state function (static state), (2) acceleration and deceleration (dynamic state) testing, and (3) caloric stimulation (stimulated state).

Resting state function is evaluated by observing the patient for nystagmus, or movement of the eyes. This movement is horizontal, vertical, or rotary and is characterized by rhythmic slow and quick components. Although the direction of the nystagmus is determined by the direction of the quick component, this is compensatory motion. It is the slow component that represents the action of the vestibular system. The ability to observe nystagmus is heightened by electronystagmography (Chap. 18) or by placing Frenzel (+20 diopter) glasses on the patient to magnify the eyes and to eliminate "fixation" (focusing on a distant object) as a means of overcoming or suppressing the nystagmus. In general, the presence of nystagmus is abnormal.

Evaluation of the resting state function also includes an assessment of the patient's posture and balance as part of the general physical examination.

Dynamic function of the vestibular system is evaluated by observing gait (balance and posture while walking). For more specific tests, rapid alternating movement is required, such as finger-nose-finger or heel-to-shin, past-pointing, or optokinetic tests.

One method of showing past-pointing is instructing the patient to touch the examiner's finger with his index finger, to raise his extended arm above his head, and then to return his finger to the examiner's finger. The test is done on both sides. In the presence of a cerebellar lesion, past-pointing tends to occur on the side of the lesion. The test can be "sharpened" by having the patient close his eyes.

Finger-nose-finger or heel-to-shin tests assess fine degrees of cerebellar control. In the finger-nose-finger test, the patient alter-

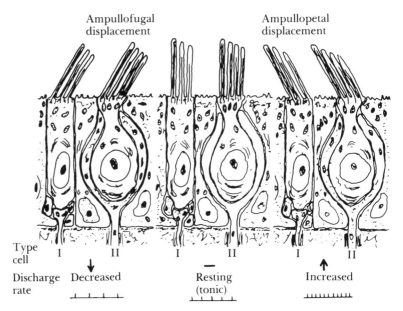

Figure 1-10. Hair cells of the crista. Both types I and II respond to ampullofugal displacement with a decrease in the resting discharge rate, and both produce an increase in the discharge rate in response to ampullopetal displacement of the cilia.

nately touches his or her nose and the examiner's fingertip with his or her index finger. The test is sharpened by randomly moving the examiner's finger and by instructing the patient to move as rapidly and accurately as possible. In the heel-to-shin procedure, the patient is instructed to run the heel of one foot up and down the shin of the other leg from ankle to knee as rapidly and accurately as possible, which provides a similar assessment of lower limb control.

An example of rapid alternating movement testing is provided by asking the patient to pat alternately the surface of one hand with the dorsal and ventral surfaces of the other as rapidly as possible. The two sides are compared, taking into consideration handedness as well as general coordination. Cerebellar dysfunction causes the activity to disintegrate and is termed *dysdiadochokinesia.*

In the Romberg test the patient is instructed to put his feet together, gain balance, and close his eyes. It can be sharpened by instructing the patient to walk "in tandem" by placing the heel of one foot to the toe of the other. With cerebellar dysfunction, the patient tends to fall to the side of the lesion.

During gait and balance evaluation, the patient tends to fall toward the side of the cerebellar pathology. With peripheral ves-

tibular hypofunction, the gait is wide-based, especially in the absence of other orienting input. With vestibular malfunction, gait or balance and posturing may be impossible.

In general terms of vestibular dysfunction, the slow component of spontaneous nystagmus, past-pointing, and direction of fall all tend to be in the same direction.

Optokinetic nystagmus involves observation of the rapidly alternating movement of the eyes that occurs when they are fixed on one object after another in rapid succession. Special rotary drums with alternating black and white stripes are available for comprehensive testing in conjunction with electronic recording. The optokinetic test evaluates both the vestibulo-ocular and visual systems, centrally and peripherally, and is therefore somewhat less useful than other vestibular tests.

New refinements in swing and rotational tests as well as platform tests should provide additional information in the evaluation of the vestibular system. These tests are somewhat less useful at this time in that they generally test the bilateral system, simultaneously, and are quite expensive and difficult to interpret.

EUSTACHIAN TUBE FUNCTION

If the tympanic membrane is intact, the patient is instructed to squeeze the nose tightly and blow "to pop the ears" (the Valsalva maneuver) while the eardrum is observed under magnification. If the eustachian tube opens, the tympanic membrane may be seen to "balloon." The patient is then instructed to swallow, causing the ballooning to disappear as the eustachian tube opens to equalize the positive middle ear pressure previously created.

Alternatively, if the tympanic membrane is not intact, the patient is instructed to occlude one nostril while "atomized" oil is puffed into the other nostril through a nasal olive-tip as the patient is instructed to say "K-K-K" or "kick-kick-kick." The oil droplets pass through the nasopharynx under the positive pressure and then up to the eustachian tube (which opens as the "K" attempt tenses the tensor veli palatini) and out the perforation. The drops may be visualized under magnification in the ear canal to verify tubal function.

It is recognized that none of the aforementioned eustachian tube tests validly test normal eustachian tube function. The tests are helpful in assessing patency and providing a helpful office screening method.

The otologic examination may be tedious, time-consuming, and even inconclusive. On the other hand, it may be completed rapidly, leading to a straightforward diagnosis that lends itself to complete surgical correction. A complete patient work-up often includes laboratory tests as described in Chapter 6 and radiographic studies as described in Chapter 7. It is important to be thorough and logical in the completion of the examination, as well as sensitive to the patient's needs, limitations, and feelings.

SUGGESTED READING

Adams, G. L., Boies, Jr., L. R., and Paparella, M. M. *Boies' Fundamentals of Otolaryngology* (5th ed.). Philadelphia: Saunders, 1978.

DeWeese, D. D., and Saunders, W. H. *Textbook of Otolaryngology* (6th ed.). St. Louis: Mosby, 1981.

English, G. M. *Otolaryngology*. Hagerstown, Md.: Harper & Row, 1976.

Goodhill, V. *Ear Diseases, Deafness and Dizziness*. Hagerstown, Md.: Harper & Row, 1979.

Johnson, E. W. Tuning forks to audiometers and back again. *Laryngoscope* 80:49, 1970.

Shambaugh, G. E., Jr., and Glasscock, M. E., III. *Surgery of the Ear* (3rd ed.). Philadelphia: Saunders, 1980.

Sheehy, J. L. The Otologic Hearing Examination. In J. Northern (Ed.), *Hearing Disorders*. Boston: Little, Brown, 1976. Pp. 3–9.

Wood, R. P., II, Northern, J. L., and Jafek, B. W. *Manual of Otolaryngology: A Symptom-Oriented Text*. Baltimore: Williams & Wilkins, 1979.

2

The Basic Audiologic Evaluation

Robert W. Keith

The basic audiologic evaluation has several purposes including diagnosing conductive versus sensorineural site of lesion, determining the need for nonsurgical rehabilitation, deciding subsequent audiologic test battery approaches, and determining disability and compensation.

In this chapter, the audiologic evaluation refers to pure-tone air-conduction (AC) and bone-conduction (BC) threshold tests, speech-reception threshold tests (SRT), and speech discrimination (SD) tests. These audiometric tests are usually thought of as routine or the basic test battery. Because of the significance of the decisions that result from the basic audiologic evaluation, these tests must be carefully done, the underlying assumptions of the tests must be clearly understood, and the results properly interpreted.

Jerger [15] notes that critics of clinical audiology assert that basic audiometry can be delegated to a minimally trained technician. The reason for Jerger's statement is that these tests appear to be quite simple to administer; therefore, the assumption seems to follow that they can be administered by someone with minimal training and understanding of the underlying principles. Price [25] states that many inaccurate audiograms exist because of the assumption that little training is required to do basic audiometry. The purpose of this chapter is to describe some of the principles necessary for the administration and interpretation of basic audiometric tests.

PURE-TONE AUDIOMETRY

Pure-tone audiometry has developed from the basic principles of the tuning fork tests that were introduced during the 1800s. These tests were named after the men who first described them and include the Weber test introduced in 1834, the Rinne test in 1855, and the Schwabach test in 1885.

The Weber test is most useful when a unilateral hearing loss is present. This test is conducted by placing the stem of a vibrating tuning fork on the midline of the patient's skull. If the sound cannot be heard on the forehead or vertex, the tuning fork may be placed on the teeth for maximum loudness. The patient is asked to indicate the ear in which the sound is heard. Localization of the sound toward the poorer hearing ear indicates the presence of a conductive hearing loss on that side. Localization to the better ear indicates that the hearing loss in the opposite ear is sensorineural.

The Rinne test was originally described as placing the stem of a vibrating tuning fork on the mastoid process of the patient's temporal bone. When the bone-conducted sound is no longer heard, the tuning fork is moved quickly to approximately 1 inch from the ear canal, and the patient is asked if he hears the sound again. Currently, many examiners ask the patient to compare the loudness of the bone- and air-conducted sound as the tuning fork is moved from mastoid to near the ear. If bone conduction is heard louder or longer than air conduction (a "negative Rinne"), then a conductive hearing loss is present. A sensorineural loss is present if air conduction is heard louder or longer than bone conduction (a "positive Rinne"). To a degree, the examiner can determine the magnitude of any conductive loss by using a series of tuning forks in octaves from 256 Hz through 4096 Hz. In general, the higher the frequency at which a negative Rinne (BC > AC) is obtained, the greater the conductive hearing loss [27].

Another simple method for determining the presence of a conductive versus sensorineural hearing loss is through the Bing test. With the tuning fork in the midline position, the examiner gently occludes the patient's external auditory canal with his or her finger. When middle ear function is normal, the occlusion of the ear canal results in an increase in loudness of the tuning fork with a shift of the sound toward the occluded ear. When there is a greater than 5 to 10 dB conductive hearing loss present, occluding the external ear canal will have no noticeable effect.

The Schwabach test is a method of determining whether the patient's hearing by bone conduction is normal or impaired. The test is conducted by presenting a bone-conducted sound to the patient's mastoid process. When the patient no longer hears the sound, the tuning fork is moved quickly to the examiner's mastoid. Assuming that the examiner's bone-conduction hearing is known, the Schwabach test determines whether the patient's bone-conduction hearing is better than, equal to, or worse than the examiner's and is therefore normal or impaired.

Using these tuning fork tests, the examiner can determine whether the patient's hearing loss is conductive or sensorineural, and whether a hearing loss by bone conduction exists. Although tuning fork tests enjoy widespread application, there are in reality many problems inherent in their use. For example, a calibrated signal is lacking, decay rates differ among tuning forks, overtones are generated by striking the tuning fork too hard, and vibrotactile sensations can be mistaken for sound.

One difficulty with the Weber test is that some children and adults find it difficult to report where they hear a tone. In addition, patients who have long-standing unilateral sensorineural hearing loss have lost the ability to localize sound and are apt to give tuning fork results that are inconsistent with their hearing losses. One of the biggest problems with the Rinne test is that the examiner fails to recognize that the sound emanating from the stem of a tuning fork will be conducted by the bones of the skull to both cochlea. Therefore, a patient with a "dead" ear can easily hear the sound in the better ear by cross conduction of the bone-conduction stimulus. This phenomenon is called *crossover*. When unrecognized crossover occurs, the examiner will report a negative Rinne (BC > AC), indicating the presence of a conductive hearing loss when, in fact, a false-negative Rinne has occurred. To avoid crossover, it is necessary to mask the nontest ear with noise. With tuning fork tests, this is usually done by presenting a Bárány Noise Box to the nontest ear.

The value of understanding tuning fork tests is that the principles underlying those tests exists in modern audiometry. Every audiometer used in diagnostic testing has the capacity to present tones by air conduction through earphones and by bone conduction through a "bone-conduction vibrator" that is placed on the skull. The comparison of air-conduction thresholds to bone-conduction thresholds provides the basis for determining if middle ear dysfunction and conductive hearing loss exist. When bone conduction is better than air conduction, it is said that an *air-bone gap* exists, which is similar to a negative Rinne (BC > AC) result. On the other hand, when there is no air-bone gap, it is the same as a positive Rinne (AC > BC), and middle ear function is normal. Any existing hearing loss is sensorineural.

The *threshold* of hearing is defined as the minimum effective sound pressure of a signal that is capable of evoking an auditory sensation. In audiometry, threshold is recorded as the intensity of a tone at which the patient will respond approximately 50% of the time. Hearing thresholds obtained with an audiometer are reported in *decibels* (dB) with 0 dB hearing level (HL) being the average hearing level of a group of young adults with no otologic pathology or history of noise trauma. Therefore, comparison of the patient's bone-conduction threshold to 0 dB HL is the same principle involved in the Schwabach tuning fork test when the patient's bone conduction is compared to the examiner's who serves as the reference.

The pure-tone audiogram is obtained by testing air conduction and bone conduction at several frequencies, especially 500, 1000, 2000, and 4000 Hz. Most examiners include 250 Hz and either 6000 or 8000 Hz, and many test at 3000 Hz, especially for patients with histories of noise exposure or high-frequency hearing loss at 4000 Hz.

Several techniques for establishing pure-tone thresholds have been suggested. They include going from an inaudible to an audible stimulus (ascending method) or achieving threshold by going from an audible to an inaudible stimulus (descending method). Carhart and Jerger [6], recommend presentation of a series of tone pulses ascending in 5 dB steps until the patient responds. Threshold is usually achieved in three or four ascents. The patient responds usually by raising an index finger or lighting a signal light when the tone is heard. Audiometric results are graphed with intensity on the ordinate and frequency on the abscissa.

The audiogram system recommended by the American Speech-Language-Hearing Association [3] is compared to a system recommended by Jerger [4] in Figure 2-1.

A direct comparison of tuning fork test findings to an audiometric test result is shown in Figure 2-2. The results indicate a mild sensorineural hearing loss in both ears (shortened Schwabach) with a 30 dB conductive hearing loss superimposed on the right ear (negative Rinne). The Weber lateralization to the poorer ear indicates a conductive loss on that side.

There are several problems unique to the measurement of bone conduction. The foremost problem is the lack of effective acoustic separation of the two cochleae. That is, when a stimulus is applied to the skull by bone conduction, it activates both cochlea simultaneously and nearly equally. Therefore, it is necessary to mask the non-test ear to eliminate it from the testing situation. The simplest rule to decide if masking is necessary is to "apply masking to the opposite ear during bone-conduction testing whenever an air-bone gap is observed" [28]. There is no need to mask during bone-conduction testing when no air-bone gap is present in either ear.

Another rule for determining when to mask during bone-conduction testing is based on results of the Weber test. When the signal lateralizes to one ear it is probably safe to test that ear without using masking. When the other ear is tested, masking must be applied to the ear to which the tone lateralized. This rule requires careful interpretation of the Weber lateralization reports. When lateralization reports seem inconsistent or improbable they should be disregarded, and masking should then be used.

In testing bone conduction, the vibrator must be applied to the skull with a force of at least 400 gm. Failure to apply that amount of force will result in poorer bone-conduction thresholds than actually exist [20]. The bone-conduction vibrator can be applied to the mastoid portion of the temporal bone or to the midline of the forehead. Various investigators [12, 24, 29] have reported that frontal placement yields increased reliability of results on test-retest measurements. On the other hand, frontal placement results in limiting the output of the audiometer because 10 to 15 dB more energy is needed in the low frequencies to reach threshold when compared to mastoid placement [9].

An additional variable in bone-conduction testing is the improvement in thresh-

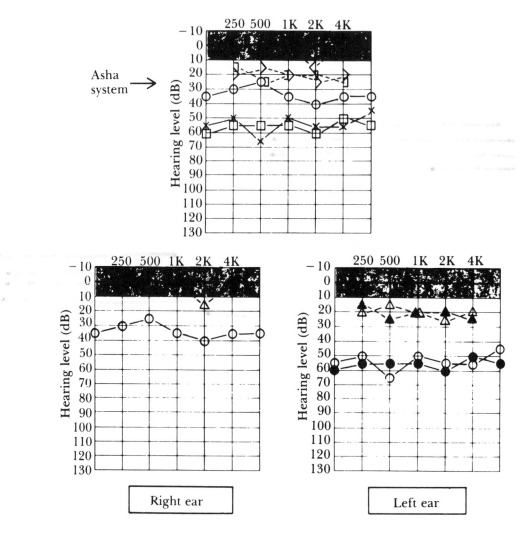

Audiometric symbol system—Jerger

Figure 2-1. Comparison of Asha *recommended audiogram format* [3] *with a proposed audiometric symbol system recommended by Jerger* [14]. *Shown is a hypothetical case of bilateral conductive loss. The Jerger format uses a right and left ear audiogram for better visualization of results. Note better visualization of AC and BC gaps for each ear, and effect of contralateral masking of AC and BC thresholds for left ear in graph at bottom right.* ([14] *Copyright 1976, American Medical Association.*)

old about by occlusion of the external auditory meatus, described previously in the discussion of the Bing test. This occlusion effect is present only when the middle ear is normal; it is reduced or absent depending on the amount of the conductive impairment. The magnitude of the effect can be as much as 25 dB in the low frequencies, with little or no effect above 1500 Hz [10]. The primary problem resulting from the occlusion effect is the enhancement of the BC signal in the ear on which the earphone is placed during masking. The improved BC threshold from the occlusion requires increased masking noise to be effective and requires different amounts of

masking depending on whether the middle ear function on the ear to be masked is normal or abnormal. Because the amount of the occlusion effect varies from person to person, the amount of noise required to properly mask is also different.

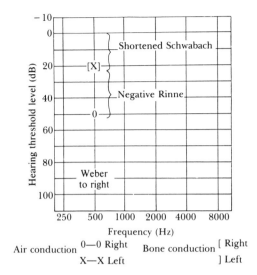

Figure 2-2. Comparison of tuning fork results and audiometric test results.

When the possibility of crossover exists during pure-tone testing, masking is introduced into the nontest ear to rule out a response from that side. It is best to assume that a bone-conduction signal stimulates both cochlea simultaneously and that masking is required whenever an air-bone gap is observed. During air-conduction testing, it is best to assume that an earphone signal reaches the opposite cochlea by passing through the bones of the head. Therefore, it is necessary to mask when the air-conduction threshold of the test ear exceeds the bone-conduction threshold of the nontest ear by 40 dB or more [28].

The amount of masking used in any situation is determined by many factors. There are different types of noise available in different audiometers. White noise, with approximately equal acoustic energy at all frequencies between 100 and 6000 Hz, is commonly used. Complex noise, with more acoustic energy concentrated in the low frequencies, is frequently used on old audiometers and is generally an unsatisfactory masker. Narrow band noise is the most efficient and desirable masker for pure-tone testing because, as a variable frequency source, it contains acoustic energy only in a narrow band of frequencies around the test signal. Because unnecessary energy is eliminated, narrow band noise is not as loud and therefore is less distract-

ing to the patient. Narrow band masking is presently available in many small portable audiometers. Speech noise has energy distribution for masking speech and is used solely for that purpose. It is important for the reader who is new to this subject to realize that except for special situations, masking noise is always presented by air conduction, even when pure-tone thresholds are being tested by bone conduction.

The amount of masking noise used in any given situation is affected by many factors. It is necessary to present the noise several decibels above the air-conduction threshold for it to be an effective masker. That is, a certain level of noise above threshold is necessary for *minimum masking*. If a hearing loss exists in the ear to be masked, the amount of noise must be increased by the amount of the hearing loss to achieve *effective masking*. On the other hand, if too much masking is used, the noise will crossover to the test ear and elevate the thresholds obtained on that side. This is known as *overmasking*.

The trick in masking is to know precisely the kind of noise that is being used and the amount of noise that will achieve minimum and maximum masking. When hearing loss is bilateral, masking becomes more difficult because there may not be enough noise available in the audiometer to overcome the loss and reach minimum masking levels. When a conductive hearing loss is present, as soon as minimum masking levels have been achieved, the masker can also be at crossover levels, causing an artificial shift in threshold on the test ear. In these situations, other diagnostic tests are used to determine the amount of air-bone gap and cochlear function. Methods of determining proper masking levels are described in almost every audiology textbook.

PURE-TONE AUDIOMETRY IN ASSESSING HEARING HANDICAP AND DISABILITY

The terms *hearing impairment, handicap,* and *disability* should convey different meanings. Hearing impairment is intended to mean a deviation in auditory structure or function, usually meaning poorer than normal. Hearing handicap means the disadvantage imposed by a hearing loss on a person's daily communication. Hearing disability is the determination of compensation for the loss of function caused by a hearing impairment that is sufficient to cause a hearing handicap. In general, the size of the hearing disability award should be in direct proportion to the extent of the hearing handicap [3].

For purposes of discussing test results with patients, many clinicians use adjective descriptions to designate the degree of hearing impairment. Although their terms are not standardized and do not take into account speech discrimination ability and other factors, a commonly used scale is shown in Table 2-1. When computing the average hearing level in decibels, the air-conduction pure-tone thresholds obtained at 500, 1000, and 2000 Hz are used.

Many different formulas have been used for assigning percentage loss of hearing handicap for disability determination. The American Academy of Otolaryngology (AAO) and the American Council of Otolaryngology (ACO; now known as the American Academy of Otolaryngology-Head and Neck Surgery) have proposed a "Guide for the Evaluation of Hearing Handicap" [1]. Their formula is based on the patient's average hearing level for thresholds at 500, 1000, 2000, and 3000 Hz. The monaural percentage loss is computed by taking that average minus 25 dB (the low "fence" where handicap presumably begins) multiplied by 1.5%.

Table 2-1. Scale of Hearing Impairment

Average hearing level (dB) (1969 ANSI)	Hearing loss label
0–15	Normal hearing
16–25	Slight hearing loss
26–40	Mild hearing loss
41–55	Moderate hearing loss
56–70	Moderately severe hearing loss
71–90	Severe hearing loss
91+	Profound hearing loss

Source: J. G. Clark, Uses and abuses of hearing loss classification. *Asha* 23:493, 1981.

An American Speech-Language-Hearing Association Task Force on Hearing Handicap [3] has recommended the assumption of a 2% linear growth in hearing handicap over the range of average hearing levels at 1000, 2000, 3000, and 4000 Hz between 25 and 75 dB for both the AAO-ACO and ASHA formulas. A binaural hearing handicap is determined by using a 5 : 1 better ear-poorer ear weighting scale. After considering these formulas, it should be clear to the reader that it is inappropriate to equate the average hearing level in decibels to percentage of hearing loss when counseling patients.

SPEECH AUDIOMETRY

The assessment of hearing using speech as a stimulus is probably the oldest hearing test known. Any time a clinician talks with his or her patient, the patient's ability to hear and understand speech is informally assessed. The quantification of these tests began in the mid-1800s when examiners began attempts to classify hearing disorders based on ability to hear various vowels, consonants, phonemes, words, or numbers. In addition, estimates of hearing were based on ability to hear whispered speech or speech at normal and moderate intensity levels. The classic spoken—and whispered—voice tests were an attempt to determine the amount of hearing loss a patient had and were quantified as 20/20 feet for normal conversational voice and 15/15 feet for normal whispered voice. These tests lack precision for many reasons, one of which is the difficulty of monitoring voice levels.

Modern speech audiometry attempts to measure two clinical quantities: speech reception thresholds (SRT) and speech discrimination (SD) ability. Speech reception thresholds are usually obtained by asking patients to repeat words presented by air conduction through earphones. The intensity of the words is varied to determine the level, in decibels, at which the words are intelligible approximately 50% of the time. The word list most frequently used for this test is the Central Institute for the Deaf (CID) Auditory Test W-1 [13]. This list comprises 36 familiar spondee words (two-syllable words with equal stress on both syllables) that are homogeneous with respect to intelligibility at any intensity. (Some examples of spondee words are: *hotdog, cowboy,* and *airplane.*) The intelligibility of these words rises from 20 to 80% with an 8 dB increase in intensity so that the SRT is clinically easy to establish and reliable on test-retest measurements.

When speech audiometry was introduced, the sound pressure produced by speech audiometers was calibrated so that SRT would be approximately equal to the pure-tone average (PTA) of thresholds obtained at the frequencies 500, 1000, and 2000 Hz. Today, the PTA-SRT comparison is used as a measure of test reliability. When the PTA-SRT comparison is not within a few decibels, one or another of the threshold measurements is suspect. One of the first indications of a nonorganic hearing loss is a large discrepancy between the PTA and the SRT, often with the SRT being substantially better than the PTA. Another use of the SRT is in the assessment of hearing levels in children who are too young to respond to pure-tone audiometry.

All the tests mentioned thus far are threshold tests, that is, the examiner seeks to determine the lowest level at which the air-conduction or bone-conduction pure tone can be heard or the spondee word understood. Speech discrimination tests, on the other hand, are suprathreshold tests. Several different approaches have been attempted in an effort to develop a speech discrimination test that (1) is reliable on test-retest measurements; (2) separates normal from hearing-impaired patients; and further, (3) separates patients with different types and etiologies of hearing loss. Another application of speech discrimination scores is in estimating how well a person functions in a social or vocational setting.

SPEECH DISCRIMINATION IN SITE-OF-LESION TESTING

Most speech discrimination tests consist of lists of 50 monosyllables, representing familiar words, that are equally difficult to understand. The 50-word lists are also phonetically balanced (PB) to represent the frequency of occurrence of sounds in everyday English. Lists of commonly used words include the Central Institute for the Deaf Auditory Test W-22, lists 1 through 4 [13]. These lists were developed to improve on the Harvard PAL PB-50 test materials that contained many unfamiliar words. Many other suitable word lists exist, including those compiled by Peterson and Lehiste [23]; Tillman, Carhart, and Wilbur [30]; Fairbanks [11]; and others. Standardized word lists are also available in Spanish and other languages. According to Carhart [5], it appears that "as long as the test items are meaningful monosyllables and the phonetic distribution is appropriately diversified, one 50-word compilation is relatively equivalent to another." The reader must understand that undistorted word discrimination tests presented in quiet at comfortable loudness levels are not sensitive measures of disorders of the auditory system. In fact, the original authors of the CID W-22 Auditory Test [13] point out in a footnote that "experience to date (in clinical trials) indicates that . . . the W-22 does not satisfactorily separate patients with mixed deafness from patients with pure conductive deafness." It is ironic that, in spite of this early warning, clinicians have used the W-22 test extensively for more than 20 years.

Even with their weaknesses, speech discrimination test results can be very useful for diagnostic purposes. In general, patients with normal hearing and purely conductive loss have high speech discrimination scores, between 96 and 100%. Patients with high-frequency or mild, flat cochlear hearing loss can also be expected to yield high discrimination scores. Usually, the greater the cochlear hearing loss, the poorer the speech discrimination score with the degree of discrimination compatible with the magnitude and slope of the pure-tone hearing loss [22]. A neural lesion, on the other hand, will often yield speech discrimination scores that are relatively poorer than may be expected on the basis of examining the pure-tone thresholds. In Figure 2-3 a patient with a 35 dB cochlear hearing loss has a bilateral speech discrimination score of 90%. In Figure 2-4, however, a patient with a 30 dB hearing threshold and a neural lesion (eighth nerve tumor) on the right side shows speech discrimina-

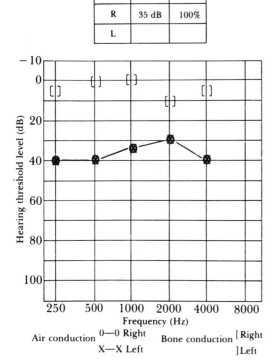

Ear	SRT	PB-Max
R	35 dB	100%
L		

Air conduction 0—0 Right   Bone conduction [Right
                X—X Left   ] Left

Figure 2-3. Patient audiogram with 35 dB bilateral conductive hearing loss; note air-bone gap and good speech discrimination for right ear.

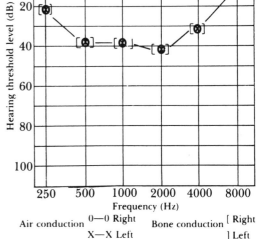

Ear	SRT	PB-Max
R	35 dB	70%
L	35 dB	70%

Air conduction 0—0 Right   Bone conduction [Right
                X—X Left   ] Left

Figure 2-4. Patient audiogram with 35 dB bilateral cochlear hearing loss; note reduced speech discrimination scores.

tion of only 76%. In summary, speech discrimination scores that are poorer than predicted from pure-tone thresholds should alert the examiner to the possible presence of a retrocochlear lesion. In these cases additional diagnostic tests described in other chapters should be administered.

Several investigators have studied ways of increasing the diagnostic efficiency of speech discrimination tests by making them more difficult. Common modifications include low-pass filtering [4] and Speech in Noise Testing [8]. Performance-intensity (PI) functions appear to have diagnostic value with performance decrements observed at high intensities when eighth nerve and low brain stem lesions are present [16, 17]. An example of PB rollover is shown in Figure 2-5, in which the discrimination score in the involved ear falls to 56% at a high intensity.

A different approach to speech audiometry has been developed by Jerger and associates [19]. These speech materials contain ten "synthetic" sentences that are identified by number by the patient rather than repeated. An example of a synthetic sentence is, "Small boat with a picture has become." The authors state that when presented with a competing speech message at various signal-to-noise ratios or when performance intensity functions are obtained, the Synthetic Sentence Identification test can be a useful adjunct in the evaluation of site of lesion in auditory system. In fact, Jerger and Jordan [18] claim that unless more sensitive speech audiometric measures are used, a significant number of patients with retrocochlear auditory dysfunction will be incorrectly classified as "audiometrically normal."

SPEECH DISCRIMINATION IN ASSESSING SOCIAL EFFICIENCY
At the present time, there are no speech discrimination tests available that can ade-

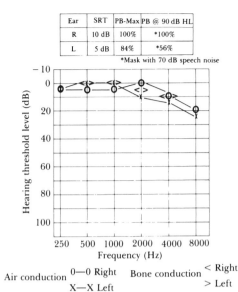

Ear	SRT	PB-Max	PB @ 90 dB HL
R	10 dB	100%	*100%
L	5 dB	84%	*56%

*Mask with 70 dB speech noise

Air conduction 0—0 Right   Bone conduction < Right
                X—X Left   > Left

Figure 2-5. Patient audiogram with left-side acoustic tumor; note speech discrimination score of 84% with normal hearing, and 56% at high intensities.

quately predict how well a patient hears and understands speech in everyday situations. Attempts at predicting social efficiency for purposes of establishing rehabilitation programs or for vocational or educational counseling must be based on qualitative interpretation of the speech discrimination score. Because a patient yields a 72% speech discrimination score on the CID W-22 test does not mean that he will understand 72% of what is said at home, at school, or at work. Speech discrimination tests are usually administered in quiet, whereas most people live in a relatively noisy environment, and noise can often decrease a person's ability to understand speech. On the other hand, speech discrimination scores are obtained by presenting words in isolation when, in a normal environment, the context of what is being said (contextual clues) will enable persons to understand what may be missed in isolation. In addition, the extent to which a person communicates depends on his level of motivation, how well he uses visual clues, how familiar he is with the context of the discussion, how good he may be at filling in the blank spaces (how well he guesses), and many other factors.

Therefore, the insightful clinician will attempt to combine what he sees in the test scores with what he observes in the patient to arrive at an estimate of the patient's social efficiency.

VARIABLES IN SPEECH DISCRIMINATION TESTING

Certain factors within the test situation, such as using live voice instead of recorded stimulus materials for presenting word lists, will affect the final results. Using live voice increases the probability that a word will be poorly articulated and therefore difficult for the patient to understand. In addition, live-voice testing introduces such variables as different voices, articulatory patterns, and stresses on words; regional, dialectal, or foreign accents; and male and female voices. The use of recorded speech, on the other hand, ensures that exactly the same stimulus is presented on test-retest conditions, test results are standardized, and comparison of results obtained on different days by different examiners and different clinics is facilitated.

Another factor in speech discrimination testing is the number of errors introduced by monitoring spoken responses. A complex communication process goes on between patient and examiner when speech discrimination tests are administered. The speech stimulus is presented to the patient who interprets it and repeats it to the examiner who interprets the response and decides whether it is correct or erroneous. When comparing scores obtained by verbal versus written responses, significant errors in results can be introduced by the examiner as a listener [22]. Nevertheless, a written response cannot always be obtained. Not all patients can read and write, and the additional time required for a written response is sometimes impractical. Consequently, talk-back communication systems in testing rooms should be of the highest quality to ensure that the spoken response can be clearly heard.

Another factor in interpreting the speech discrimination score is the level at which the stimulus word is presented. In the normal ear, W-22 word lists achieve 100% intelligibility at approximately 25 dB above the patient's threshold (25 dB sensation level). Therefore, most examiners give speech discrimination tests at 30, 40, or 50 dB sensation levels or at the most comfortable listening level (MCL). In attempting to determine the maximum speech discrimination score (PB-Max), it is sometimes difficult to predict the level at which the PB-Max score can be achieved. The difficulty, then, of obtaining discrimination scores at only one intensity is that the examiner can be sure that the maximum speech discrimination score is obtained only if the score approximates 100%. For a lesser score, the clinician must determine whether the patient might have achieved a better score for the materials if they were presented at a lower or higher intensity. The best way to obtain this information is to obtain speech discrimination scores at several levels to plot the intensity versus speech discrimination function. Although this procedure is clinically time-consuming, it is sometimes necessary and fruitful.

OTHER FACTORS IN AUDIOLOGIC EVALUATION

Reger [26] lists 11 factors that influence the reliability of audiometric test results. They include the following:

1. The accuracy of the calibration of the audiometer. Audiometers should be given daily biologic checks of calibration and laboratory or electroacoustic checks annually.
2. The magnitude of the masking effect of ambient noise in the testing environment. Audiometric testing must be done in a noise-free environment. Audiometric tests obtained in noisy environments can be invalid and unreliable. They fail to identify minimally hearing-impaired patients with either sensorineural or conductive hearing loss and, especially during hearing screening programs, give a false sense of security that children with hearing loss are being identified when, in fact, they may be missed.
3. Failure to use effective masking to avoid shadow curves (crossover).
4. Position and pressure of the earphone or bone-conduction oscillator.

5. Physical conditions within the test situation that influence body comfort, including temperature, humidity, and time of day.
6. Age, intelligence, reaction time, and previous test experience of the patient. It is necessary for the examiner to adjust his audiometric test procedure to fit the patient's ability to respond. With the use of play audiometric techniques, operant conditioning, and other techniques, it is possible to obtain pure-tone thresholds on children younger than 2 years. When it is not possible to obtain threshold measurements through conventional pure-tone or speech audiometry, other techniques are available for the assessment of hearing level, and no child is too young to refer for audiologic evaluation.
7. Physiologic condition and mental attitude of the patient (alert, interested, relaxed, cooperative, drowsy, indifferent, fatigued, depressed, tense, or apprehensive).
8. Training, experience, insight, and personality of the audiometrist.
9. Complexity of the stimulus presentation techniques used in determining auditory sensitivity.
10. Ambiguity of response instructions to the patient.
11. The use of complex reporting techniques.

Other factors can also affect audiometric results, such as tinnitus, often described by patients as a "ringing" or "buzzing" sound in their ears. Tinnitus may result in inconsistent patient responses or in elevated thresholds because of its similarity to the pitch of pure-tone stimuli. The use of a pulsed or warble tone often helps the patient identify a pure-tone stimulus as separate from the tinnitus [2].

The patient may appear to have a conductive hearing loss in two situations when, in fact, none is present. The first occurs when the pressure of the earphones collapses the external ear canal giving an invalid 30 to 40 dB air-bone gap. This finding can be detected when there is a discrepancy between the tuning fork tests and audiometric results, a discrepancy between hearing tests results and the patient's history, or a discrepancy between the audiometric and otologic examinations. Methods to determine if the threshold is affected by a collapsed ear canal include obtaining a free-field SRT, testing with earphones held slightly away from the head, or with an ear mold or polyethylene tubing in the external auditory canal to hold it open during testing [10].

A second invalid air-borne gap is frequently seen in patients who have severe hearing losses with air-conduction thresholds at 90 to 100 dB and bone-conduction responses at 250 and 500 Hz at approximately 25 and 50 dB, respectively. This air-bone gap is a result of vibrotactile response and is not an auditory response [21]. Vibrotactile responses are seldom, if ever, observed at frequencies higher than 500 Hz on audiometers with conventional maximum bone-conduction output.

When results of the basic audiologic evaluation have been obtained, they should be compared to observations of the patient's auditory behavior, to the patient's history, and to findings of the otologic examination. Significant discrepancies among these findings should require the examiner to ask why they exist, what additional procedures are necessary, and which indicator is most sensitive for assessing hearing levels.

REFERENCES

1. American Academy of Otolaryngology and American Council of Otolaryngology. Guide for the evaluation of hearing handicap. *J.A.M.A.* 241:2055, 1979.
2. Alpiner, J. G. Some aspects of tinnitus aurium as related to hearing impairment. *Maico Audiological Library Series* Vol. 5, 1968.
3. American-Speech-Language-Hearing Association. On the definition of hearing handicap. *Asha* 23:293, 1981.
4. Bocca, E., Calearo, C., and Cassinari, V. A new method for testing hearing in temporal lobe tumors. Preliminary report. *Acta Otolaryngol.* 44:219, 1954.
5. Carhart, R. Problems in the Measurement of Speech Discrimination. In I. M. Ventry, J. B. Chaiklin, and R. F. Dixon (Eds.), *Hearing Measurement: A Book of Readings.* New York: Appleton-Century-Crofts, 1971. P. 267.
6. Carhart, R., and Jerger, J. Preferred method for clinical determination of pure-tone thresholds. *J. Speech Hear. Disord.* 24:330, 1959.
7. Clark, J. G. Uses and abuses of hearing loss classification. *Asha* 23:493, 1981.
8. Cohen, R. L., and Keith, R. W. The use of low-pass noise in speech discrimination of pure tone thresholds. *J. Speech Hear. Res.* 19:48, 1976.
9. Dirks, D. D. Factors related to bone-conduction reliability. *Arch. Otolaryngol.* 78:551, 1964.
10. Elpern, B., and Naunton, R. F. The stability of the occlusion effect. *Arch. Otolaryngol.* 77:376, 1963.
11. Fairbanks, G. Test of phonemic differentiation: The rhyme test. *J. Acoust. Soc. Am.* 30:596, 1958.
12. Hart, C. W., and Naunton, R. F. Frontal bone-conduction tests in clinical audiometry. *Laryngoscope* 71:24, 1961.
13. Hirsh, I. J., et al. Development of materials for speech audiometry. *J. Speech Hear. Disord.* 17:321, 1952.
14. Jerger, J. A proposed audiometric symbol system for scholarly publications. *Arch. Otolaryngol.* 102:33, 1976.
15. Jerger, J. The future of audiology (letter to the editor). *Asha* 16:249, 1974.
16. Jerger, J., and Jerger, S. Auditory findings in brainstem disorders. *Arch. Otolaryngol.* 99:342, 1974.
17. Jerger, J., and Jerger, S. Diagnostic significance of PB word functions. *Arch. Otolaryngol.* 93:573, 1977.
18. Jerger, J., and Jordan, C. Normal audiometric findings. *Am. J. Otol.* 1:157, 1980.
19. Jerger, J., Speaks, C., and Trammell, J. L. A new approach to speech audiometry. *J. Speech Hear. Disord.* 3:318, 1968.
20. Konig, E. Variations in bone conduction as related to force of pressure exerted on the vibrator. *Trans. Beltone Inst. Hear. Res.* 6:1, 1957.
21. Nober, E. H. Pseudo-auditory bone conduction thresholds. *J. Speech Hear. Disord.* 29:469, 1964.
22. Northern, J. L., and Hattler, K. W. Evaluation of four speech discrimination test procedures on hearing impaired patients. *J. Aud. Res.* (Suppl. 1), 1974.
23. Peterson, G. E., and Lehiste, I. Revised CNC lists for auditory tests. *J. Speech Hear. Disord.* 27:62, 1962.
24. Pohlman, A. G., and Kranz, F. W. Monaural tests on bone acuity under various conditions with some general comments on bone acuity. *Arch. Otolaryngol.* 35:632, 1926.
25. Price, L. L. Pure Tone Audiometry. In D. Rose (Ed.), *Audiological Assessment.*

Englewood Cliffs, N.J.: Prentice-Hall, 1971. P. 167.

26. Reger, S. N. Pure-Tone Audiometry. In A. Glory (Ed.), *Audiometry: Principles and Practices*. Baltimore: Williams & Wilkins, P. 108.

27. Shambaugh, G. E., Jr. *Surgery of the Ear*. Philadelphia: Saunders, 1959. P. 64.

28. Studebaker, G. A. Clinical masking of the non-test ear. *J. Speech Hear. Disord.* 37: 360, 1967.

29. Studebaker, G. A. Placement of vibrator in bone conduction testing. *J. Speech Hear. Res.* 5:31, 1962.

30. Tillman, T. W., Carhart, R., and Wilbur, L. A test for speech discrimination composed of CNC monosyllabic words. *Technical Documentary Report No. SAM-TDR-62.135.* U.S. Air Force School of Aerospace Medicine, Brooks Air Force Base, Texas, 1963.

SUGGESTED READING

Jerger, S., and Jerger, J. *Auditory Disorders*. Boston: Little, Brown, 1981.

Katz, J. *Handbook of Clinical Audiology* (2d ed.). Baltimore: Williams & Wilkins, 1978.

Keith, R. W. (Ed.). *Audiology for the Physician*. Baltimore: Williams & Wilkins, 1980.

Newby, H. *Audiology* (4th ed.). Englewood Cliffs, N.J.: Prentice-Hall, 1979.

Paparella, M., and Shumrick, D. A. *Otolaryngology Volume II: The Ear* (2nd ed.). Philadelphia: Saunders, 1980.

Rintlemann, W. F. *Hearing Assessment*. Baltimore: University Park Press, 1979.

3

Diagnostic Audiology

Jay W. Sanders

Diagnostic audiology is the application of specialized auditory tests designed to evaluate various aspects of the response. The tests are qualitative rather than quantitative, in that they are concerned with the nature of the response—the manner in which the system responds—rather than the degree of hearing loss. The specialized stimuli and manner of stimulus presentation of these tests elicit responses that permit a determination of the presence and location of a pathologic condition in the auditory system. Essentially, the site of lesion can be determined as being the middle ear, the cochlea, the eighth nerve, or the central auditory nervous system. This information, the site of the lesion in the system, is of great value to the physician in the diagnosis of the disorder.

Specifying a middle ear disorder is primarily the role of pure-tone audiometry and impedance measurement, and these procedures are presented in Chapters 2 and 4, respectively. Special tests for central disorders are included in Chapter 16. This chapter, then, is concerned with special auditory tests for sensorineural hearing impairment of the peripheral auditory system—the cochlea and the eighth nerve. Because the symptoms and the hearing loss in various cochlear disorders may mimic those of an eighth nerve lesion such as an acoustic tumor, the distinction between these two sites of lesion is of great importance. The seriousness of the eighth nerve pathology and the premium placed on the earliest possible diagnosis lend additional importance to the development and application of special auditory tests designed to distinguish between cochlear and eighth nerve sites of lesion.

THE DEVELOPMENT OF SPECIAL AUDITORY TESTS

The concept and application of special auditory testing in sensorineural hearing loss began with the discovery that a specific loudness response, a phenomenon that has come to be called *loudness recruitment*, is present in ears with cochlear pathology but absent in ears with normal hearing, middle ear disorders, or eighth nerve lesions. The discovery generated great interest, because it had not been possible previously with audiologic testing to make the distinction between cochlear and eighth nerve pathology. Intensive study was directed toward recruitment, and additional special tests were developed in the search for recruitment test methods. The study led during the 1950s to the development of a series of qualitative tests designed to assess auditory response in three areas: suprathreshold loudness, auditory adaptation, and speech discrimination. Through research and usage, these tests have come to constitute a classic battery of diagnostic tests. Although the efficacy of at least some of the tests is now in question [76], the battery is still in widespread use for site-of-lesion testing in sensorineural hearing impairment.

THE CLASSIC SPECIAL TEST BATTERY
Suprathreshold Loudness Response
The classic special auditory test battery includes two different tests of suprathreshold loudness response. One of these is the loudness balance test for loudness recruitment and the other is a test of differential sensitivity for intensity.

Loudness Recruitment. The ear with loudness recruitment exhibits a more rapid increase in loudness with increase in intensity than is shown by the normal ear when loudness growth is measured in sensation level. One of the earliest observations of recruitment was made by Pohlman and Kranz [69] in 1924. These investigators noticed that some impaired ears experienced normal loudness when stimuli were at suprathreshold intensity. In a later report, Fowler [14] found that in some patients with unilateral hearing loss, equal loudness in the two ears could be achieved at a suprathreshold level by presenting the stimulus at a much greater sensation level to the normal ear. He reasoned that the growth of loudness must be much more rapid in the impaired ear, requiring a lesser intensity increase. On the basis of these findings, he developed a test procedure that compared loudness growth in the impaired ear with that in the opposite normal ear [15]. In a later report [16], Fowler coined the term *recruitment* to describe the phenomenon.

Fowler's test for recruitment is the alternate binaural loudness balance test (ABLB). In this test, a tone is presented alternately to the good ear and the poor ear of a person with a unilateral hearing loss. The signal intensity is maintained at a constant level in one ear and varied in the other until the subject reports an experience of equal loudness in the two ears. The sensation levels required for equal loudness are then compared. A significantly smaller sensation level in the impaired ear suggests a more rapid growth of loudness in that ear and indicates the presence of recruitment. Jerger [33] has suggested that the results of the ABLB be interpreted as follows:

No recruitment: equal loudness at equal sensation levels ±10 dB
Complete recruitment: equal loudness at equal hearing levels ±10 dB
Partial recruitment: equal loudness at sensation levels between those for no recruitment and those for complete recruitment

Although several reports [27, 33, 35] have suggested various modifications and refinements, the essentials of the test are unchanged from those of Fowler.

Fowler's ABLB test is limited in application in that it can be used only with patients having unilateral hearing loss. This problem was overcome with the development by Reger [70] of a loudness balance procedure that can be used in patients with bilateral hearing loss. In the Reger test, called the monaural bi-frequency loudness balance test (MBFLB), loudness growth is compared between a normal frequency and an impaired frequency in the same ear. That is, tones at the two test frequencies are alternated in the test ear. Intensity is held constant at one frequency and varied at the other to achieve the equal loudness experience. As with the ABLB, a comparison is made of the sensation levels required for equal loudness. Jerger's criteria for interpretation of the ABLB can also be used with the MBFLB.

Although the loudness balance tests developed by Fowler and Reger in 1936 were excellent techniques for the demonstration of recruitment, the phenomenon appeared to have no significant application, and little attention was given it until the landmark study in 1948 by Dix, Hallpike, and Hood [12]. With Fowler's ABLB, Dix and associates demonstrated that recruitment is characteristically present in Meniere's disease and absent in pathology of the eighth nerve. They also described a fourth result on the ABLB in addition to no recruitment, partial recruitment, and complete recruitment. This result, called *decruitment,* is a slower than normal growth of loudness in the impaired ear. Equal loudness in the two ears requires a greater sensation level to the impaired ear, the opposite of recruitment. Dix and associates noted decruitment in acoustic tumors, and subsequent studies [9, 17, 23, 90] have shown that decruitment occurs only with pathology of the eighth nerve, which suggests a transmission loss in the impaired nerve.

The findings of Dix and associates generated tremendous interest in the phenomenon of loudness recruitment, because it appeared to permit the important distinction between cochlear and eighth nerve site of lesion in ears with sensorineural impairment. As noted earlier, this distinction had not been previously possible with audiologic testing. Follow-up studies of recruitment with the loudness balance tests [13, 20, 50, 84, 92, 94] confirmed the findings of Dix and associates, and recruitment came to be recognized as directly related to cochlear pathology.

Since the early work of Fowler and the subsequent studies by others, the following definition of recruitment has evolved into a classic: *Loudness recruitment is an abnormally rapid growth of loudness with increase in intensity.* The loudness growth in the impaired ear is described in the definition as "abnormally" rapid because it differs from the loudness growth in the normal ear with which it is compared, and "different from normal" has been interpreted as "abnormal." Actually, the growth of loudness in the impaired ear is not abnormal but is entirely normal at the high intensity at which it is measured. On the ABLB in a patient having a unilateral hearing loss, loudness growth is compared at low intensity in the normal ear and high intensity in the impaired ear, and the difference in loudness growth is a result of the different intensity levels used. If the ABLB

is done in a masked normal ear, permitting a comparison of loudness growth at high and low intensity levels in normal ears, the result is a classic recruitment function [74].

This way of looking at recruitment raises the question of why the ear with sensorineural hearing loss from eighth nerve pathology does not show recruitment on the ABLB, as that ear is also tested at high intensity. The only plausible answer to the absence of recruitment in ears with eighth nerve pathology (and the presence of decruitment in some such ears) is a transmission loss in the impaired nerve. Thus, the pathologic result on the ABLB is not the presence of recruitment but rather its absence. Recruitment is a normal loudness response at high intensity. A *slow* loudness growth at high intensity, characterized by no recruitment or by decruitment, is the abnormal result on the ABLB test and is consistent with pathology of the eighth nerve [74, 75].

Differential Sensitivity to Intensity. Although the loudness balance tests of Fowler and Reger are excellent methods for the demonstration of loudness recruitment, they are encumbered by various limitations. The patient must have normal hearing in the opposite ear (ABLB) or at least at one frequency in the impaired ear (MBFLB). Further, they require special equipment, they are time-consuming, and some patients have difficulty performing the required tasks. These problems led investigators to seek a simpler, more widely applicable test for recruitment, and the search turned to the difference limen for intensity (DLI). The rationale for use of the DLI was the assumption that if loudness growth is abnormally rapid in the recruiting ear then the DLI must be abnormally small. A test that would reveal an abnormally small DLI in a suspect ear would thus give an indirect indication of the presence of loudness recruitment. From 1948 to 1955 several methods were proposed for the measurement of the DLI at suprathreshold levels as an indirect test of loudness recruitment [10, 28, 29, 55], all of which were to some degree successful in distinguishing cochlear and eighth nerve pathology. At the same time, however, other investigators [25, 52, 54] were finding that the DLI tests did not always agree with the results of the loudness balance tests and concluding that the DLI tests did not measure loudness recruitment. Finally, in 1961, Jerger [32] pointed out that the DLI procedure, while perhaps not a measure of recruitment, was a second and different test for distinguishing cochlear and eighth nerve pathology, a procedure that could be used in addition to, rather than in place of, the loudness balance tests for recruitment. With this proposal Jerger began the concept of a battery of tests for site-of-lesion determination.

The DLI procedure that was accepted as part of the test battery was the short increment sensitivity index (SISI), described by Jerger, Shedd, and Harford in 1959 [41]. The SISI is not actually a measure of difference limen for intensity but is rather a test of the patient's ability to hear short duration intensity increments of 1 dB superimposed on a continuous tone presented at a 20 dB sensation level. Larger increments, beginning at 5 dB, are used to orient the patient to the task, and the test consists of a series of twenty 1 dB increments. The patient's score on the test is the percentage of 1 dB increments heard. Jerger and associates found that patients with cochlear pathology heard the increments quite easily and consistently obtained high scores on the test, always 70% or higher. Scores were always low, however, never more than 15% in patients with normal ears and with ears with conductive impairment or eighth nerve pathology.

Follow-up studies [22, 95] have confirmed the findings of Jerger and associates, and SISI results are now described in terms of the following score categories:

0–30%	Negative for cochlear pathology
35–65%	Questionable
70–100%	Positive for cochlear pathology

On the basis of these early reports, the SISI became widely accepted as a special auditory test that could be used in addition to the loudness balance tests for recruitment in ears with sensorineural hearing impairment.

Unfortunately, as happened with the loudness balance test for recruitment, "different from normal" on the SISI was equated with "abnormal," and positive scores on the test came to be regarded as abnormal and pathologic. Cochlear pathology was thought, somehow, to render the ear more sensitive to small changes in intensity, resulting in a high score on the test. Low SISI scores were regarded as the normal response. Again, however, as with the recruitment tests, the results obtained on the SISI for patients with cochlear pathology is a normal loudness response at the high intensity at which the test is given in an ear with hearing loss. Although the SISI is not a measure of the difference limen for intensity, scores on the test are related to the patient's DLI at the intensity level of the test presentation. Earlier studies have shown that for patients with normal ears [72, 89] and with ears with cochlear pathology [89], the DLI is 2 to 3 dB at low intensity levels and less than 1 dB at high intensities. When the SISI is presented at a 20 dB sensation level to a patient with cochlear pathology with a 50 dB hearing loss, the test presentation level is 70 dB hearing level. At that intensity, the normal ear obtains scores at or near 100% [66, 67, 96].

If a positive score on the SISI is a direct result of the high intensity at which the test is presented, the question arises as to why the patient with hearing loss from eighth nerve pathology, also tested at high intensity, obtains a negative score. Here again, the only plausible answer is a transmission loss in the impaired nerve, a kind of neural "conductive" impairment. This answer will also explain the occasional patient with eighth nerve pathology who cannot hear increments of 2 or even 3 dB on the SISI, a situation akin to a result of decruitment on the loudness balance test.

Again, as with the loudness balance tests for recruitment, the pathologic result on the SISI is not the positive score observed in cochlear pathology but rather the negative score obtained from the ear with a hearing loss resulting from eighth nerve pathology. The positive score is a normal loudness response at high intensity; the failure to obtain a positive score at high intensity is the abnormal result on the test, consistent with a lesion of the eighth nerve [75].

Auditory Adaptation

Auditory adaptation, sometimes called *per-stimulatory fatigue*, is a decrease in auditory sensitivity during stimulation as a result of the stimulation. Two different tests of adaptation receive wide acceptance and have become components of the classic special auditory test battery.

The Tone Decay Test. On the basis of earlier reports [24, 26] of abnormal adaptation in patients with Meniere's disease, Carhart in 1957 [5] proposed the threshold tone decay test (TDT) of abnormal auditory adaptation for use in conjunction with recruitment testing to identify cochlear pathology. The procedure of the TDT is simple, and the only equipment required is a pure-tone audiometer. The patient is instructed to signal when he hears a tone and to maintain the signal as long as he hears the tone. The test is begun at the patient's threshold of sensitivity, and intensity is increased without interruption in 5 dB steps whenever necessary to determine the least intensity at which the patient can maintain response for 60 seconds. With the TDT, Carhart observed threshold shifts, defined as *tone decay,* of 20 to 30 dB in patients with cochlear pathology. He also discovered, however, that some patients with sensorineural loss of unknown origin showed tone decay of 50 to 60 dB and even beyond the limits of the audiometer. In a follow-up study of auditory adaptation in patients with sensorineural loss, Jerger, Carhart, and Lassman [34] found that patients with cochlear pathology did indeed show moderate amounts of abnormal auditory adaptation, but that the excessive adaptation observed by Carhart in a few cases was limited to patients with eighth nerve pathology. Subsequent studies confirmed the findings of Jerger and associates, and the results of the Carhart TDT are now interpreted according to the following criteria:

TONE DECAY RANGE (dB)		INTERPRETATION
Mild	0–10	Normal or conductive
Moderate	15–30	Cochlear
Excessive	35 or more	Eighth nerve

Although several modifications of tone decay testing have been proposed [21, 62, 65, 73], comparative studies [62, 68] have shown that the greatest accuracy in predicting the site of lesion is obtained with the original Carhart procedure, or with the modification suggested by Olsen and Noffsinger [62]. The Olsen and Noffsinger modification is only a slight change from the original Carhart method, in that the test is begun at a 20 dB sensation level rather than at threshold.

Bekesy Audiometry. A second procedure for the evaluation of auditory adaptation was proposed by Jerger [30] in 1960, using the Bekesy self-recording, automatic audiometer. Although the Bekesy audiometer had been used in several previous studies of adaptation [49, 53, 71], Jerger's report was a much more detailed analysis, in that he examined response tracings to a continuous and to an interrupted tone for sweep frequency and fixed frequency tests in 434 patients with conductive, cochlear, and eighth nerve pathology, as well as normal hearing. The rationale for the use of the Bekesy audiometer in the evaluation of auditory adaptation is that the adapting ear will show a threshold shift in response to the continuous tone but not to the interrupted tone. A comparison of threshold responses to the two stimuli permits a determination of the presence and magnitude of adaptation. From his analysis of the audiograms, Jerger proposed the following categorization and interpretations:

TYPE	INTERPRETATION
I	Interrupted and continuous tone-response tracings interweave throughout the frequency range. Consistent with normal hearing or a conductive impairment
II	Interrupted and continuous tone-response tracings interweave at low frequencies but separate in the midfrequency range, with the continuous tone tracing paralleling that for the interrupted tone at a hearing level 8 to 10 dB greater. The continuous tone tracing may also become much narrower in the high frequencies. Consistent with cochlear pathology
III	Continuous tone-response tracing shows an immediate break-away from that for the interrupted tone and drops rapidly to the limits of the audiometer. Consistent with eighth nerve pathology

IV   Continuous tone-response tracing shows an immediate break-away from that for the interrupted tone, but then parallels the interrupted tone tracing at a hearing level that is greater by 25 dB or more. Consistent with eighth nerve pathology

In a later study of diagnostic audiometry, Jerger [32] reported a predictive accuracy of 94% for Bekesy audiometry in a patient group that included conductive, cochlear, and eighth nerve pathologies.

Although the Bekesy test requires special equipment, the procedure is widely accepted as another measure of auditory adaptation, and Bekesy audiometry has been given a prominent place in the classic special auditory test battery.

The Test Battery Approach
The 1948 study by Dix, Hallpike, and Hood [12], using loudness recruitment to distinguish between cochlear and eighth nerve pathologies, was described as a landmark study. A second landmark study in the development of diagnostic audiology was that reported by Jerger in 1961 [32]. In this report, Jerger described the results obtained on Bekesy audiometry, the SISI, and the ABLB in 52 patients with known sites of lesion. The predictive accuracy of each test in each site-of-lesion category is reported in Table 3-1. As shown, the predictive accuracy of the tests range from 71 to 100% for the individual patient subgroups, and from 86 to 94% across the subgroups. As pointed out by Jerger, no one test perfectly predicts the site of lesion: for each test,

there are false-negatives in one or more diagnostic categories. Jerger went on to point out, however, that when the test results are considered in combination and interpretation is based on the *pattern* of results from the battery of tests, predictive accuracy improves to 100%. On the basis of Jerger's compelling data, clinicians adopted the concept of a test battery, and that approach to diagnostic audiology is generally found in most clinics today.

Studies of the results of the classic special auditory test battery since the original report by Jerger [32] have continued to show a high predictive accuracy for the various tests in patients with cochlear pathology. Table 3-2 reports the results obtained from patients with cochlear lesions in three later studies compared with Jerger's 1961 findings. As shown, the predictive accuracy has decreased very little, if at all, over the time span covered. With predictive accuracies as high as these for the individual tests, it can be expected that the pattern of results from the test battery would yield an even higher accuracy. For the 1974 study, for example, the predictive accuracy of clinical judgments based on the test battery approach was 96% [78].

It may be noted that three of the studies reported in Table 3-2 include the speech discrimination score as a site-of-lesion indicator. Following several earlier reports of extremely poor speech discrimination scores in ears with eighth nerve pathology [20, 51, 81, 93], Jerger suggested in 1960

Table 3-1. The predictive accuracy* of three special auditory tests in 52 patients with known site of lesion

| Test | Site of lesion | | | |
	Conductive (n = 21)	Cochlea (n = 20)	Eighth nerve (n = 11)	Overall accuracy
SISI	71%	100%	91%	86%
Bekesy	90%	95%	100%	94%
ABLB	100%	75%	82%	86%

* Number of ears in percent in which the test result is consistent with the known site of lesion.
Source: J. Jerger, Recruitment and allied phenomena in differential diagnosis. *J. Aud. Res.* 1:145, 1961.

Table 3-2. The predictive accuracy* of five special auditory tests in ears with cochlear pathology from four reports

Test	1961 [32] (n = 20)	1969 [90] (n = 23)	1973 [46] (n = 89)	1974 [78] (n = 100)
ABLB	75%	100%		87%
SISI	100%	91%	92%	88%
Bekesy	95%	100%	83%	93%
TDT		96%		82%
Speech discrimination			83%	83%	71%

* Number of ears in percent in which the test result is consistent with cochlear pathology.

Table 3-3. The predictive accuracy* of five special auditory tests in patients with eighth nerve pathology from eight reports

Test	1961 [32] (n = 11)	1965 [44] (n = 110)	1969 [90] (n = 23)	1969 [45] (n = 157)	1973 [46] (n = 321)	1974 [78] (n = 28)	1976 [6] (n = 121)	1977 [47] (n = 500)
ABLB	82%	60%	52%			67%	57%	50%
SISI	91%	60%	50%	76%	63%	48%	60%	55%
Bekesy	100%	73%	70%	67%	60%	51%	47%	57%
TDT		76%	80%			69%	77%	78%
Speech discrim- ination		71%	57%	66%	55%	44%	50%	56%

* Number of ears in percent in which the test result is consistent with eighth nerve pathology.

[31] that pathology of the eighth nerve interferes with the transmission of complex information such as speech and that an excessive deterioration of speech discrimination ability is another indicator of pathology of the eighth nerve. Since that time, many clinicians have included the speech discrimination test as part of the classic special auditory test battery.

Unfortunately, for patients with eighth nerve pathology, the predictive accuracy of the classic special auditory tests has not held up nearly as well as for patients with lesions of the cochlea. Table 3-3 reports the results of the special tests from seven later studies in comparison with the 1961 data of Jerger [32]. As shown in the table, the accuracy of most of the tests has dropped rapidly and markedly to little better than chance. A notable exception is the tone decay test (TDT). In four of the five studies using the TDT, predictive accuracy for that test has continued in the 76 to 80% range.

The decreased predictive accuracy of the tests for eighth nerve pathology is probably attributable to a greatly increased awareness and suspicion of acoustic tumor, leading to a referral for audiologic testing at a much earlier stage in the development of the lesion. Several studies [42, 44, 45, 47] have suggested a direct relationship between tumor size and auditory test accuracy—that is, for small acoustic tumors the predictive accuracy of the classic special auditory tests is quite low. The welfare of the patient is closely associated with the earliest possible diagnosis of an acoustic tumor, and it is in the earliest stages of the development of the lesion that the classic special

auditory tests are least sensitive. These results strongly suggest the need for the development and application of new and different diagnostic tests with much greater sensitivity to eighth nerve pathology in the earliest stages of its development.

ADDITIONAL SPECIAL AUDITORY TESTS
A number of qualitative auditory tests have been described and proposed as additions to, or replacements for, the tests now included in the classic special auditory test battery. Several of these tests have proved to be far more sensitive to eighth nerve pathology than are the classic special tests. High priority should be given to these procedures in the selection of a special test battery for site-of-lesion determination in patients with sensorineural hearing impairment.

The Auditory Brain Stem Response
The auditory brain stem response measurement (ABR), although a relatively new procedure, has rapidly proved to be an extremely sensitive and accurate test for determining site of lesion in patients with sensorineural impairment. Several investigators [60, 76, 91] have described the ABR as the most sensitive indicator available for distinguishing between cochlear and eighth nerve pathologies.

The ABR is an electrophysiologic procedure for recording the average electrical activity generated in the eighth nerve and brain stem by an auditory stimulus. In response to auditory stimulation at a suprathreshold level, the ABR in the normal auditory system is a series of five to seven waves numbered I through VII according to latency. Wave V, the fifth peak in the series, is a particularly prominent and strong response, and attention is given to it in the analysis of the response. The indications of a retrocochlear lesion are a complete absence of wave V in the presence of a clearly audible signal or the presence of wave V at abnormally prolonged latencies. The latter may take the form of an abnormally increased absolute wave V latency, increased interwave latency differences (I–III, III–V, I–V), and an increased interaural wave V latency difference.

ABR measurement is not a test for acoustic tumor, but rather it is an assessment of the integrity of the auditory nervous system from the cochlea through the brain stem. Nevertheless, it is an extremely useful procedure in patients suspected of eighth nerve pathology. A number of studies [3, 7, 19, 48, 59, 82, 91] have reported predictive accuracy of 90 to 100% in patients with eighth nerve pathology. Other studies [18, 86–88] have shown an unusual sensitivity for the procedure for pathology in other portions of the auditory nervous system from the cochlea through the brain stem.

When compared to other tests, new procedures, and the classic auditory tests, ABR measurement does indeed appear to be the most sensitive and accurate special auditory test currently available for the qualitative assessment of sensorineural hearing loss (see Chap. 5).

The Acoustic Reflex Test
The acoustic reflex (AR) is a contraction of the stapedius muscle in response to a loud acoustic stimulus, observed as an increase in the acoustic impedance at the eardrum. Measurement of the AR is an integral part of the impedance test battery for the assessment of middle ear disorders, but it also has an important application in the evaluation of sensorineural hearing loss. When the acoustic reflex test (ART) is used in site-of-lesion testing, the earphone ear is the test ear. Concern is with whether a reflex can be elicited and with the sensation level and hearing level required for an observable response. The ART in its present form has developed from two different reports and evaluates two aspects of auditory response—suprathreshold loudness and auditory adaptation.

The Metz Test. The earliest proposal for use of the AR in the evaluation of sensorineural hearing impairment was presented by Metz in 1952 [58]. Metz suggested that the ART is actually a direct test for loudness recruitment. He pointed out that in the recruiting ear the AR occurs at the same hearing levels as in the normal ear as a result of loudness recruitment. Because of the elevated sensitivity thresholds in these ears, however, the AR is at a reduced sensation level. Later studies [1, 50, 92] have found a close agreement between the presence of loudness recruitment and the AR at reduced sensation levels in patients with cochlear pathology, and further reports [40, 63, 80] have also found that patients with cochlear pathology have AR thresholds at reduced sensation levels. Northern [61] has suggested a cutoff of 60 dB sensation level, and this level appears to be an accurate dividing line. Using the 60 dB sensation level cutoff point, Sanders, Josey, and Glasscock [79] found a predictive accuracy for the ART of 99% in 105 cochlear pathologic ears.

Whether the Metz test is a direct measure of loudness recruitment may be of academic interest but does not affect the clinical utility of the procedure. The important fact is that the test is highly successful in determining the presence of cochlear pathology.

The Acoustic Reflex Decay Test. An important and valuable new addition to the ART was presented in 1970 by Anderson, Barr, and Wedenberg [2]. These investigators found that the ear with eighth nerve pathology gives a response on the ART that is different from that seen in the normal ear or in the ear with cochlear pathology and is consistent with the nature of eighth nerve disorder. In 17 ears with confirmed acoustic tumors, the AR threshold was elevated to hearing levels greater than those for normal ears. In some of these patients, the reflex could not be obtained with stimuli to 120 dB hearing level. When the AR was present, Anderson and associates also observed a rapid decay of the reflex as

Table 3-4. The predictive accuracy in percent of the acoustic reflex test in patients with eighth nerve pathology and the numbers of ears with elevated reflex and abnormal reflex decay from seven reports of the acoustic reflex test

	1970 [2] (n = 17)	1974 [43] (n = 30)	1975 [63] (n = 28)	1976 [83] (n = 24)	1976 [79] (n = 84)	1977 [47] (n = 75)	1981 [80] (n = 152)
Percent positive for eighth nerve pathology	100	87	86	79	76	85	77
Number of ears with:							
Elevated reflex	17	22	19	11	55	39	106
Abnormal decay	10	4	6	8	9	25	17

a result of abnormal auditory adaptation in the earphone ear when a continuous stimulus was presented 10 dB above the AR threshold. They noted further, however, that reflex decay may occur when the normal ear is tested at frequencies of more than 1000 Hz, and recommended that the decay test be done only at 500 and 1000 Hz. The procedure for the test was to determine the half-life of the reflex—that is, the time in seconds required for the reflex to decrease in amplitude to one half its original magnitude. In all cases the half-life was less than 5 seconds, and a recent report [64] has recommended 5 seconds as a criterion.

Further studies of the ART in patients with eighth nerve pathology have continued to demonstrate a good predictive accuracy for the test. Table 3-4 summarizes the results of six later reports compared with the findings of Anderson et al. Although the percent positive has decreased somewhat, it has continued reasonably well in the 75 to 85% range. It may be noted from the table that in almost all of the reports, elevation of the AR threshold was the predominant indicator of eighth nerve pathology, with decay of the reflex occurring relatively seldom.

In a recent study, Sanders and associates [80] have suggested a modification of the interpretation categories for the ART. In previous studies, ART results have been interpreted as either positive or negative for a given site of lesion. Sanders and associates have suggested adding a third category of "questionable." Their rationale for this category was that when the procedures of Metz and Anderson and colleagues are combined, it is possible to obtain results that are in conflict. For example, the AR may be at a reduced sensation level but at an elevated hearing level, or the AR may be at a reduced sensation level and a normal hearing level but show abnormal decay. In both of these examples, one aspect of the result suggests cochlear pathology whereas another is consistent with a lesion of the eighth nerve. In the classification system suggested by Sanders and associates, these results would be described as questionable—neither confirming nor ruling out a suspect site of lesion. In their study of the ART with the category of questionable, they found that although the positive rate was reduced from 97 to 83% for cochlear lesions, the false-negative rate continued to be quite low. In patients with acoustic tumors, the positive rate of 77% was unchanged, and, importantly, the false-negative rate was reduced from 23% to only 9%. This is a significant improvement in the overall accuracy of the ART in patients with eighth nerve pathology.

The Ipsilateral Reflex Test. A valuable addition to the ART procedure has been the capability for an ipsilateral measurement of the reflex. The stimulus is presented through the probe tube, and the AR is observed in the stimulated ear. The ipsilateral AR measurement permits the clinician in some instances to rule out one or more possible causes for an abnormal response. For example, if a stimulus to a right ear suspected of eighth nerve pathology fails to elicit a reflex in the left ear on contralateral measurement, any of the following could be the reason:

1. Middle ear impairment in the left ear
2. Seventh nerve lesion on the left side
3. Brain stem lesion affecting the crossing pathways
4. Eighth nerve lesion in the right ear

The presence of an ipsilateral reflex in the left ear would rule out the first two possibilities, bringing the clinician closer to a definitive interpretation.

Quantification of the Acoustic Reflex. A further modification of the ART proposed in several recent studies [8, 56, 57, 97] demonstrating an even greater sensitivity of the test for eighth nerve pathology is the precise quantification of the various parameters of the reflex, such as the latency, rise-decay times, and amplitude. Quantification is accomplished by recording the reflex for off-line computer analysis or by directly measuring with a storage oscilloscope [8] or an averaging computer [77, 97]. In a study of 21 patients, all suspect for acoustic tumor on the basis of previous tests, Mangham, Lindeman, and Dawson [56] distinguished between patients with tumors and patients without with a predictive accuracy of 100% on the basis of the quantified AR. Although further data are needed, quantification shows great promise for the improvement of an already excellent diagnostic auditory test.

Difficult Speech Tests

The speech discrimination score, a test included among the classic special auditory tests, has rapidly become one of the least sensitive measures of the battery. A more recent and much more sensitive use of speech discrimination measurement in site-of-lesion testing is the performance-intensity function.

The PI-PB Function. The performance-intensity (PI) function obtained with phonetically balanced (PB) monosyllabic words was described as a site-of-lesion test by Jerger and Jerger in 1971 [37]. In this test, discrimination scores are obtained with 25-word lists of PB words at a sufficient number of sensation levels to establish a function. Testing does not cease with the establishment of a plateau but is carried to intensity levels of 90 to 100 dB hearing level. Normal patients and patients with cochlear pathology tend to maintain a reasonably stable plateau even at high intensity levels; whereas the patient with an eighth nerve lesion may achieve a reasonably high PB-Max but then show a precipitous decrease in discrimination—called a *rollover effect*—as intensity is increased to high levels. Rollover may also be seen in some patients with cochlear pathology, however, and the significant result on the test is neither the presence nor the degree of rollover but rather the rollover relative to the best score. The magnitude of the rollover (best score minus poorest score after rollover) is divided by the best score to obtain what Jerger and Jerger called the PI-PB index [37]. An index of 0.45 was found by Jerger and Jerger and later by Dirks and associates [11] to provide the clearest separation between cochlear and eighth nerve pathologies. In a still later study using different test materials, Bess, Josey, and Humes [4] obtained the sharpest separation with an index of 0.25. In all three studies, however, cochlear and eighth nerve pathologies were clearly separated by the PI-PB index, with the eighth nerve disorder tending strongly toward much higher indexes than those for the cochlear lesions. In all three studies, the predictive accuracy for both sites of lesion was 90 to 100%.

Synthetic Sentence Tests. A second difficult speech test that is a useful adjunct to the PI-PB test is the performance intensity–synthetic sentence identification (PI-SSI) function [36]. In this test, a function is obtained with the synthetic sentence material of Speaks, Jerger, and Tramell [85]. The sentences are presented against a competing message of continuous discourse at a message-to-competition ratio of 0 dB. The PI-PB and PI-SSI tests used in combination permit allowances for the audiometric configuration, in that the PB material is more affected by high-frequency loss; whereas the sentences are more sensitive to loss in the low frequencies. Also, because a lesion in the central auditory system is more likely to affect the sentence material, the two tests in combination may suggest distinctions among cochlear, eighth nerve, and central lesions.

Modifications of Bekesy Audiometry
In recent years, several modifications have been proposed in the application of Bekesy audiometry as a test of auditory adaptation in sensorineural hearing impairment. Although clinical data are still sparse on these techniques, they appear to be promising procedures and are worthy of continued consideration.

The Forward-Backward Discrepancy. The forward-backward discrepancy test is carried out in the same way as Jerger's original procedure for Bekesy audiometry [30], but with an additional task. After the patient has traced a threshold response to the interrupted and continuous tones across the frequencies from low to high, a threshold response is obtained to the continuous tone backward—that is, from high to low frequency. The result is then interpreted in terms of the relationship between the interrupted and continuous tone but also as to any discrepancy between the continuous tone forward and backward. Significant discrepancies between the forward and backward continuous tone tracings are regarded as suggestive of eighth nerve pathology. In a detailed study of the procedure, Jerger, Jerger, and Mauldin [39] found a predictive accuracy of 99% in 121 cases of cochlear pathology and 78% in 23 cases of retrocochlear pathology. In a recent analysis of the predictive accuracy and clinical feasibility of several test methods, Musiek and associates [60] recommended the forward-backward Bekesy test for inclusion in a test battery for the detection of eighth nerve disorders.

The Bekesy Comfortable Loudness Test. Based on the hypothesis that the audiologic signs of eighth nerve pathology occur earliest at high intensity, Jerger and Jerger [38] have proposed that Bekesy audiometry should be done at a suprathreshold level rather than at threshold. Accordingly, they obtained response tracings to the continuous and interrupted tones at the patient's most comfortable loudness level in a procedure called the Bekesy Comfortable Loudness (BCL) test. Interpretation was based on the auditory adaptation shown by the relationship of the response tracings to the interrupted and continuous tones. If this was negative for eighth nerve pathology, the patient then traced a most comfortable loudness response to the continuous tone from high to low frequency—combining the concept of the forward-backward discrepancy with the suprathreshold measure. In an analysis of BCL results in 148 cases without retrocochlear pathology (normal, conductive, cochlear), Jerger and Jerger [38] reported that results were negative for retrocochlear pathology in 90%, positive in 2%, and unclassifiable in 8%. In 16 patients with retrocochlear pathology, results were positive for that site of lesion in 69%, negative in 2%, and unclassifiable in 19%. The predictive accuracy of these results is excellent, not only in terms of the high percentage of correct identifications in each diagnostic category, but also especially in terms of the extremely low false-negative of only 2% for each group.

The results that have been reported for both the Bekesy forward-backward test and the BCL test show a marked improvement in diagnostic accuracy over threshold Bekesy audiometry, and both procedures show promise as special auditory tests. For both, however, further clinical data are needed.

RECOMMENDATIONS FOR A SPECIAL AUDITORY TEST BATTERY
The analysis presented here of the predictive accuracy of the classic special auditory test battery clearly indicates the need to replace at least some of these tests with measures more sensitive to eighth nerve pathology in the early stages of its development. On the basis of information available at this time, the following tests are recommended:

1. The auditory brain stem response (ABR). Although a relatively new procedure, this

test has already proved to be the most sensitive measure presently available for site-of-lesion testing in sensorineural impairment. A major drawback is the expense of the equipment, and the test does not have to be available in every center. It should be available, however, directly or through referral, to every patient in whom retrocochlear pathology is suspected.

2. The acoustic reflex test (ART). This test has also demonstrated a very high predictive accuracy in patients with eighth nerve as well as cochlear pathologies. It is a relatively simple procedure that can be carried out in a short time with equipment that should be readily available in every hearing clinic.

3. Difficult speech audiometry. The combination of the PI-PB and PI-SSI function tests, while perhaps not quite as definitive as the ABR and ART, is nevertheless an excellent addition to those procedures. Special equipment is not required.

4. The tone decay test (TDT). This is the one procedure from the classic special auditory test battery that has continued to demonstrate an acceptable predictive accuracy, at least when it is carried out with the Carhart procedure or with the Olsen and Noffsinger modification of the Carhart method. Again, special equipment is not required.

It may be noted that the recommendation is still for a battery of tests. In spite of the excellent predictive accuracy of some of the tests listed, as yet none are perfect. A higher probability of success will still be obtained when clinical judgment is based on the pattern of results obtained from a battery of tests rather than on the results of any one test. The clinician should, of course, keep in mind the relative accuracy of the various procedures and weigh a decision accordingly. Finally, it should be repeated that these tests are recommended on the basis of information available at this time. Diagnostic audiology is a highly dynamic facet of the profession. New discoveries are occurring daily, and the clinician must keep up with these and be ready to modify clinical practice accordingly.

REFERENCES

1. Alberti, P. W., and Kristensen, R. The clinical application of impedance audiometry. *Laryngoscope* 80:735, 1970.
2. Anderson, H., Barr, B., and Wedenberg, E. Early diagnosis of VIIIth nerve tumors by acoustic reflex tests. *Acta Otolaryngol.* [Suppl.] 263:232, 1970.
3. Bauch, C. D., Rose, D. E., and Harner, S. G. Auditory brainstem response results from 255 patients with suspected retrocochlear involvement. *Ear Hear.* 3:83, 1982.
4. Bess, F., Josey, A. F., and Humes, L. Performance intensity functions in cochlear and eighth nerve disorders. *Am. J. Otol.* 1:27, 1979.
5. Carhart, R. Clinical determination of abnormal auditory adaptation. *Arch. Otolaryngol.* 65:32, 1957.
6. Clemis, J. D., and Mastricola, P. G. Special audiometric test battery in 121 proved acoustic tumors. *Arch. Otolaryngol.* 102:654, 1976.
7. Clemis, J. D., and McGee, T. Brain stem electric response audiometry in the differential diagnosis of acustic tumors. *Laryngoscope* 89:31, 1979.
8. Clemis, J. D., and Sarno, C. N. The acoustic reflex latency test: clinical application. *Laryngoscope* 90:601, 1980.
9. Davis, H., and Goodman, A. C. Subtractive hearing loss, loudness recruitment and decruitment. *Ann. Otol.* 75:87, 1966.
10. Denes, P., and Naunton, R. F. The clinical detection of auditory recruitment. *J. Laryngol. Otol.* 64:375, 1950.
11. Dirks, D., et al. Use of performance-intensity functions for diagnosis. *J. Speech Hear. Disord.* 42:408, 1977.
12. Dix, M. R., Hallpike, C. S., and Hood, J. D. Observations upon the loudness recruitment phenomenon, with especial reference to the differential diagnosis of disorders of the internal ear and VIIIth nerve. *J. Laryngol. Otol.* 62:671, 1948.
13. Eby, L. G., and Williams, H. L. Recruitment of loudness in the differential diagnosis of end-organ and nerve fiber deafness. *Laryngoscope* 61:400, 1951.
14. Fowler, E. P. Marked deafened areas in normal ears. *Arch. Otolaryngol.* 8:151, 1928.
15. Fowler, E. P. A method for the early detection of otosclerosis. *Arch. Otolaryngol.* 24:731, 1936.
16. Fowler, E. P. The diagnosis of disease of the neural mechanism by the aid of sounds well above threshold. *Trans. Am. Otol. Soc.* 27:207, 1937.
17. Fowler, E. P. Some attributes of "loudness

recruitment" and "loudness decruitment." *Trans. Am. Otol. Soc.* 53:78, 1965.

18. Gilroy, J., and Lynn, G. E. Computerized tomography and auditory-evoked potentials. *Arch. Neurol.* 35:143, 1978.

19. Glasscock, M. E., et al. Brain stem evoked response audiometry in clinical practice. *Laryngoscope* 89:1021, 1979.

20. Goodman, A. C. Some relations between auditory function and intracranial lesions with particular reference to lesions of the cerebellopontine angle. *Laryngoscope* 67:987, 1957.

21. Green, D. S. The modified tone decay test (MTDT) as a screening procedure for eighth nerve lesions. *J. Speech Hear. Disord.* 28:31, 1963.

22. Griffing, T. A., and Tuck, G. A. Split-half reliability of the SISI. *J. Aud. Res.* 3:159, 1963.

23. Hallpike, C. The loudness recruitment phenomenon: its clinical significance and neurological basis. *Proc. R. Soc. Med.* 58:190, 1965.

24. Hallpike, C., and Hood, J. D. Some recent work on auditory adaptation and its relationships to the loudness recruitment phenomenon. *J. Acoust. Soc. Am.* 23:270, 1951.

25. Hirsh, I. J., Palva, T., and Goodman, A. C. Difference limen and recruitment. *Arch. Otolaryngol.* 60:525, 1954.

26. Hood, J. D. Auditory fatigue and adaptation in the differential diagnosis of end-organ disease. *Ann. Otol. Rhinol. Laryngol.* 64:507, 1955.

27. Hood, J. D. Basic audiological requirements in neuro-otology. *J. Laryngol. Otol.* 83:695, 1969.

28. Jerger, J. A difference limen recruitment test and its diagnostic significance. *Laryngoscope* 62:1316, 1952.

29. Jerger, J. Differential intensity sensitivity in the ear with loudness recruitment. *J. Speech Hear. Disord.* 20:183, 1955.

30. Jerger, J. Bekesy audiometry in analysis of auditory disorders. *J. Speech Hear. Res.* 3:275, 1960.

31. Jerger, J. Audiological manifestations of lesions in the auditory nervous system. *Laryngoscope* 70:417, 1960.

32. Jerger, J. Recruitment and allied phenomena in differential diagnosis. *J. Aud. Res.* 1:145, 1961.

33. Jerger, J. Hearing tests in otologic diagnosis. *Asha* 4:139, 1962.

34. Jerger, J., Carhart, R., and Lassman, J. Clinical observations on excessive threshold adaptation. *Arch. Otolaryngol.* 68:617, 1958.

35. Jerger, J., and Harford, E. R. Alternate and simultaneous binaural balancing of pure tones. *J. Speech Hear. Res.* 3:15, 1960.

36. Jerger, J., and Hayes, D. Diagnostic speech audiometry. *Arch. Otolaryngol.* 103:216, 1977.

37. Jerger, J., and Jerger, S. Diagnostic significance of PB word functions. *Arch. Otolaryngol.* 93:573, 1971.

38. Jerger, J., and Jerger, S. Diagnostic value of Bekesy comfortable loudness tracings. *Arch. Otolaryngol.* 99:351, 1974.

39. Jerger, J., Jerger, S., and Mauldin, L. The forward backward discrepancy in Bekesy audiometry. *Arch. Otolaryngol.* 96:400, 1972.

40. Jerger, J., Jerger, S., and Mauldin, L. Studies in impedance audiometry: I. Normal and sensorineural ears. *Arch. Otolaryngol.* 96:513, 1972.

41. Jerger, J., Shedd, J. L., and Harford, E. R. On the detection of extremely small changes in sound intensity. *Arch. Otolaryngol.* 69:200, 1959.

42. Jerger, J., and Waller, J. Some observations on masking and the progression of auditory signs in acoustic neuroma. *J. Speech Hear. Disord.* 27:140, 1962.

43. Jerger, J., et al. The acoustic reflex in eighth nerve disorders. *Arch. Otolaryngol.* 99:409, 1974.

44. Johnson, E. W. Auditory test results in 110 surgically confirmed retrocochlear lesions. *J. Speech Hear. Disord.* 30:307, 1965.

45. Johnson, E. W. Audiologic diagnosis of acoustic neuromas. *Arch. Otolaryngol.* 89:280, 1969.

46. Johnson, E. W. Clinical application of special hearing tests. *Arch. Otolaryngol.* 97:92, 1973.

47. Johnson, E. W. Auditory test results in 500 cases of acoustic tumor. *Arch. Otolaryngol.* 103:152, 1977.

48. Josey, A. F., Jackson, C. G., and Glasscock, M. E. Brain stem evoked response audiometry in confirmed eighth nerve tumors. *Am. J. Otol.* 1:285, 1980.

49. Kos, C. M. Auditory function as related to the complaint of dizziness. *Laryngoscope* 65:711, 1955.

50. Kristensen, H. K., and Jepsen, O. Recruitment in otoneurological diagnosis. *Acta Otolaryngol.* 42:553, 1952.

51. Liden, G. Speech audiometry: An experimental and clinical study with Swedish language materials. *Acta Otolaryngol.* [Suppl.] 114:145, 1954.

52. Liden, G., and Nilsson, G. Differential audiometry. *Acta Otolaryngol.* 38:521, 1950.

53. Lierle, D. M., and Reger, S. N. Experimen-

tally induced temporary threshold shifts in ears with impaired hearing. *Ann. Otol. Rhinol. Laryngol.* 64:263, 1955.

54. Lund-Iversen, L. An investigation on the difference limen determined by the method of Luscher and Zwislocki in normal hearing and in various forms of deafness. *Acta Otolaryngol.* 42:219, 1952.

55. Luscher, E., and Zwislocki, J. A simple method for indirect monaural determination of the recruitment phenomenon (difference limen in intensity in different types of deafness). *Acta Otolaryngol.* 78:156, 1948.

56. Mangham, C. A., Lindeman, R. C., and Dawson, W. R. Stapedius reflex quantifications in acoustic tumor patients. *Laryngoscope* 90:242, 1980.

57. McPherson, D. L., and Thompson, D. Quantification of the threshold and latency parameters of the acoustic reflex in humans. *Acta Otolaryngol.* Suppl. 353, 1977.

58. Metz, O. Threshold of reflex contraction of muscles of the middle ear and recruitment of loudness. *Arch. Otolaryngol.* 55:536, 1952.

59. Miller, G. W., and Josey, A. F. Acoustic neuroma: Results of brain stem evoked response audiometry. *South. Med. J.* 71:1062, 1978.

60. Musiek, F. E., et al. Audiologic test selection in the detection of eighth nerve disorders. *Am. J. Otol.* 4:281, 1983.

61. Northern, J. L. Clinical Management Procedures. In J. Jerger and J. Northern (Eds.), *Clinical Impedance Audiometry* (2nd ed.). Acton, Mass.: American Electromedics Corp. 1980.

62. Olsen, W. O., and Noffsinger, D. Comparison of one new and three old tests of auditory adaptation. *Arch. Otolaryngol.* 99:94, 1974.

63. Olsen, W. O., Noffsinger, D., and Kurdziel, S. Acoustic reflex and reflex decay. *Arch. Otolaryngol.* 101:622, 1975.

64. Olsen, W. O., Stach, B., and Kurdziel, S. Acoustic reflex decay in 10 seconds and in 5 seconds for Meniere's disease patients and for VIIIth nerve tumor patients. *Ear Hear.* 2:180, 1981.

65. Owens, E. Tone decay in eighth nerve and cochlear lesions. *J. Speech Hear. Disord.* 29:14, 1964.

66. Owens, E. The SISI test and VIIIth nerve versus cochlear involvement. *J. Speech Hear. Disord.* 30:252, 1965.

67. Owens, E. Differential Intensity Discrimination. In W. F. Rintelmann (Ed.), *Hearing Assessment.* Baltimore: University Park Press, 1979.

68. Parker, W., and Decker, R. L. Detection of abnormal auditory threshold adaptation. *Arch. Otolaryngol.* 94:1, 1971.

69. Pohlman, A. G., and Kranz, F. W. Binaural minimum audition in a subject with ranges of deficient acuity. *Proc. Soc. Exp. Biol. Med.* 20:335, 1924.

70. Reger, S. N. Differences in loudness response of the normal and hard-of-hearing ear at intensity levels slightly above threshold. *Ann. Otol. Rhinol. Laryngol.* 45:1029, 1936.

71. Reger, S. N., and Kos, C. M. Clinical measurements and implications of recruitment. *Ann. Otol. Rhinol. Laryngol.* 61:810, 1952.

72. Riesz, R. R. Differential intensity sensitivity of the ear for pure tones. *Physiol. Rev.* 31:867, 1928.

73. Rosenberg, P. E. Rapid clinical measurement of tone decay. Presented to the National Convention of the American Speech and Hearing Association. New York, 1958.

74. Sanders, J. W. Recruitment. In W. F. Rintelmann (Ed.), *Hearing Assessment.* Baltimore: University Park Press, 1979.

75. Sanders, J. W. Diagnostic Audiology. In N. J. Lass, L. V. McReynolds, J. L. Northern, and D. E. Yoder (Eds.), *Speech, Language and Hearing.* Philadelphia: Saunders, 1982.

76. Sanders, J. W., and Bess, F. H. Special auditory testing: Review and update. *Am. J. Otol.* 3:172, 1981.

77. Sanders, J. W., and Humes, L. A direct method for quantification of the acoustic reflex. Presented to the Convention of the American Speech-Language-Hearing Association, Detroit, Michigan, 1980.

78. Sanders, J. W., Josey, A. F., and Glasscock, M. E. Audiologic evaluation in cochlear and eighth nerve disorders. *Arch. Otolaryngol.* 100:283, 1974.

79. Sanders, J. W., Josey, A. F., and Glasscock, M. E. The acoustic stapedial reflex test in cochlear and eighth nerve disorders. Presented to the Third International Symposium on Impedance Audiometry. American Electromedics Corp., Dobbs Ferry, New York, 1976.

80. Sanders, J. W., et al. The acoustic reflex test in cochlear and eighth nerve pathology ears. *Laryngoscope* 91:787, 1981.

81. Schuknecht, H., and Woellner, R. C. Hearing loss following partial section of the cochlear nerve. *Laryngoscope* 63:441, 1953.

82. Selters, W. A., and Brackmann, D. E. Acoustic tumor detection with brain stem electric response audiometry. *Arch. Otolaryngol.* 103:181, 1977.

83. Sheehy, J. L., and Inzer, B. E. Acoustic re-

flex test in neurootologic diagnosis. *Arch. Otolaryngol.* 102:647, 1976.

84. Simonton, K. M. End organ deafness. *Arch. Otolaryngol.* 63:262, 1956.

85. Speaks, C., Jerger, J., and Tramell, J. Comparison of sentence identification and conventional speech discrimination scores. *J. Speech Hear. Res.* 13:755, 1970.

86. Starr, A., and Achor, J. Auditory brain stem responses in neurological disease. *Arch. Neurol.* 32:761, 1975.

87. Stephens, S. D., and Thornton, A. R. D. Subjective and electrophysiologic tests in brain stem lesions. *Arch. Otolaryngol.* 102: 608, 1976.

88. Stockard, J. J., and Rossiter, V. S. Clinical and pathologic correlates of brain stem auditory response abnormalities. *Neurology* 27:316, 1977.

89. Swisher, L. P. Response to intensity change in cochlear pathology. *Laryngoscope* 76: 1706, 1966.

90. Tillman, T. W. Special hearing tests in otoneurologic diagnosis. *Arch. Otolaryngol.* 89:25, 1969.

91. Thomsen, J., Terkildsen, K., and Osterhammel, P. Auditory brain stem response in patients with acoustic neuromas. *Scand. Audiol.* 7:179, 1978.

92. Thomsen, K. A. The Metz recruitment test and a comparison with the Fowler method. *Acta Otolaryngol.* 45:544, 1955.

93. Walsh, T. E., and Goodman, A. Speech discrimination in central auditory lesions. *Laryngoscope* 65:1, 1955.

94. Yantis, P. A. Locus of the lesion in recruiting ears. *Arch. Otolaryngol.* 62:625, 1955.

95. Yantis, P. A., and Decker, R. L. On the short increment sensitivity index (SISI test). *J. Speech Hear. Disord.* 29:231, 1964.

96. Young, I. M., and Harbert, F. Significance of the SISI test. *J. Aud. Res.* 7:303, 1967.

97. Zito, F., and Roberto, M. The acoustic reflex pattern studied by the averaging technique. *Audiology* 19:395, 1980.

4

Impedance Audiometry

Jerry L. Northern

Acoustic impedance measurements provide efficient, objective, and often illuminating information to the routine audiometric evaluation and otologic examination. Some clinicians use acoustic impedance information initially with each patient to predict audiometric findings; others use acoustic impedance measures to confirm audiometric results on difficult-to-test patients. Acoustic impedance measurements may be used to obtain diagnostic information concerning the site of auditory lesion, the nature of hearing loss, and as a substitute for some of the advanced psychophysical behavioral audiometric tests. Impedance audiometry has established itself as an important part of the hearing evaluation and as an essential element in otologic diagnosis.

The utilization of acoustic impedance in otologic diagnosis has been advocated for many years. In 1946, Metz, a Scandinavian, published a monograph [31] in which he described many of the acoustic impedance applications used today. A mechanical impedance device was introduced into the United States in the mid-1960s with the potential of being a valuable diagnostic tool [34]. However, it was never widely accepted because of difficulties in its routine clinical use. Therefore, the device, along with the notion of acoustic impedance measurement, fell into general disuse in North America.

Publications in 1970 by Liden, Peterson, and Bjorkman [28], Jerger [20], and Alberti and Kristensen [2] stimulated new clinical interest in the electroacoustic technique of measuring acoustic impedance. Subsequently, interest in acoustic impedance measurements has resulted in numerous clinical applications that will have long-term, important influence on audiometric and otologic evaluation [43]. Complete textbooks on impedance audiometry have recently been published by Jerger and Northern [22] and Feldman and Wilber [15].

BASIC IMPEDANCE CONSIDERATIONS

The theory of operation of the electroacoustic impedance meter is relatively simple, and the technical manipulations of the

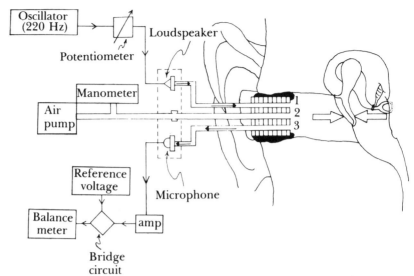

Figure 4-1. Schematic diagram of an electro-acoustic impedance meter with the probe tip sealed in external auditory meatus. The probe tip has three holes: (1) to emit 220 Hz probe tone, (2) to control cavity air pressure, and (3) pick-up microphone to compare SPL in ear canal cavity with reference SPL in impedance meter. (From J. Jerger, Clinical experience with impedance audiometry, Arch. Otolaryngol. 92:311, 1970. Copyright 1970, American Medical Association.)

equipment to perform the test procedures can be learned in a few hours. Interpreting test results, however, requires the knowledge of a skilled clinician who understands and appreciates the subtle diagnostic patterns and acoustic impedance test battery relationships.

By definition, *impedance audiometry* is an objective means of assessing the integrity and function of the peripheral auditory mechanism. The electroacoustic impedance technique relies on the principle that intensity is a function of cavity size. A signal of fixed intensity introduced into a large cavity and a small cavity will produce two different sound pressure levels. The large cavity will have a lower sound pressure level; a higher sound pressure level will exist in the small cavity.

The schematic diagram of the impedance meter (Fig. 4-1) illustrates a closed cavity between a probe tip in the external auditory canal and the tympanic membrane. The electroacoustic impedance meter simply measures the sound pressure level in this closed cavity by emitting a probe signal through one probe tip hole and measuring its intensity with a pick-up microphone from another one of the probe tip holes. The third hole in the probe tip is connected to an air manometer capable of varying the air pressure conditions within the closed cavity. A description of the principles of electroacoustic impedance

measurement is provided by Northern and Grimes [39].

In essence, the electroacoustic impedance meter is a miniature sound pressure level measurement device. The sound pressure level of the probe tone in the ear canal cavity is determined by the compliance of the tympanic membrane and middle ear system. The pick-up microphone quantifies the sound pressure level (or intensity) of acoustic energy that is reflected into the external auditory canal. A high amount of reflected energy is measured when the middle ear system is stiff or heavy, as in ossicular fixation or otitis media. In contrast, discontinuity of the middle ear system creates a flaccid tympanic membrane that absorbs much of the probe-tone sound energy and reflects very little into the external auditory canal. The impedance meter measures the reflected sound energy for clinical determinations regarding the compliance of the tympanic membrane and middle ear mechanism.

The middle ear is a stiffness-dominated mechanical system; and, as noted in "stiffness"-type audiograms, the stiffness factors are sensitive to low-frequency pure tones. Thus, most electroacoustic impedance meters use a low-frequency probe tone of 220 Hz. Some researchers advocate the use of higher frequency probe tones such as 660 or 800 Hz in addition to the 220 Hz signal. Alberti and Jerger [1] evaluated 1143 ears with probe tones of 220 and 800 Hz and concluded that no additional significant diagnostic information is obtained with probe-tone frequencies higher than 220 Hz.

THE IMPEDANCE TEST BATTERY

The basic impedance test battery includes tympanometry, static compliance, the physical volume test, and the acoustic reflex measurement. Although each test provides some information about the function and integrity of the auditory mechanism, the information becomes more meaningful when relationships among the three tests are considered. Diagnostic judgments can be made with greater assurance with the overall configuration of the entire impedance test battery. Though tympanometry is useful to a limited degree, static compliance norms are too variable for accurate diagnosis, and absence of the acoustic reflex may be due to several possible factors.

Tympanometry

Tympanometry is an objective method for evaluation of the mobility of the tympanic membrane and the functional condition of the middle ear. Tympanometry is the measurement of eardrum compliance change as air pressure is altered in the external auditory canal. These measurements are recorded on a graph known as a *tympanogram,* which represents the compliance–air pressure function. Tympanometry is similar to the task of the clinician who blows air against the eardrum (pneumatic otoscopy) and makes subjective visual judgments about the mobility of the tympanic membrane. However, pneumatic otoscopy often uses air pressures from ±700 to 1000 mm H_2O; tympanometry uses amounts of air pressure ranging between +200 mm H_2O and −400 mm H_2O.

The tympanic membrane is at *maximum compliance* when the air pressure in the middle ear is equal to the air pressure in the external ear canal. Tympanometry can thereby provide an indirect measure of existing middle ear pressure through the identification of the air pressure in the external auditory canal at which the eardrum shows its maximum compliance. By deduction, this pressure is also the existing middle ear pressure. Patients who have intact tympanic membranes, no middle ear pathology, and adequate eustachian tube function will show tympanic membrane maximum compliance at atmospheric pressure. Patients with intact eardrums and poorly functioning eustachian tubes show tympanic membrane maximum compliance at negative air pressure values. Research has shown the accuracy of tympanometric measurements of middle ear pressure to be within 15 mm H_2O of the actual middle ear pressure [13].

Tympanograms have been classified into patterns related to various conditions of the middle ear system by Jerger [20], Liden and associates [29], and Paradise and associates [40]. The Jerger classification of tympanograms is summarized in Figure 4-2. The type A curves are found in patients with intact, mobile eardrums and good eustachian tube function, as indicated by normal (or near-atmospheric) middle ear pressure. The type A_S curve represents slightly stiffened tympanic membrane compliance, whereas the A_D pattern represents the abnormally flaccid tympanic membrane. Type A tympanograms are generally found in patients with normal hearing or sensorineural loss; type A_S patterns are generally associated with otosclerosis, tympanosclerosis, fixed malleus, or a heavily thickened or scarred tympanic membrane. The A_D pattern is most often associated with a discontinuity of the middle ear ossicular chain. An exception to these tympanogram generalizations has been shown in which a comparison of tympanograms from normal and otosclerotic ears shows the average pattern to be virtually indistinguishable [27].

The type B tympanogram represents a nonmobile tympanic membrane characterized by little change in compliance of the tympanic membrane as air pressure in the

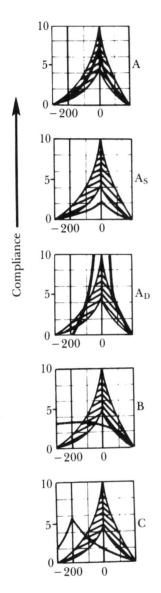

Figure 4-2. General classification of tympano-grams. Type A tympanogram, with normal compliance and normal middle ear pressure, is noted in normal hearing patients, patients with sensorineural hearing loss, and some otosclerotic patients. Type A_S tympanogram, with reduced compliance and normal middle ear pressure, is noted in patients with otosclerosis, thickened or heavily scarred tympanic membranes, or tympanosclerosis. Type A_D tympanogram, representing very flaccid or hypermobile tympanic membrane, is noted in patients with discontinuity of middle ear ossicles. Type B tympanogram shows poorly mobile tympanic membrane. This type of curve is noted when patients have tympanic membrane perforations, otitis media, ear canal totally occluded with cerumen, or a

external ear canal is varied. This condition may be noted in patients with otitis media, perforations, tympanic membrane ventilation tubes, excessive cerumen, or some congenital fixations.

The type C tympanogram represents an intact, mobile tympanic membrane with poor eustachian tube function demonstrated by excessive negative middle ear pressure. This curve may or may not be related to the presence of middle ear effusion. Bluestone, Beery, and Paradise [7] report a low incidence of middle ear fluid with type C tympanograms, but other authors find a high incidence of effusion with negative middle ear pressure [38].

Static Compliance

Static compliance is also a measure of middle ear mobility. The factors of compliance include mass, friction, and stiffness, which work together in a complex manner to facilitate or impede motion of the middle ear system. Historically, this test procedure is referred to as *acoustic impedance.* Currently, however, *compliance* seems to be a more favorable term than *impedance.* Considerable controversy exists in the United States concerning the clinical contribution of static compliance to otologic and audiologic diagnosis. Unfortunately, because a wide range of compliance values exist for various otologic pathologies that overlap with normal middle ear mechanisms, diagnosis of ear pathology based only on the static compliance measure must be considered with extreme caution.

Static compliance is measured in terms of equivalent volume in cubic centimeters based on two volume measurements. The first volume measurement (C_1) is made with the tympanic membrane clamped in a position of poor compliance with +200 mm H_2O air pressure. The second volume measurement (C_2) is made with the tympanic membrane at the maximum compliance pressure. Because sound is more easily transmitted by the tympanic mem-

patent ventilation tube inserted in tympanic membrane. Type C tympanogram, with near normal compliance but abnormally negative middle ear pressure. This curve may or may not be accompanied by middle ear effusion.

brane during the second volume measurement (C_2), the probe-sound pressure in the enclosed cavity of the external canal is lower than noted in the first volume measurement (C_1), and a larger "equivalent volume" will be indicated.

The static compliance measure is contaminated by the compliance of the air in the external canal itself. Static compliance is calculated by subtracting C_1 from C_2, which cancels out the external ear canal compliance and leaves a final compliance value that is the amount of compliance of the middle ear mechanism. Thus, $C_2 - C_1$ equals the static compliance of the ear in units of equivalent volume in cubic centimeters. In general clinical use, static compliance is abnormally low when the value is smaller than 0.28 cc and abnormally high when the value is larger than 2.5 cc. The major clinical contribution of the static compliance measurement is to differentiate between the fixated middle ear and the middle ear with an ossicular discontinuity. Only static compliance values that clearly exceed the 0.28 or 2.5 cc norms should be considered diagnostically significant.

Middle ear compliance is influenced by many variables including patient age, sex, and pathologic state [39]. The static compliance measure is corroborative information following tympanometry because both of these tests measure "compliance." The static compliance measure is considered by many to be the least valuable test in the impedance battery, and many clinicians omit it in routine clinical assessment. Indeed, Feldman [14] indicates that the static compliance measure is only appropriate when the patient's tympanic membrane is devoid of any abnormalities.

The Physical Volume Test (PVT)
An interesting application of the C_1 measure is to identify a perforation of the eardrum. If the tympanic membrane is not intact and has a hole from a perforation or a ventilating tube, the probe tone circulates sound into the entire middle ear space, and the C_1 volume measure will be quite large, often exceeding 4.0 cc or 5.0 cc in an adult. The C_1 measure in an adult with an intact eardrum is 1.0 to 1.5 cc. Thus, the static compliance C_1 measurement can be used to identify nonobservable perforations of the tympanic membrane or for the evaluation of patency of ventilating tubes in the eardrum.

Application of the physical ear canal volume in cubic centimeters will help in differentiating among the various causes of flat, type B tympanograms. A nonmobile tympanic membrane with a volume larger than 2.5 cc is usually associated with a tympanic membrane perforation or patent ventilation tube; a flat tympanogram with a normal physical ear canal volume is usually associated with middle ear effusion or middle ear ossicular abnormality. Physical volume values less than 1.0 cc may be related to cerumen occluding the external auditory canal or may indicate that the probe tip itself is occluded with debris or pressed against the ear canal wall [36].

Acoustic Reflex Threshold
The stapedial muscle contracts reflexively when the ear is stimulated with a sufficiently loud sound. This contraction occurs bilaterally, even when only one ear is stimulated. Researchers have consistently documented that the necessary loudness range is 70 dB hearing threshold level (HTL) to 100 dB HTL (median value 82.2 dB HTL) for pure-tone signals and approximately 65 db HTL for white noise [24].

In the demonstration of the acoustic reflex, the electroacoustic impedance technique uses the sudden change in the relative compliance of the middle ear system as the muscles contract. The acoustic signal is introduced through an earphone attached to the impedance audiometer headset. If the signal is sufficiently loud to the earphone ear to elicit the bilateral acoustic reflex, the contraction of the stapedius muscle in the ear containing the probe tip will suddenly decrease the compliance of that eardrum synchronously with the presentation of the stimulating earphone signal. The lowest signal intensity capable of eliciting the acoustic reflex is recorded as the acoustic reflex *threshold* for the *stimulated* ear. Under some circumstances the clinician is interested in the presence or absence of the acoustic reflex in the probe ear; on other occasions, the ear of interest is the earphone or stimulated ear. Regardless of which ear is under examination, it is standard clinical practice to record the acoustic reflex for the stimulated ear.

CLINICAL DIAGNOSIS WITH THE ACOUSTIC REFLEX

The diagnostic implications of the acoustic reflex considerably outweigh the contributions of tympanometry and static compliance measurements. An understanding of the acoustic reflex function in normal ears, ears with cochlear or eighth nerve pathology, as well as conductive loss pathology will enable the clinician to achieve considerable diagnostic information.

Cochlear Hearing Loss

The acoustic reflex function for 515 patients with cochlear sensorineural hearing loss as related to the level of hearing loss and the reflex sensation level is shown in Figure 4-3. The median acoustic reflex sensation level decreases from approximately 70 dB for patients with a 20 dB sensorineural hearing loss to approximately 25 dB sensation level for patients with an 85 dB sensorineural hearing loss. The acoustic reflex functions at 500, 1000, and 2000 Hz are quite similar and show a decibel for decibel decrease in the sensation level of the acoustic reflex threshold as a function of increase in hearing loss. The acoustic reflex function at 4000 Hz does not follow the exact pattern of the other stimulus frequencies. Because the acoustic reflex is often absent for no clear reason at 4000 Hz, clinicians should be cautious in interpreting reflex findings at this test frequency. The dotted square lines in Figure 4-3 represent the 50% presence level of the acoustic reflex. That is, with 85 dB of hearing loss, the clinician can only expect to observe the acoustic reflex at 25 dB above the auditory threshold of about half the patients with cochlear sensorineural hearing loss.

Jerger and colleagues [21] conclude that as long as the cochlear hearing loss is less than 60 dB, there is a 90% likelihood of observing the acoustic reflex when the earphone is over the ear with the hearing loss with a normal tympanogram in the probe ear. As the cochlear sensorineural loss increases to more than 60 dB, the chance of observing the acoustic reflex decreases. At 85 dB, the chance of observing the acoustic

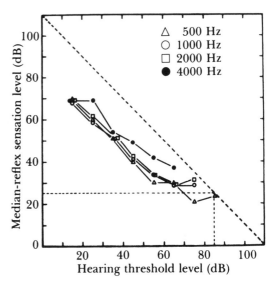

Figure 4-3. Acoustic reflex sensation level as a function of hearing loss severity in 515 patients with sensorineural hearing loss. (From J. Jerger et al., Studies in impedance audiometry: I. Normal and sensorineural ears. Arch. Otolaryngol. 96:513, 1972. Copyright 1972, American Medical Association.)

reflex is only 50%; if the loss is 100 dB HTL, only a 5 to 10% chance exists of the reflex being present. Thus, the presence of acoustic reflex thresholds at a sensation level of 60 dB or less, in light of a hearing loss less than 85 dB, provides a powerful indication for a cochlear site of lesion.

Conductive Hearing Loss

A valuable clinical tool is the fact that the acoustic reflex is obscured *bilaterally* in the presence of a *unilateral* conductive hearing loss that exceeds 30 dB HL. This occurs because when the stimulating sound is presented to the conductive loss ear, the +30 dB hearing loss is sufficient to prevent the signal from being perceived loudly enough to elicit the acoustic reflex. When the earphone is on the normal ear and the probe is in the unilateral conductive loss ear, the mechanism causing the conductive loss prevents the eardrum from showing a change in compliance. Naturally, in a bilateral conductive loss, the acoustic reflexes will be absent bilaterally because the pathology in *each* ear prohibits the probe from noting a compliance change when the opposite ear is stimulated with sound [25].

Other types of unilateral hearing loss do not obscure the reflex bilaterally. A unilateral cochlear sensorineural loss will have bilateral reflexes present as long as the hearing loss does not exceed 85 dB HL. A unilateral "dead" ear with a contralateral normal hearing ear will show reflexes when the normal hearing ear is stimulated and no reflex when the "dead" ear is stimulated. Thus, proper interpretation of acoustic reflexes in unilateral hearing loss can suggest the degree and nature of the hearing loss.

The acoustic reflex function for 154 patients with unilateral conductive hearing loss is shown in Figure 4-4. These patients were selected so that each "bad" ear had an air-bone gap and an abnormal tympanogram, whereas the normal ear showed no air-bone gap with a normal tympanogram. Figure 4-4 shows acoustic reflex results when the good ear was stimulated with sound and the probe was in the conductive loss ear (open triangles), and with sound stimulation of the conductive loss ear with the probe in the normal ear (solid circles).

The solid circle (straight line) function shows the effect of loudness attenuation by the conductive loss ear. The likelihood of absence of the acoustic reflex increases as the magnitude of the air-bone gap increases. Thus, when the earphone is over the unilateral conductive loss ear, the reflex has only a small chance of being absent as long as the air-bone gap is less than 30 dB. When the air-bone gap exceeds 30 dB, the stimulating tone can no longer be perceived loudly enough to cause the acoustic reflex to contract. The dotted line in Figure 4-4 indicates that with 27 dB unilateral air-bone gap, the acoustic reflex has only a 50% chance of being present when the probe is in the normal ear.

The open-triangle curve shows data for the condition when the stimulating sound was presented to the normal hearing ears with the probe tip inserted into the ear with the air-bone gap. Because the sound

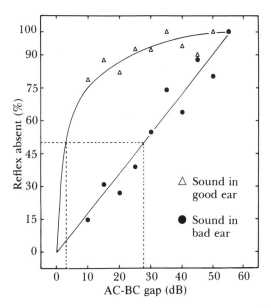

Figure 4-4. Percentage of absent acoustic reflexes as a function of air-bone gap in 154 patients with unilateral conductive hearing loss. (From J. Jerger et al., Studies in impedance and audiometry: III. Middle ear disorders. Arch. Otolaryngol. 99:165, 1974. Copyright 1974, American Medical Association.)

can easily be heard loudly enough by the normal ear, absence of the acoustic reflex on the probe ear must be caused by the air-bone gap. It should be clearly noted that a small air-bone gap of only 10 dB is sufficient to obscure the acoustic reflex as much as 80% of the time. The dotted line indicates that the 50% chance of acoustic reflex presence in the probe ear is coincident with an air-bone gap of less than 5 dB! This finding is extremely important to validate the presence of very mild conductive hearing loss. The acoustic reflex can be expected to be absent when the probe is in a conductive loss ear regardless of how small an air-bone gap exists. Conversely, if acoustic reflexes can be noted in the probe ear, it is virtually impossible for a conductive hearing loss to exist in that ear.

The acoustic reflex in patients with otosclerosis has a unique and characteristic pattern as reported by Terkildsen, Osterhammel, and Bretlau [45]. These researchers examined 34 ears with otosclerosis and found that patients with long-standing disease symptoms show low static compliance values and complete absence of the acoustic reflexes. In cases of early otosclerosis, the middle ear muscle pattern shows a slight negative movement as an on-off effect. When acoustic reflexes are present in early otosclerosis, there is a momentary negative deflection at the start of the reflex and again at the end of the reflex as the stimulating signal is shut off. Jerger and associates [23] found the acoustic reflex absent in 80% of 95 otosclerotic ears with normal tympanograms. In the remaining 20% of otosclerotic ears, normal reflexes were present in half the cases, whereas the other half showed the unique brief negative deflection at both the onset and termination of the stimulating sound. Otosclerotics have the only conductive hearing losses with normal tympanograms and absent acoustic reflexes.

Eighth Nerve Pathology
Careful interpretation of the acoustic reflexes can also supply diagnostic information about the presence of acoustic or eighth nerve tumors. Anderson and associates [4] suggested a technique known as the acoustic reflex decay test. These researchers evaluated the acoustic reflex in 17 patients with retrocochlear lesions. Of these patients, 7 showed no acoustic reflexes. In the remaining 10 patients, the acoustic reflex thresholds were elevated and could not be sustained at full magnitude for 10 seconds in the presence of an ongoing pure-tone stimulus.

Acoustic reflex decay occurs when the amplitude of the reflex declines more than half its initial magnitude in less than 5 seconds under continuous pure-tone stimulation at 10 dB reflex sensation level. Accordingly, acoustic nerve tumors have two possible positive reflex findings: (1) the acoustic reflex is absent when one would expect it to be present, or (2) the acoustic

reflex shows reflex decay under prolonged stimulation.

Researchers at Northwestern University and Baylor College of Medicine [24] combined efforts to evaluate acoustic reflex findings in 30 patients with eighth nerve disorders. Acoustic reflexes were absent at all test frequencies in 19 patients, present but elevated or with decay in 4 patients, and normally present in 7 patients. Strosser and Sheehy found similar acoustic reflex results in 56 cases of acoustic tumors (Table 4-1). According to Sanders [43], the acoustic reflex test continues to show a considerably greater predictive accuracy than the more conventional diagnostic auditory procedures.

Figure 4-5 shows the relationship between degree of hearing loss and the likelihood of reflex absence in patients with conductive, cochlear, and eighth nerve hearing disorders. These data represent absence of the acoustic reflex when the earphone is stimulating the unilateral pathologic ear. A clear demarcation of each pathologic group is evident from the acoustic reflex response of the impaired ear. When the earphone is stimulating an ear with 30 dB or greater unilateral conductive loss, with a nonpathologic ear on the contralateral side, the acoustic reflex has a high chance of being absent. Pathologic ears with cochlear involvement seldom have absent acoustic reflexes until the hearing loss exceeds 85 dB HL.

The intriguing fact, evidenced from these data, is that the acoustic reflex is absent 30% of the time in patients with *normal hearing* who have eighth nerve lesions. This likelihood of absent reflexes quickly rises to 70% with a mild 30 dB hearing loss. The absence of the acoustic reflex, in light of normal or near-normal hearing levels, must be considered suspicious until an acoustic tumor is ruled out. The rela-

Table 4-1. Acoustic Reflex Response in Retrocochlear Lesions

Studies	Number of cases	Positive response (%)	Type of positive response		
			Present and normal (%)	Absent (%)	Present but abnormal (%)
Jerger et al. [24]	30	87	23	63	13
Strosser and Sheehy [44]	56	82	18	55	27

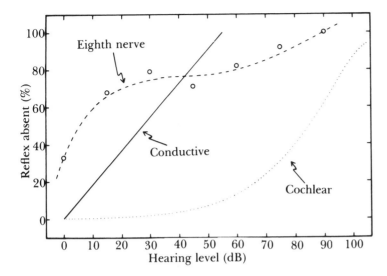

Figure 4-5. The relationship between degree of hearing loss and likelihood of acoustic reflex absence in patients with conductive, cochlear, and eighth nerve disorders. (From J. Jerger et al., The acoustic reflex in eighth nerve disorders. Arch. Otolaryngol. 99:409, 1974. Copyright 1974, American Medical Association.)

tive incidence of the various acoustic reflex findings associated with acoustic tumors may ultimately relate closely to the stage at which the tumor is detected. The conclusions in this study were that acoustic reflex findings were more sensitive to the retrocochlear pathology than Bekesy tracings, speech discrimination scores, tone decay test results, or the shape of the performance-intensity function for phonetically balanced monosyllables [24].

THE RELATION OF ACOUSTIC IMPEDANCE TO OTHER AUDIOMETRIC TESTS

Impedance audiometry is not a test of hearing, and accordingly is not a substitute for pure-tone air-conduction hearing tests. Although impedance audiometry is used clinically to identify the nature of a patient's hearing impairment, behavioral pure-tone audiometry is still the procedure of choice to represent hearing thresholds. On the other hand, impedance audiometry, because of its simplicity and objectivity, provides clinical information with more accuracy, in less time, and often with

more patient and clinician comfort than traditional behavioral-site-of-lesion procedures.

In the typical clinical setting one soon begins to see relationships between impedance measurements and audiometric behavioral tests. Our tradition in audiometric testing suggests that the more results that are available with which to affirm an otologic diagnosis, the stronger the conclusion may be.

The short increment sensitivity index (SISI), the alternate binaural loudness balance (ABLB), the monaural loudness balance (MLB), and the simultaneous midline loudness balance (SMLB), are used to localize pathology to the cochlea. These procedures rely on a patient's ability to detect small changes in signal intensity or to equate the loudness of various tones. Nonexperienced patients often find these listening tasks confusing and difficult to perform accurately.

Metz [32] suggested the use of the acoustic reflex as an indicator of cochlear pathology by identifying the presence of loudness recruitment. In cochlear hearing loss, acoustic reflexes are generally present at normal levels, and the "gap" between air-conduction thresholds and acoustic reflex thresholds is dramatically reduced. Excellent agreement exists between behavioral tests of loudness recruitment and the Metz acoustic reflex recruitment test. Obviously the Metz test is much simpler and quicker to administer than the complex listening

Table 4-2. Steps in Clinical Evaluations

Pure-tone air-conduction audiometry

Speech audiometry
↓
Impedance audiometry
↓

1-Tympanometry	Normal	Normal	Abnormal
↓			
2-Static compliance	Normal	Normal	Abnormal
↓			
3-Acoustic reflex	Normal	Absent	Absent
	Probable normal hearing or Mild to moderate sensori- neural hearing loss	Probable severe bi- lateral sensorineural hearing loss ↓	Probable conductive hearing loss ↓
	Bone-conduction test optional	Bone-conduction test optional	Proceed with bone- conduction testing

tasks involved in the loudness-balance techniques.

The pure-tone decay test (TDT) was devised as a technique to identify the presence of eighth nerve lesions. The use of the acoustic reflex in identifying retrocochlear tumors has several obvious advantages over the tone decay test. Research with acoustic tumors suggests that "positive" acoustic reflex findings are more sensitive to the presence of retrocochlear pathology than the tone decay test.

The main implementation of pulsed and continuous Bekesy tracings is to differentiate normal hearing and cochlear-impaired hearing loss patients from patients with retrocochlear lesions. A critical drawback to the Bekesy technique is that it is extremely time-consuming in routine clinical practice. Careful interpretation of pure-tone audiometry and impedance audiometry will provide similar clinical differentiation in considerably less time.

Table 4-2 is a clinical paradigm that suggests initial pure-tone air conduction and speech audiometry followed by evaluation with the impedance test battery for all patients. Patients with sensorineural hearing loss and normal hearing have bone-conduction thresholds equal to their air-conduction thresholds. Bone-conduction measurement is imperative only for those patients with conductive pathology to determine the amount of the air-bone gap and to evaluate the cochlear reserve or hearing sensitivity of the inner ear. Deletion of bone-conduction measurement on patients with normal hearing and sensorineural hearing loss will result in significant time-saving for routine clinical practice. The lack of standardized bone-conduction testing techniques and the need for careful application of masking during bone-conduction measurements make the bone-conduction test one of the most difficult testing procedures. Audiologists disagree about many aspects of bone-conduction measurement, including placement of the bone oscillator on the mastoid or frontal bone, procedures for calibration of the bone oscillator, masked or non-masked bone-conduction testing techniques, and recording of bone-conduction responses. In our practice, bone-conduction testing is performed on patients with known conductive hearing losses as identified through abnormal tympanometry, abnormal static compliance measures, accompanied by the absence of the acoustic reflex. The clinician, however, must beware the otosclerotic patient, whose impedance findings may look like a profound sensorineural hearing loss, with a normal tympanogram, normal static compliance, and absent acoustic reflexes.

It seems likely that as clinicians gain

more experience and confidence with impedance audiometry, the many advantages of the impedance measurements may outweigh behavioral tests for the identification of normal hearing, conductive hearing loss, cochlear pathology, and retrocochlear lesions.

IMPEDANCE AUDIOMETRY WITH CHILDREN

The audiometric evaluation of children has changed considerably with the use of impedance audiometry. The impedance technique is well suited for use with children because it requires little cooperation, provides objective results, and is quick and easy to administer. Often impedance audiometry may be accomplished with children who refuse to perform play conditioning tasks with pure-tone audiometry. In addition, impedance audiometry may often supply information about the hearing mechanism in very young children even when otologic or audiologic examination proves to be difficult or impossible to carry out [35]. Readers interested in additional applications of impedance audiometry with children are referred to *Hearing in Children* [38].

Otitis media with effusion is a widespread cause of hearing disorders in young school-age children. Pure-tone screening hearing tests fail to identify a large percentage of children with otologic disease. Cohen and Sade [11] report that 50% of 408 ears in children with serious otitis media passed as "normal" on school hearing tests conducted at a screening level of 25 dB HL. Brooks [8, 9] has long and often advocated the use of acoustic impedance measurement as a supplement to the standard pure-tone hearing screening test in mass populations of school children. Conventional screening of auditory functioning with pure tones is often inefficient and unsatisfactory because it is time-consuming and the results depend on too many uncontrollable variables. Extensive data now exist indicating that hearing levels as such do not necessarily identify otologic pathology—a fact pointed out in the classic Pittsburgh study [12].

A number of investigators have conducted studies to compare the efficacy of impedance audiometry with otoscopy and pure-tone screening. Von Wagoner and Harker [46] screened 1300 ears in Alaskan school children and found that 10.2% of the ears identified as pathologic with impedance and verified with otoscopy passed the pure-tone hearing screening test as "normal." McCandless and Thomas [30] employed middle ear pressure measurement and the presence of the acoustic reflex as a screening technique in a school-age population of 730 Indians. They report a 93% overall agreement between impedance screening and otoscopy findings. They report only 61% overall agreement between pure-tone screening and otoscopy.

In Scandinavia, investigators compared screening audiometry with results from otoscopy and impedance audiometry in 200 ears of 7-year-old children who had failed two pure-tone hearing screening tests at school [41]. Otoscopy identified pathology in 85% of the group, while impedance measurements of tympanometry and acoustic reflexes identified pathology in 97% of the failure sample. The major cause of disagreement between pure-tone screening and impedance screening techniques appears to be the presence of fluid in the middle ear, which does not create sufficient hearing loss to cause failure of the school hearing test. The sensitivity of tympanometry to identify the presence of middle ear fluid and tympanic membrane perforations is a valuable supplement to pure-tone screening programs.

The routine use of impedance measurements in school screening programs, however, has been a controversial issue. Clinicians active in hearing screening are well aware of the inadequacies of pure-tone screening audiometry, and thus welcome the opportunity to supplement their test protocol with impedance screening. They argue that the use of impedance in school health programs increases the overall accuracy of the screening program, reduces the number of children who must be retested prior to referral, and in fact, increases assurance that children who are referred for additional work-up have legitimate otologic problems [37, 42]. Opponents to the use of impedance in screening programs call for further research in the natural history and medical management of middle ear disease, as well as the educational and linguistic complications of middle ear disease [5]. Two sets of guidelines for impedance screening have been generated for use with preschool and school-age children, and special populations [3, 18].

OTOLOGIC APPLICATIONS OF ACOUSTIC IMPEDANCE MEASUREMENTS

Postoperative Surgical Evaluation

Impedance audiometry may provide significant information concerning post-operative results in patients who have undergone ear surgery [36]. Tympanometry can provide objective evidence concerning the healing and mobility of tympanoplasty grafts. Early tympanograms after tympanoplasty typically show the graft to be immobile. As the healing process thins the graft, the mobility of the tympanic membrane returns to normal. For middle ear surgical procedures performed in stages, some surgeons use the stability of a normal tympanogram after the initial surgical operation as an objective time lapse indication for the second surgical procedure. Postsurgical air-bone gaps that persist or that grow progressively greater with time may be evaluated with the impedance test battery. Interpretation of the tympanogram, the static compliance measure, and the presence or absence of the acoustic reflex can shed light on whether the postsurgical air-bone gap is caused by refixation of the middle ear system or by some discontinuity.

Eustachian Tube Function

The impedance technique has proved useful in the evaluation of eustachian tube function. Many extensive clinical procedures have been recommended for determining eustachian tube physiology. Eustachian tube function in patients with intact tympanic membranes is evidenced quite simply by the tympanogram and the measurement of middle ear pressure. When middle ear pressure is less than -150 mm H_2O, it may be concluded that the eustachian tube is not functioning normally.

Most clinicians are interested in documenting eustachian tube function in patients with perforations of the tympanic membrane. Because the eustachian tube is normally closed, it is possible to achieve an airtight seal with the probe tip and to build up positive or negative pressure in patients with tympanic membrane perforations. These patients should be instructed not to swallow or otherwise cause their eustachian tubes to open until instructed to do so during the test. Only the air pressure system is used in evaluating eustachian tube function in patients with eardrum perforations. Positive pressure is first introduced through the tympanic membrane perforation into the patient's middle ear until sufficient increase in pressure causes the patient's eustachian tube to suddenly open spontaneously at approximately $+280$ to $+350$ mm H_2O. If it does not open with as much as $+400$ mm H_2O, it is an indication of a poorly functioning eustachian tube. If the patient's eustachian tube opens under positive pressure, this initial step clears mucus or other debris that may be partially blocking the eustachian tube that could influence results of the following negative pressure evaluation.

The next step in evaluating eustachian tubes in patients with tympanic membrane perforations is to establish negative pressure of -200 mm H_2O in the external ear canal and middle ear cavity. The patient is then asked to swallow, yawn, or perform some action to make his eustachian tube open to equalize the negative pressure from the middle ear cavity. The clinician observes the air pressure meter during the patient's swallow, yawn, or other maneuver and notes changes in air pressure if the eustachian tube functions properly. If the patient is able to achieve some equalization of air pressure between his nasopharynx and middle ear cavity, the air pressure system will slowly adjust from -200 mm H_2O toward atmospheric pressure. Normal eustachian tube function may be inferred if the patient is able to reduce the -200 mm H_2O in his middle ear cavity to only -75 or -50 mm H_2O.

Patulous Eustachian Tube.
A patulous eustachian tube is disturbing to many patients and, at times, difficult to document objectively. Patients with abnormally open eustachian tubes complain of hearing their own breathing and vocalization and of the inability to converse at the dinner table

while chewing. The impedance meter can provide an objective diagnosis by establishing the presence of a normal tympanogram with normal middle ear pressure. The patient should inspire and expire through his mouth only, then breathe through his nose with his mouth closed, and finally stop breathing momentarily. The patient with a patulous eustachian tube will show an increase in tympanic membrane compliance with each inspiration and a corresponding decrease in tympanic membrane compliance with expiration; tympanic membrane compliance changes will be greater during the period of nasal breathing than during the period of mouth breathing alone; momentarily stopping breathing discontinues the abrupt changes in tympanic membrane compliance. When the impedance meter is in its most sensitive position it is often possible to observe compliance changes that are in synchrony with the patient's breathing, which verifies the presence of a patulous eustachian tube even when the changes are so small as to be nonobservable by otoscopy.

A thorough and complete discussion of eustachian tube function and evaluation has been published by Bluestone [6].

Fistula Test
In the fistula test, direct, positive pressure is applied to the fluids of the inner ear. If a fistula exists, the positive pressure results in a nystagmus and creates a sensation of vertigo in the patient. The impedance audiometer air pressure system provides a means by which a clinician can subtly and carefully create positive air pressure against the intact tympanic membrane or through a perforated tympanic membrane until the initial vestiges of dizziness are observed. In some clinics, the fistula test with the impedance audiometer is carried out with the patient hooked up to the electronystagmograph recorder to permit objective determination of nystagmus from positive air pressure.

Glomus Tumor
A glomus tumor is a vascular tumor of the middle ear, which is usually associated with symptoms of pulsatile tinnitus, possible hearing loss, and possible facial paralysis. This middle ear tumor is often difficult to observe otoscopically until it is rela-

tively large. The pulsations of blood through the tumor make early detection with the impedance technique possible. The air pressure system is set at slight positive air pressures up to +150 mm H_2O. The presence of a glomus tumor may be noted if the compliance change meter pulsates in synchrony with the patient's pulse. Confirmation of the diagnosis is provided when the pulsing of the compliance change meter decreases in amplitude as the carotid artery of the neck on the involved side of the patient is depressed by the clinician's thumb.

Peripheral Facial Nerve Test
Because the stapedial muscle is innervated by a small branch of the seventh cranial nerve, the presence or absence of the stapedial reflex in a patient with facial paralysis may be used to help locate the site of lesion. If the patient has facial palsy and the stapedial reflex is present, then it may be concluded that the site of lesion is distal, or at a lower level than the innervation of the stapedial muscle. With facial paralysis and no stapedial reflex present, the site of lesion may then be inferred to be proximal, or at a higher level than the takeoff of the twig innervating the stapedial muscle. When using impedance audiometry to evaluate peripheral facial nerve function, the efferent nervous system is under investigation, and interpretation of test results is based on compliance changes in the probe ear. Regularly monitoring the presence or absence of the acoustic reflex as well as the magnitude and briskness of the acoustic reflex in patients with active degeneration of the facial nerve may be a valuable technique in considering the necessity of surgical intervention. Observation of the return of the stapedial muscle reflex in patients with degenerative facial nerve disease is often seen some 10 days prior to the onset of facial muscle function return [10].

SPECIAL APPLICATIONS OF
THE ACOUSTIC REFLEX
Prediction of Hearing Level
One of the most practical clinical applications of the acoustic reflex is a procedure to estimate a patient's level of hearing sen-

sitivity. The technique, known as sensitivity prediction from the acoustic reflex (SPAR), is based on a procedure developed in Germany in 1972 [33]. The test is based on the fact that normal acoustic reflex thresholds are some 25 dB better with a broadband noise stimulus than with a pure-tone stimulus. This 25 dB difference in apparent loudness between the noise and pure-tone stimulus decreases in an orderly relationship in patients with sensorineural hearing loss. Patients with mild to moderate sensorineural hearing loss have only a 10 to 20 dB difference between the two types of stimuli; patients with severe sensorineural hearing loss have equal thresholds, or less than a 10 dB difference; patients with profound sensorineural loss will have no acoustic reflexes.

Jerger simplified the original German technique and developed the most widely used clinical procedure [25]. He recommends averaging acoustic reflex thresholds at 500, 1000, and 2000 Hz and comparing this value with the broadband noise reflex threshold to estimate *degree* of sensorineural hearing level.

This technique has tremendous implications for the auditory evaluation of young children and patients with nonorganic hearing loss. The degree of hearing loss and slope of audiometric configuration can now be reasonably predicted with only six objective acoustic reflex thresholds.

Limitations of the test include the necessity for normal middle ear function in the patient so that acoustic reflexes are not absent owing to the presence of conductive hearing pathology. Persons with suspected brain injury are also poor candidates for SPAR. With these two limiting qualifications in mind, the test has significant promise in the hearing evaluation of difficult-to-test patients. An excellent review and discussion of the prediction of hearing loss from the acoustic reflex has recently been published by Hall [17].

Ipsilateral Acoustic Reflex Measurement
Recent equipment designs now enable many impedance meters to measure the presence of the acoustic reflex in an ipsilateral mode. In the ipsilateral condition, the stimulus is presented through the probe tip and reflex response is monitored in the same ear. A major advantage of the ipsilateral technique is that the confusion regarding which ear is being tested is eliminated.

The initial clinical application for the ipsilateral reflex test was in the differential diagnosis of brain stem lesions [16]. Brain stem lesions that interrupt the crossed acoustic reflex pathways cancel the presence of contralaterally measured reflexes, but the ipsilateral reflex is bilaterally present. Additional clinical applications of the ipsilateral reflex include validation of unilateral mild conductive hearing loss and mild disorders of the peripheral facial nerve. Comparison of crossed and uncrossed (contralateral vs ipsilateral) reflex thresholds provides an important diagnostic tool for differentiating pathology of the eighth nerve from lesions of the central auditory tracts in the brain stem [19, 26].

DIAGNOSTIC IMPLEMENTATION OF IMPEDANCE AUDIOMETRY
Impedance audiometry offers much to the practice of audiology and otology in the diagnosis of clinical problems. The impedance audiometer is an indispensable tool when fully utilized by an experienced clinician. This instrument was originally developed to evaluate conductive hearing impairment, but its utility has now been extended so that evaluations of inner ear, retrocochlear, and brain stem problems are common practice. The impedance technique has proved valuable in predicting or confirming audiometric findings regarding the nature of conductive or sensorineural hearing loss, the differentiation of various types of conductive hearing impairment, the elucidation of sensorineural hearing loss into problems of the cochlear or eighth nerve, the quantification of degree and slope of sensorineural hearing loss, as well as the integrity of intact auditory reflex pathways in the brain stem.

Maximum diagnostic implementation of impedance audiometry requires careful consideration and caution. The powerful diagnostic implications of impedance audiometry may give clinicians an unwarranted sense of security, particularly when used by naive clinicians. For example, absence of the acoustic reflex may not be due to a single simple cause, but rather a complex combination of unsuspected conductive hearing impairment not identified in routine audiometry or otoscopy, a subtle peripheral facial nerve problem, or an undetected eighth nerve or brain stem problem. Audiologists must learn to play the percentages in impedance diagnosis and be aware that results from any clinical patient may be the exception to the rule. Physicians, on the other hand, must learn through experience the value of impedance findings in the final diagnosis.

1. *Learn to recognize overall patterns in the impedance test battery.* Do not use any *single* test in the battery to reach diagnostic conclusions; avoid specific clinical interpretations based solely on one element of the impedance test battery. Impedance measurements are strongest when combined with other evaluation procedures including otoscopy, audiometry, and behavioral observations.

2. *Pay little attention to the absolute value of any of the impedance test battery results.* Little useful information is obtained from the absolute value of the amplitude or height of the tympanogram; static compliance should be regarded as being within normal limits, below normal limits, or above normal limits—there is little importance in exact knowledge of the static compliance; and it is often sufficient to know that the acoustic reflex is present or absent, within normal limits, elevated, or at a reduced sensation level. Finicky clinicians may overlook the clinical impedance picture if they are too concerned with the absolute numbers involved in each impedance battery element.

3. *Beware of implicit diagnostic conclusions based only on the impedance test battery.* No test is infallible; few otologic problems have one, and only one, cause. The clinician must realize that several reasons may cause an abnormal tympanogram, and all these reasons may influence the measurement of the acoustic reflex threshold. The impedance test battery results from a patient with otosclerosis may be the same as the impedance results obtained for a patient with profound sensorineural hearing loss. The impedance technique is a strong diagnostic tool, but the sophisti-

cated clinician bases final decisions on the total patient presentation of complaint, history, audiometry, physical examination, and impedance test battery.

REFERENCES

1. Alberti, P. W., and Jerger, J. F. Probe-tone frequency and the diagnostic value of tympanometry. *Arch. Otolaryngol.* 99:206, 1974.
2. Alberti, P. W., and Kristensen, R. The clinical application of impedance audiometry. *Laryngoscope* 80:735, 1970.
3. American Speech and Hearing Association. Guidelines for acoustic immitance screening of middle ear function. *Asha* 21:283, 1978.
4. Anderson, H., Barr, B., and Wedenberg, E. Early diagnosis of VIIIth nerve tumors by acoustic reflex tests. *Acta Otolaryngol.* (Suppl.) 263:232, 1970.
5. Bess, F. H. Impedance screening for children: A need for more research. *Ann. Otol. Rhinol. Laryngol.* [Suppl. 68] 89:229, 1980.
6. Bluestone, C. D. Assessment of Eustachian Tube Function. In J. Jerger and J. Northern (Eds.), *Clinical Impedance Audiometry* (2d ed.). Acton, Mass.: American Electromedics Corp., 1980.
7. Bluestone, C. D., Beery, Q. C., and Paradise, J. L. Audiometry and tympanometry in relation to middle ear effusions in chidren. *Laryngoscope* 89:594, 1974.
8. Brooks, D. N. The use of the electroacoustic impedance bridge in the assessment of middle ear function. *Int. Audiol.* 8:563, 1969.
9. Brooks, D. N. Hearing screening: A comparative study of an impedance method and pure-tone screening. *Scand. Audiol.* 2:67, 1973.
10. Citron, D., and Adovr, K. Acoustic reflex and loudness discomfort in acute facial paralysis. *Arch. Otolaryngol.* 104:303, 1978.
11. Cohen, D., and Sade, J. Hearing on secretory otitis media. *Can. J. Otolaryngol.* 1:27, 1972.
12. Eagles, E. L. Selected findings from the Pittsburgh study. *Trans. Am. Acad. Ophthalmol. Otolaryngol.* 76:343, 1972.
13. Eliachar, I., Sando, I., and Northern, J. L. Measurement of middle ear pressure in guinea pigs. *Arch. Otolaryngol.* 99:172, 1974.
14. Feldman, A. S. Eardrum abnormality and the measurement of middle ear function. *Arch. Otolaryngol.* 99:211, 1974.
15. Feldman, A. S., and Wilber, L. A. (Eds.) *Acoustic Impedance and Admittance—The Measurement of Middle Ear Function.* Baltimore: Williams & Wilkins, 1976.
16. Greisen, O., and Rassmussen, P. E. Stapedius muscle reflexes and otoneurological exam-

inations in brainstem tumor. *Acta Otolaryngol.* 70:366, 1970.

17. Hall, J. Predicting Hearing Loss From the Acoustic Reflex. In J. Jerger and J. Northern (Eds.), *Clinical Impedance Audiometry* (2d ed.). Acton, Mass.: American Electrometrics Corp., 1980. P. 141.

18. Harford, E. R., et al. (Eds.). *Impedance Screening for Middle Ear Disease in Children.* New York: Grune & Stratton, 1978.

19. Hayes, D., and Jerger, J. Patterns of acoustic reflex and auditory brainstem response abnormality. *Acta Otolaryngol.* 92:199, 1981.

20. Jerger, J. Clinical experience with impedance audiometry. *Arch. Otolaryngol.* 92:311, 1970.

21. Jerger, J., Jerger, S., and Mauldin, L. Studies in impedance audiometry: I. Normal and sensorineural ears. *Arch. Otolaryngol.* 96:513, 1972.

22. Jerger, J., and Northern, J. (Eds.). *Clinical Impedance Audiometry* (2d ed.). Acton, Mass.: American Electromedics Corp., 1980.

23. Jerger, J., et al. Studies in impedance audiometry: III. Middle ear disorders. *Arch. Otolaryngol.* 99:165, 1974.

24. Jerger, J., et al. The acoustic reflex in VIIIth nerve disorders. *Arch. Otolaryngol.* 99:409, 1974.

25. Jerger, J., et al. Predicting hearing loss from the acoustic reflex. *J. Speech Hear. Disord.* 39:1, 1974.

26. Jerger, S., and Jerger, J. Diagnostic value of crossed vs. uncrossed acoustic reflexes: Eighth nerve and brain stem disorders. *Arch. Otolaryngol.* 103:445, 1977.

27. Jerger, S., et al. Studies in impedance audiometry: II. Children less than six years old. *Arch. Otolaryngol.* 99:1, 1974.

28. Liden, G., Peterson, J. L., and Bjorkman, G. Tympanometry. *Arch. Otolaryngol.* 92:248, 1970.

29. Liden, G., Peterson, J. L., and Bjorkman, G. Tympanometry: A method for analysis of middle ear function. *Acta Otolaryngol.* 263:218, 1970.

30. McCandless, G. H., and Thomas, G. K. Impedance audiometry as a screening procedure for middle ear disease. *Trans. Am. Acad. Ophthalmol. Otolaryngol.* 78:2, 1974.

31. Metz, O. The acoustic impedance measured on normal and pathological ears. *Acta Otolaryngol.* Suppl. 63, 1946.

32. Metz, O. Threshold of reflex contractions of muscles of the middle ear and recruitment of loudness. *Arch. Otolaryngol.* 55:536, 1952.

33. Niemeyer, W., and Sesterhenn, G. Calculating the hearing threshold from the stapedius reflex threshold for different sound stimuli. *J. Audit. Communic.* 11:84, 1972.

34. Nilges, T. C., Northern, J. L., and Burke, K. Zwislocki acoustic bridge: Clinical correlations. *Arch. Otolaryngol.* 89:69, 1969.

35. Northern, J. L. Acoustic Impedance in the Pediatric Population. In F. Bess (Ed.), *Childhood Deafness: Causation, Assessment and Management.* New York: Grune & Stratton, 1977a. Pp. 136–152.

36. Northern, J. L. Impedance audiometry for otologic diagnosis. In *Proceedings of the Shambaugh Fifth International Workshop on Middle Ear Microsurgery and Fluctuant Hearing Loss.* Chicago: Strode, 1977b. Pp. 75–83.

37. Northern, J. Impedance screening: An integral part of hearing screening. *Ann. Otol. Rhinol. Laryngol.* [Suppl. 68] 89:233, 1980.

38. Northern, J. L., and Downs, M. P. *Hearing in Children* (2nd ed.). Baltimore: Williams & Wilkins, 1978.

39. Northern, J. L., and Grimes, A. M. Introduction to Acoustic Impedance. In J. Katz, (Ed.), *Handbook of Clinical Audiology* (2nd ed.). Baltimore: Williams & Wilkins, 1978. Pp. 344–355.

40. Paradise, J. L., Smith, C. G., and Bluestone, C. D. Tympanometric detection of middle ear effusion in infants and young children. *Pediatrics* 58:198, 1976.

41. Renvall, V., et al. Impedance audiometry as a screening method in school children. *Scand. Audiol.* 2:133, 1973.

42. Roeser, R., and Northern, J. Screening for Hearing Loss and Middle Ear Disorders. In R. Roeser and M. Downs (Eds.), *Audiotory Disorders in School Children.* New York: Thieme-Stratton, 1981. Pp. 120–150.

43. Sanders, J. N. W. Diagnostic Audiology. In Lass, et al. (Eds.), *Speech, Language and Hearing.* Philadelphia: Saunders, 1982. Pp. 944–967.

44. Strosser, J., and Sheehy, J. Otologic applications of acoustic impedance. Presented to Second International Symposium on Impedance. Houston, Texas, 1973.

45. Terkildsen, K., Osterhammel, P., and Bretlau, P. Acoustic middle ear muscle reflexes in patients with otosclerosis. *Arch. Otolaryngol.* 98:152, 1973.

46. Harker, L., and Von Wagoner, R. Application of impedance audiometry as a screening instrument. *Acta Otolaryngol.* 77:198, 1974.

5

Auditory Evoked Potentials

Kurt Hecox
John T. Jacobson

The audiologic evaluation of difficult-to-test patients continues to present a major challenge to the hearing specialist. This group includes the very young, the uncooperative adult, and the multihandicapped. Dissatisfaction with the validity and repeatability of behavioral measures in these groups has been a major impetus for the development of electrophysiologic measures of auditory function. Although the strengths and limitations of routine behavioral procedures for these populations are a source of continued debate, there is a general consensus that the use of "adjunctive" measures to confirm the results of traditional behavioral tests is desirable. The relative importance of behavioral, impedance, and evoked potential audiometry in the overall test battery is not yet resolved and is likely to attract the attention of clinical researchers for years to come. This chapter introduces the reader to the principles and clinical applications of auditory evoked potentials and emphasizes the importance of auditory brain stem response (ABR) audiometry in the diagnosis of unsuspected or unconfirmed hearing loss.

To date, the primary application of evoked response audiometry has been to diagnose hearing impairment in the infant and multihandicapped patient. Another important, but less critical, contribution (in comparison to the adequacy of available alternative tests) has been to identify retrocochlear disorders, including acoustic neuromas [26, 36].

A second role played by the auditory evoked potentials is to facilitate anatomic localization of the disease process. As will be noted in subsequent sections, evoked potentials can often separate the contribution of conductive, sensory, and neuropathology elements of hearing loss [30, 32]. Although many diagnostic tools are available to the audiologist for site-of-lesion testing, few are applicable to the difficult-to-test patient. The ease and repeatability with which evoked potentials are obtained

The authors would like to acknowledge the technical support of the many persons who were involved in the collection of the data discussed herein, and Nancy Henderson for her technical support during the writing of this manuscript. The work was supported in part by NINCDS Grant NS-16436 and Health and Welfare Canada, #6603-1114-44.

makes site-of-lesion testing achievable regardless of age.

The final contribution of evoked potential audiometry is an improved nosology and an increased sensitivity to central auditory disorders. This last application remains speculative but may prove to have as great an impact on audiologic practice as the more widely accepted application—the detection of peripheral hearing loss. Using evoked potentials, it is possible to separate the many peripheral pathologies from intrinsic brain stem lesions and to contrast both of these disorders with cortical dysfunction. The behavioral correlates of central auditory abnormality findings of the evoked potentials are not completely understood. Recent investigations have been quite promising, however, in that central abnormalities on the auditory evoked potentials have been reflected in psychophysical tests not ordinarily included in the diagnostic audiology battery [15].

In summary, evoked response audiometry contributes to the detection of hearing loss in the difficult-to-test patient, aids in the localization of underlying pathology, and offers the possibility of an improved basis for the study of the process of central auditory disorders. The impact of ABR audiometry has increased so rapidly over the past 5 years that this test has become available in virtually every metropolitan area in North America. Thus, familiarity with both its strengths and weaknesses must become more generally appreciated to prevent indiscriminate overuse.

HISTORICAL DEVELOPMENT

The evolution of electroencephalographic recordings (EEG) can be logarithmically conceptualized. That is, the most significant contributions to the field have occurred both recently and simultaneously with advances in computer technology and recording techniques. When considering the technical limitations of the day, it was no small achievement when electrical potentials were initially recorded from the exposed cortex of animals [2]. However, more than half a century elapsed before spontaneous EEG activity was monitored from the human scalp [1]. Following the extensive work of Hans Berger, distinct patterns in human EEG activity to sensory stimulation were first reported by Loomis and colleagues [29]. Thereafter, Davis and associates [6] described a series of auditory evoked cortical potentials in human beings. These series of observations led to what is now referred to as the "V" or vertex potential reflecting the scalp location from which the response was most robust. Since the discovery of auditory evoked potentials, research has been directed toward the development of its clinical applications to the diagnosis of auditory and neurologic abnormalities.

Early research was plagued by the fact that the amplitude of the ongoing background noise (spontaneous EEG activity) was greater than that of the stimulus related event. Although this problem was partially solved by Dawson [8] using a superimposed photographic technique to "add" EEG tracings, it was the development of an electronic averaging process [3, 5] that revolutionized the field of electrophysiologic measurement. Clark [3] devised a stimulus "time-locked" computer principle that converted analogue data into digital values. Using this principle, he was able to algebraically sum events and thereby separate stimulus-related electrical potentials from the larger nontime-locked spontaneous EEG activity.

Several series of auditory evoked potentials can be monitored from the human scalp. Although the recording techniques are similar, these far-field potentials differ in their latency, amplitude, wave morphology, and underlying generators. Picton and colleagues [31] have described three types of auditory evoked potentials: the transient, the sustained, and the perceptual responses. For the purposes of this chapter, comments are restricted to the transient response. Transient responses are elicited by stimuli with rapid onsets (such as a click) and are usually categorized on the basis of their latencies in milliseconds. The early (10 msec), middle (10–50 msec), and late (50–500 msec) components have received considerable attention clinically. Each epoch of the evoked potential can provide clinical information at several levels of the auditory system.

Although early clinical investigation focused on electrical events generated in the primary and association areas of the auditory cortex, their clinical applicability to assess and to identify hearing impairment in all but normal hearing adults proved questionable. More recently, ABR audiometry has been advocated as a clinical technique for assessing auditory and neurologic investigations. Although initially observed by Sohmer and Feinmesser [37], it was Jewett and his colleagues [22, 23, 24] who accurately identified the neural generators of the far-field recorded potentials. In adults, the ABR normally consists of five to seven vertex-positive wave peaks, each designated consecutively with Roman numerals and separated in duration by approximately 1 msec. Brain stem responses are stimulus dependent, independent of subject state, and commonly recorded within the first 10 msec after a click stimulus. Owing to the complexity of the brain stem pathway and the neural activity of the auditory system to a transient stimulus, the origin of the individual wave peaks remains a point of controversy. With the exception of wave I, which is a far-field reflection of the electrical activity of the auditory nerve, the remainder of the wave peaks are undoubtedly generated by several sources along the brain stem pathways.

NORMATIVE VALUES AND DEVELOPMENTAL DEPENDENCY

The use of auditory brain stem response audiometry as a diagnostic clinical tool has focused on two principle areas: (1) the evaluation and assessment of peripheral auditory mechanisms and related pathology and (2) the neurologic integrity of the acoustic nerve and brain stem pathway. The criteria for ABR interpretation are usually based on the latency of individual wave peaks and their interwave intervals. Although amplitude measurements have been used as supplementary evidence, they have not gained clinical popularity because of their inherent variability. Changes in the brain stem response latency, amplitude ratios, and waveform morphology have all been reported secondarily to subject differences, various stimulus and recording parameters, and pathologic conditions [39, 41]. Therefore, accurate clinical decisions must be based on a knowledge and understanding of normal response variability. Two ABR parameters—latency and amplitude ratios—lend themselves to quantitative interpretation. Interaction of these parameters often produces response morphology alterations, as shown in the following discussion. To this point, the following section discusses the influence of subject and recording variables on measurement criteria.

Response Latency

Absolute wave latency can be defined as the time period between stimulus onset and the peak of a measured response. The difference between two wave peaks is considered the interwave interval (IWI) and is a partial reflection of neural conduction time between the acoustic nerve and brain stem nuclei. Both absolute and interwave intervals are measured in milliseconds. The absolute latency of wave V has received primary attention in clinical interpretation because of its stability under varying conditions. The unique characteristic associated with wave V latency is its predictable sensitivity to intensity change. That is, as intensity decreases, the latency of wave V increases proportionally.

Response Amplitude

Amplitude is expressed in absolute values and measured in microvolts from the peak of one wave component to its following trough within a prescribed time frame. The ratio of amplitude between two wave peaks is considered the relative amplitude ratio (RAR). The RAR has been advocated for clinical use because it decreases the variability associated with absolute amplitude measures.

Wave amplitude increases with stimulus intensity, and all but wave V decrease in amplitude with increasing rate. In adults, the wave V amplitude rarely exceeds 1 μv even at moderate to intense signal intensities and remains relatively stable at increased presentation rates. The ratio of wave V to wave I amplitude varies with age but is pathologic when it is less than 0.5.

Wave Morphology

Morphology of the brain stem response usually refers to the visual appearance of the wave configuration. This aspect of interpretation is more subjective in nature and lacks quantitative precision. At least five different nomenclatures describe the various wave peaks. Jewett and Williston [25], Lev and Sohmer [28], and Thornton [46] use a chronologic order to describe sequential peak components, whereas Terkildsen and associates [45] and Davis [7] have reported waves based on the latency of the wave peak. Unfortunately, in such instances, the same wave peak may be labelled differently by each author. For example, wave V (Jewett), N_4 (Thornton), and P_6 (Davis) all refer to the identical wave peak. We suggest that the Jewett and Williston nomenclature, which uses Roman numerals to sequentially describe waves I through VII, be adopted as a standard procedure and therefore will be used throughout this chapter.

Another aspect of wave morphology, which may lead to confusing interpretation, is the polarity-convention used by different authors: that is, which direction is displayed as "up"? Most North American clinics currently display vertex-positive as an upward deflection ("positive-up" convention) while the European literature advocates the opposite (vertex-positive downward).

The morphology of the brain stem response has also been shown to be affected by age, pathology, and other stimulus-related variables [16, 42]. For example, in normal hearing subjects, as intensity is decreased, the amplitude of waves I through IV are reduced to a larger proportion than the amplitude of wave V. At higher intensities, wave I has been reported to separate into a bifid wave making accurate latency and amplitude identification difficult. In addition, the IV to V wave complex will change shape as a function of stimulus polarity [4, 11, 43].

Infant responses differ from adult potentials and change as a function of maturation. Newborn responses consist of three vertex-positive waves whose latencies and amplitudes differ significantly from the corresponding adult waves. The amplitude of wave I in newborns is twice that of adults while wave V is approximately half as large. By 4 months of age, wave IV has begun to develop, and a IV to V complex can be seen while wave II emerges as a separate wave at about this same time.

The clinical interpretation of auditory brain stem response audiometry may be influenced by various stimulus and recording techniques. Following is a brief description of those parameters that affect brain stem latency and amplitude.

Intensity. A decrease in stimulus intensity will prolong the latency of all wave components. For clinical diagnosis, wave V latency has been used most frequently for threshold determination and site-of-lesion diagnosis. The rate of change of wave V with intensity is about 40 μsec/dB. It is possible to identify replicable wave V responses to within 10 dB of normal hearing sensitivity in adults and to approximately 20 dB in newborns. If, however, ABR is to be used as a neurologic measure, suprathreshold presentation levels are necessary to identify individual waves and their latency differences. The I-to-V IWI is most often used as an index of neural conduction time. The adult I-to-V difference is approximately 4.0 msec and is relatively insensitive to intensity change. The comparable value for newborns is about 5.0 msec.

Rate. An increase in click stimulus repetition rate will increase the absolute response latency while producing negligible changes in wave V amplitude. At rates less than 10 per second, there is little effect of rate on latency whereas at higher presentation rates, wave components increase differentially. Wave V produces the largest prolongation, increasing at a rate of 0.006 msec/Hz. This differential wave increase (greater for wave V than for wave I) results in an increasing IWI with increasing rate.

Repetition rate also influences response amplitude. A decrease in wave amplitude occurs for all waves but to a lesser degree for wave V. At stimulus rates of up to 80 per second, wave V maintains approximately 85% of its original amplitude. Obviously, a reduction in amplitude will change the morphology of the brain stem response. Therefore, a thorough understanding of rate function is essential for normative comparisons.

Stimulus Envelope Characteristics. The majority of auditory and neurologic diagnostic assessments have been performed using unfiltered clicks as stimuli. Clicks have a nearly instantaneous rise-fall time and appear to provide the optimum auditory stimulus for evoking neural synchronization. It is important to recall, however, that a click reflects the resonance characteristics of the transducer and therefore initiates a high- to middle-frequency response from the cochlea. As a consequence, threshold estimates can only refer to high- or middle-frequency sensitivity.

Tone pips, tone bursts, and filtered clicks have been used to improve frequency specificity. Owing to their brief duration, these signals still result in acoustic spread of energy away from stimulus center frequency. This spread of energy may activate wide regions of the cochlea, eliciting nonspecific neural synchronization and thus introducing potentially misleading results. In an attempt to reduce the contribution of this spectral dispersion of energy, masking paradigms have been introduced. These include both high-pass noise masking [10] and octave band notched noise [33].

Stimulus Polarity. A great deal of uncertainty exists in the literature over the question of stimulus polarity. While morphologic changes in the IV/V wave response have been reported in normal hearing adults, there is less agreement about the effect of polarity on latency. Although the absolute latency of wave I has been reported to occur earlier when a rarefaction stimulus is used, waves III and V appear to be insensitive to differences in polarity [11, 43]. Caution must be exercised in wave I interpretation, however, owing to its latency variability. It has been reported [43] that approximately 17% of the normal hearing population have shorter wave I latencies to condensation clicks while 22% of the population showed no difference. Differences secondary to the use of polarity are complex and partially unresolved.

Electrode Placement. Brain stem response activity that is generated at subcortical levels is volume transmitted and monitored on the surface of the scalp as far-field potentials. Owing to this volume conduction, scalp electrode placement is not considered to be as critical as it once was. A routine three-electrode montage usually consists of an active electrode placed at either the vertex (C_z) or forehead (F_z) with the earlobe or mastoid sites as reference, although systematic studies of age interactions in scalp topography are not available.

Filter Settings. ABR characteristics are influenced by the bandpass filter cutoff frequency used in testing. A change in the filter setting will alter waveform phase resulting in latency and amplitude shifts [27]. Most clinicians, in an attempt to decrease background activity, record using an amplifier bandpass of 100 to 3000 Hz. For improved frequency specificity using lower frequency signals, low-frequency cutoffs at 20 to 30 Hz are suggested [38, 44].

Age Dependency. As previously stated, infant ABR morphology is clearly different from the adult brain stem response. In newborns, waves I, III, and V are present but each is delayed in latency with respect to similar adult tracings [19, 20, 34, 35] (Fig. 5-1). The amplitude of wave I is approximately twice the adult response whereas wave V does not reach adult amplitude until at least 9 to 12 months of age. As a consequence, the V/I amplitude ratio is much smaller in newborns than in adults.

Physiologic immaturity is also reflected in newborn and infant ABR latencies. Wave V latency decreased by 0.4 msec/week between 34 and 48 weeks' gestation [9, 19, 20, 40]. Thereafter, there is a reduction in the rate of decrease, and adult value is reached by approximately 12 months. Wave I, in contrast, approaches adult values by the second month of life [19, 34]. Thus, maturation differentially affects component latencies. Peripheral transmission, as measured by the absolute latency of wave I, matures sooner owing to an improved middle ear system, cochlear sensitivity, and acoustic nerve transmission. The improvement in central transmission is usually attributed to changes in myelination and synaptic efficiency.

Reliable ABRs have been measured in

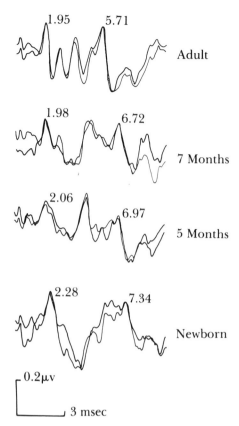

1.95   5.71

Adult

1.98   6.72

7 Months

2.06   6.97

5 Months

2.28   7.34

Newborn

0.2μv

3 msec

Figure 5-1. Brain stem auditory evoked responses vary with age. Note the increasing latency with decreasing age for all components. Positivity to the vertex is plotted upward in this and all subsequent figures. Each tracing results from the presentation of 2000 stimuli.

premature infants as early as 28 weeks' gestation [40]. Owing to maturational effects, independent norms must be established (or extrapolated) on a weekly basis if accurate diagnostic assessment is to be presumed for premature infants. Recall that infant normative data has been established using unfiltered clicks only, and the effects of alternative stimuli need further definition.

INTERPRETATIVE PRINCIPLES

There are at least two major approaches to the diagnosis of hearing loss using auditory brain stem response audiometry. The first, and more traditional, is to reduce signal intensity until a reliable wave V response is no longer detected, resulting in a threshold estimate. The discrepancy between abnormal and normal response threshold rep-

resents the amount of hearing loss. This procedure is analogous to that used in behavioral audiometry and has the common goal of using threshold evaluations to assess hearing dysfunction. Responses obtained from patients A and B are shown in Figure 5-2. For patients A and B, click-evoked thresholds appear to be about 45 dB nHL. In normal hearing adults, the electrophysiologic threshold is usually 10 dB nHL greater than behavioral threshold. Therefore, if the discrepancy between normal and patient response is 35 dB in both cases, this difference represents the estimated hearing loss. This approach can be used for unfiltered clicks, tone pips, tone bursts, or in combination with bandpass noise. However, as outlined in the previous section, adequate age-specific normative data exist only for click stimuli.

A second approach is to characterize the latency properties of the ABR at several signal intensities (Fig. 5-3). The latency-intensity (LI) function is then compared to the norm. The absolute amount of displacement from normal and any differences in the slope of the function are used to estimate the amount of loss and determine the site of lesion, respectively. The LI functions for patients A and B (see Fig. 5-2) are plotted in Figure 5-3. Patient A, illustrated in the top panel of Figure 5-3, shows a displacement rightward of the LI function for wave V amounting to nearly 1.4 msec at each point along the curve function. As can be seen on the abscissa, this corresponds to a shift of approximately 35 dB. That is, the latencies produced by the 60 dB signal correspond to those usually seen in response to a 25 dB stimulus. This decibel displacement can also be estimated by realizing that every decibel change in intensity corresponds to a 0.04 msec latency shift. Thus, 1.4 msec/0.04 msec/dB yields a 35 dB intensity shift. A parallel but displaced LI function is usually seen in conductive pathology, although the diagnosis of a conductive disorder requires confirmation by bone conducted ABRs.

As shown in the center panel of Figure 5-3 (patient B), the displacement of the LI function is sometimes intensity dependent. This is most commonly seen when the LI function is abnormally steep, as shown in this case. The amount of latency prolonga-

Patient A   Patient B

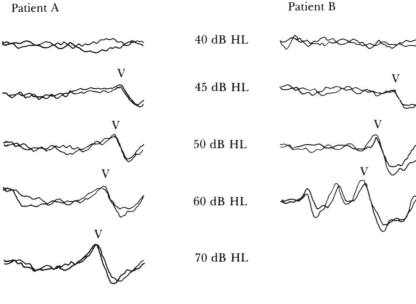

	40 dB HL	
V	45 dB HL	V
V	50 dB HL	V
V	60 dB HL	V
V	70 dB HL	

3 msec
├──┤

Figure 5-2. Responses obtained from patients whose thresholds are equivalently elevated but whose suprathreshold rate of latency decrease are different. The latencies of patient A are prolonged a constant amount with increasing latency, whereas the responses of patient B converge to normal by 60 dB nHL. Patient A has a conductive loss and patient B has a sensory loss.

tion is 1.5 msec at 45 dB, 0.6 msec at 50 dB, whereas the latency at 60 dB HL is normal. This pattern of an abnormally steep LI function is virtually pathognomonic of inner ear disease and is usually accompanied by behavioral recruitment. Quite clearly, estimates of hearing loss or site-of-lesion diagnosis obtained at a single intensity could result in major errors, as displayed by patient B. The estimated loss for this patient at 45 dB is 35 dB, a 15 dB loss at 50 dB, whereas there is no evidence of impairment at 60 dB. Thus, the use of absolute latencies to predict peripheral auditory impairment cannot be accurately accomplished by sampling at a single intensity. The third type of LI function, not illustrated with raw data tracings, has an abnormally shallow shape. This slope has a strong association with predominantly high-frequency impairment of the audiogram.

The use of the LI function to estimate

hearing loss can be further refined by projecting the LI function to a threshold value, using the intensity corresponding to the threshold latency as the patient's threshold. For example, if the LI function of patient B were projected to 8.5 msec using the slope of the patient's LI function, the estimated threshold would be approximately 42 dB. This threshold was obtained by noting that the response at 45 dB was 8 msec or 0.5 msec short of the 8.5 msec projection. The slope of the LI function is 0.2 msec/dB so that a decrease of 2.5 dB corresponds to an increase of 0.5 msec in latency (2.5 dB × 0.2 msec/dB).

The advantage of the LI technique over the threshold approach lies in the additional information inherent in the LI function. An abnormally shallow LI function is most consistent with a predominantly high-frequency hearing loss, thus providing some insight into the audiometric configuration. The absence of an abnormally steep or shallow slope does not negate recruitment or a predominantly high-frequency hearing loss, respectively. These diagnostic signs are only useful when present; their absence carries no diagnostic information.

A secondary advantage of suprathreshold measurements is that variability in waveform morphology is much greater at

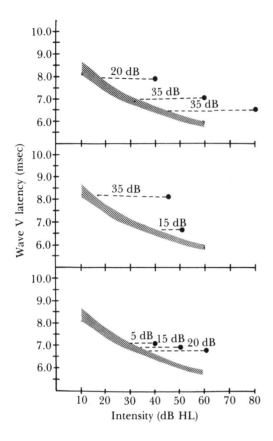

Figure 5-3. Normal (hatched areas) and three patterns of response abnormalities are plotted. The top panel (patient A) illustrates the parallel displacement of the latency-intensity function, most consistent with, although not diagnostic of, conductive impairment. The middle panel (patient B) shows a steep latency-intensity function, diagnostic of cochlear disease. The lowest panel shows a shallow latency-intensity function, diagnostic of predominantly high-frequency loss.

low intensities. Furthermore, the integration of neurologic and audiologic information can be effectively accomplished only at suprathreshold levels where the identification and separation of waveform components can be achieved. The use of the threshold and suprathreshold techniques are not mutually exclusive. Other procedures, such as using alternative stimuli as well as masking paradigms, have not been sufficiently validated, and adequate norms are not available.

An additional advantage of these tech-

niques is that unilateral impairment may be documented because testing is always performed with earphones, not in a sound-field (Fig. 5-4).

The definitive diagnosis of conductive pathology and quantification of the relative contribution of middle ear versus inner ear disease can be accomplished only by performing air- and bone-conduction ABRs. As previously discussed, such bone-conduction conditions require the generation of separate latency norms while wave form morphology, interwave intervals, and amplitude ratios are relatively independent of the mode of stimulus presentation (air vs bone). Slopes of more than 0.06 msec/dB are diagnostic of inner ear pathology, and slopes of less than 0.03 msec/dB are still diagnostic of predominantly high-frequency audiometric configurations. The general method for establishing an air-bone gap using bone-conduction ABRs is similar to that described for air-conduction signals. The discrepancy between threshold estimates is the amount of latency shift between the patient and normative data and is used to estimate the amount of hearing loss. This degree of loss is then compared to that estimated by air-conduction signals. The discrepancy between air- and bone-generated estimates of hearing impairment represents the electrophysiologic air-bone gap. Figure 5-5 illustrates the application of this procedure. Note that the air-conduction signals for patient D generate an LI function consistent with a 35 dB hearing loss whereas the response threshold is also approximately 40 dB above that seen in normal ears. Bone-conduction responses are delayed by an equivalent amount resulting in an estimate of hearing impairment of 35 dB. The discrepancy between air- and bone-conduction estimates, in this case 0 dB, is the air-bone gap.

There are many technical aspects to the application of bone-conduction ABRs and many theoretic pitfalls inherent in these procedures. For example, the spectral content of air- and bone-conduction signals is surely not the same. Furthermore, there may be significant variability in the application of the bone-conduction oscillator when compared to standard earphones. Finally, bone-conduction oscillator position is a major determinant of the thresh-

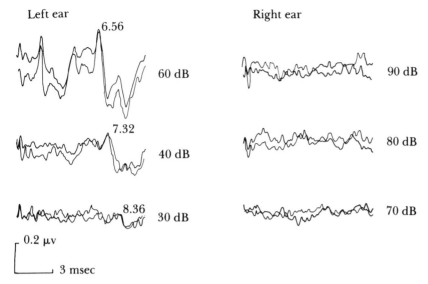

Figure 5-4. Normal wave V tracings were obtained from the left ear of a high-risk infant. With appropriate masking of the nontest ear, the right ear showed no replicable brain stem responses. At birth, this newborn passed behavioral screening (sound field) but was seen for ABR screening because she was a high-risk newborn (cytomegalovirus and hepatitis). She was identified as unilateral sensorineural impaired.

Figure 5-5. Latencies to air- and bone-conduction signals are plotted as a function of intensity in patient D. Note that air- and bone-conduction latencies are equivalently displaced from normal, implying a nonconductive disorder. Correction has been made for the difference in electrical energy required to produce equivalent HL points for bone-conduction presentation. (Normal range for latency-intensity function is represented by cross-hatched lines.)

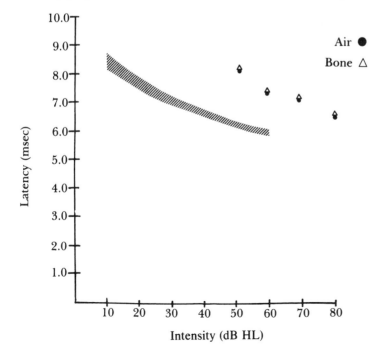

old and latency of the observed ABR. Most of these points are not unique to the use of bone-conduction signals in electrophysiologic testing and are familiar to the audiologist from bone-conduction behavioral testing. When using bone-conduction stimulus, the test ear must always be isolated from the nontest ear by noise masking, similar to conventional behavioral testing.

One of the controversial areas in the application of ABRs to audiologic and neurologic testing is the need for audiometric information prior to the initiation of electrophysiologic evaluation. We generally do not make audiometric information available to the staff responsible for completing the ABR testing before the test procedure. This approach has not, in our experience, significantly lowered our efficiency in patient evaluation. When evaluating the results of the ABR, we do not take into account audiometric results. However, at the level of generating a specific diagnosis and developing a future diagnostic and management plan, audiologic information is often crucial for the intelligent use of ABR results. These principles are especially important when evaluating the pediatric patient.

In summary, two approaches to the quantification of peripheral hearing loss have been used successfully. The first is to progressively lower stimulus intensity until the response disappears, and this is considered to be the patient's threshold. The second approach uses suprathreshold stimulus levels to estimate the patient's threshold and to make inferences regarding site of lesion. The use of bone-conduction ABRs is a useful adjunct to these procedures in making a more definitive diagnosis of conductive pathology and performing an initial quantification of the relative contribution of inner and middle ear pathology to an observed loss. These principles are not age dependent, although the values used in the construction of clinical norms must be age specific.

AUDIOLOGIC CORRELATES

The inclusion of a new clinical technique as part of a diagnostic battery cannot occur before considerable data on its validity have been collected. Establishing validity can be performed in a number of ways, but one minimum criterion must be that the measure against which validation is to be performed is more accurate than the instrument being evaluated. Because of the controversies surrounding the validity of behavioral techniques in a young patient, it is understandable that the validation procedures have been largely undertaken in the adult population where concerns regarding the reliability of the behavioral data are minimized. The degree to which the auditory brain stem potentials are able to accurately predict auditory impairment is also a function of the methodology used in applying the response [17, 19]. For example, early attempts at predicting the degree of auditory impairment refer to latencies obtained at a single intensity [21]. As illustrated in the previous section, such an approach is beset with difficulties because the accuracy of the prediction will interact with the type and locus of the pathology. To the extent that various studies have used differing methodologies in the application of ABR measurement, it is expected that discrepancies in the accuracy of predictions will also ensue.

Despite continued controversy regarding the accuracy of the technique, certain limitations have been defined and are generally accepted. There is little disagreement that the ABR poorly reflects the integrity of hearing at less than 500 Hz [13, 21]. Correlations between ABR predictions of hearing loss and audiometric patterns suggest that the ABR best approximates hearing threshold at 2000 Hz [32], and that major errors in prediction can occur at more than 4000 Hz and less than 500 Hz. Several laboratories, including Jerger and associates [21], have reported consistently accurate predictions concerning the puretone average loss in the 1000 to 4000 Hz region using the techniques described in the section Interpretative Principles. Our experience in correlating pure-tone average loss at 1000, 2000, and 4000 Hz has shown an average discrepancy of less than 5 dB, although major discrepancies can occur at other frequencies. The number of major discrepancies in predicting pure-tone average is quite limited, and in less than 1% of cooperative adults have we found serious discrepancies in predicted hearing loss.

When using click stimuli, our experience, like others, is that specific predictions about frequency dependency of the hearing loss may be incorrect a significant proportion of the time.

Because the target population for the application of this technique is generally the very young or uncooperative patient, our primary goal has been to identify patients in need of long-term follow-up with special attention to habilitation, including amplification. It is in this regard that our clinical experience is most encouraging. Most of the major discrepancies obtained in ABR audiometry either occur in audiometric patterns found primarily in adults (4 kHz notches) or are of the type that may not alter the decision to initiate hearing-aid evaluation or habilitation. For example, the ABR is quite insensitive to the audiometric pattern associated with noise-induced hearing loss, but this audiometric configuration is rare in infants and does not constitute a "significant" clinical problem. Losses restricted to frequencies less than 1000 Hz may go undiagnosed using this technique, but amplification is usually not the primary means of habilitation in this context, at least initially. Thus, the major types of discrepancy between behavioral thresholds and electrophysiologic predictions of those thresholds are fortunately encountered only rarely in the target population for ABR audiometry.

The generally good agreement between behavioral and electrophysiologic predictions of average threshold shift is somewhat surprising. The number of ways in which discrepancies can arise are multiple. For example, the duration of the signal used to evoke the electrophysiologic response is much shorter than that used for traditional behavioral audiometry. Any differences in temporal integration as a function of pathology (as suggested by several investigators of cochlear disease) can produce a discrepancy between the two techniques. The ABR certainly does not sample from all of the cell types included within each of the nuclei responsible for generating the response. The cells producing the ABR are short-time constant neurons primarily responsive to signal onset and insensitive to subtleties of the fine structure of long-duration stimuli [18]. It

is for this reason that it is often said that the ABR measures synchrony of auditory pathway function and not "hearing." In this respect, it is not surprising that patients with white matter disorders, such as multiple sclerosis, may have normal audiograms but severely compromised ABRs. Again, such abnormalities appear to be infrequent among infants, although the theoretical possibility of confusing neurologic with audiologic impairment must always be kept in mind. Such confusion can be minimized by adhering to the previously defined principles.

The follow-up results of large infant population studies are only now becoming available [12, 14]. The results of these reports are indeed encouraging. Perhaps the most impressive statistic is that no infant with normal brain stem auditory evoked potentials has been reported to have benefited from amplification. There are surely patients with significant auditory impairment, usually at the cortical level, who will have normal ABRs, yet none have responded favorably to amplification procedures. Therefore, the false-negative rate, or the number of patients missed by this procedure, appears nonexistent or negligible. The price of such sensitivity is of course an increased false-positive rate. The exact value for false-positive errors is not yet known but in some series runs as high as 80% (ours is approximately 30%). Included in these false-positive rates are all patients with transient conductive pathology and other forms of temporary hearing impairment. Whether these should be described or characterized as false-positive is a matter of debate. Long-term follow-up studies in these populations suggest that estimates of the percentage of graduates of neonatal intensive care units who have significant auditory impairment is much larger than that previously appreciated (approximately 3–5%) [14, 20]. One of the major impacts of the ABR has therefore been the increased recognition of previously underestimated numbers of hearing handicapped persons resulting in a reconsideration of the strategies needed to optimally diagnose and manage their hearing loss.

Another important application of the ABR has been the diagnosis of retrocochlear disease, especially the detection of acoustic neuromas. The evidence is quite strong that the ABR is the most sensitive single instrument in the detection of retrocochlear lesions. The findings of normal interwave intervals, amplitude ratios, and response to changing rate stimulation nearly eliminates the possibility of the presence of an acoustic neuroma. In patient samples with acoustic neuromas, accurate detection rates of surgically confirmed tumors ranged between 90 and 96%. Although the ABR is certainly a sensitive instrument in this context, it is in no way specific to acoustic neuromas; identical results can be obtained from patients with multiple sclerosis, cerebrovascular accidents, infectious disorders, and a variety of degenerative diseases.

In summary, the ABR correlation with behavioral audiometric results has been good. Pure-tone averages are reasonably well predicted by click and tone pip evoked responses. Exact information concerning the audiometric configuration is not yet available from any of the auditory brain stem evoked response procedures. A number of promising techniques exist but validation of these techniques is not yet sufficient. Prediction of patients in need of additional habilitative or amplification procedures can be accurately and rapidly made with this technique, and the ABR is probably the most sensitive instrument available in the recognition of retrocochlear disease. One of the potentially complicating factors in the estimate of hearing loss is the concurrent presence of neurologic disease.

NEUROLOGIC DISORDERS

The diagnosis of neurologic impairment is based on three criteria: (1) prolonged interwave intervals (2) abnormally small amplitude ratios (V/I), and (3) abnormal responses to changing rates of stimulation. Of the three, the IWI criterion is the most commonly used, and abnormalities of the IWI are the most often encountered. The displacement of the wave V latency-intensity function from normal can, in principle, be secondary to either peripheral or central abnormalities. Central is here designated as any disorder of the cochlea, that is, neural.

The patient results shown in Figure 5-6, illustrate that phenomenon. Note that the LI function for wave I is normal, whereas the wave V LI function is abnormal (consistent with a 25 dB loss). This patient has an abnormal LI function and no evidence of peripheral auditory dysfunction (wave I) on evoked potential testing and behavioral pure-tone audiometry. In contrast, in Figure 5-7, equally displaced latencies for both waves I and V are shown, reflecting the peripheral origin of the auditory impairment. Implicit in the use of the wave V latency-intensity function or in the use of wave V as a threshold measure is that the wave V complex faithfully reflects changes at the level of the auditory periphery (wave I).

When this assumption is in error, as in Figure 5-6, the estimates of peripheral auditory impairment will differ from pure-tone testing. Therefore, all attempts to use the brain stem auditory evoked potential as an audiologic device must begin with the application of neurologic criteria to ensure that the use of wave V as an index of peripheral auditory impairment is justified. If the patient's IWI, amplitude ratios, and response to a changing rate of stimulation are within normal limits, then the audiologic evaluations may proceed. If central abnormalities are present, then audiologic assessment must be based on an analysis of wave I.

The most significant impact of the ABR on the detection of hearing impairment has been in the newborn at risk for hearing loss, the high-risk infant graduating from the neonatal intensive care unit, and the multihandicapped. The coincidence of clinical neurologic impairment and audiologic disorders in this group is not negligible. Similarly, a significant percentage of patients with central auditory abnormalities also exhibits peripheral auditory disease. The nonrandom association of these findings is surely due to overlapping etiologies.

The implications of central auditory abnormalities for the management and habilitation of pediatric patients is poorly understood. The most extreme example is illustrated in Figure 5-8, which illustrates a relatively normal wave I input-output function but no observable wave III or wave V complex. From the behavioral standpoint, this patient was believed to have at least a

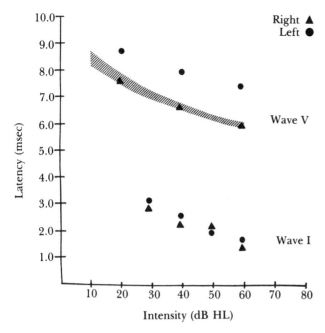

Figure 5-6. Latencies of waves I and V are plotted as a function of intensity for both ears. Note that the wave I latencies are identical on the normal (right) side and abnormal (left) side, whereas wave V latencies are markedly different *for left and right ears. This permits the diagnosis of "central" auditory pathology. (Normal range for latency-intensity function is represented by cross-hatched lines.)*

Figure 5-7. Latencies of waves I and V are plotted as a function of intensity for both ears. Note that response latencies from the pathologic ear (▲) are delayed for both waves I and V, im- *plying peripheral auditory dysfunction. (Normal range for latency-intensity function is represented by cross-hatched lines.)*

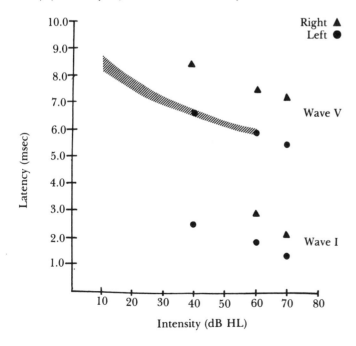

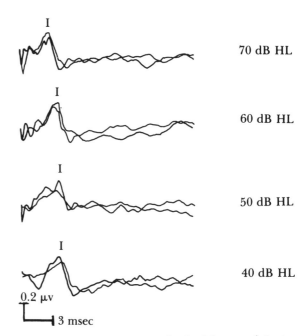

70 dB HL

60 dB HL

50 dB HL

40 dB HL

0.2 μv

3 msec

Figure 5-8. Responses obtained from an infant who suffered an episode of asphyxia. Note that only wave I is elicited at each intensity. Follow-up audiometry confirmed that the patient has severe to profound hearing loss as predicted by the evoked response. The locus of the pathology could only be inferred from the physiologic data, however.

severe hearing loss. The same patient received no benefit from an amplification device, which was not surprising, because the peripheral auditory input was normal. Therefore, the existence of central auditory disease should alert the audiologist to interpretative difficulties and suggest the need for additional neurologic evaluation to determine the etiology of the observed abnormalities.

FUTURE TRENDS

As currently performed in most centers, auditory brain stem response audiometry can closely characterize the average hearing loss from 1000 to 4000 Hz. With rare exception, detailed information concerning the frequency specificity of the loss and residual hearing at 500 Hz and less is unavailable. Although many procedures have been developed to circumvent these shortcomings (including the use of middle latency components, the SN_{10}, tone pip ABR, the 40 Hz response, and derived band pass masking techniques), clinical data are as yet insufficient to guide selection among these techniques. Judging from the intensity of current research activities in this area, it is likely that this problem will be resolved within the near future.

The second major issue likely to receive continued attention in the near future is the nature of false-positive errors using the ABR. There is cumulative evidence that middle ear pathology is common in the graduates of neonatal intensive care units. In most of these patients, the middle ear disorder is transient and can be the cause of an infant failing an initial evaluation yet showing normal sensitivity on subsequent evaluations. Although this is not a false-positive at the time of testing, it is a failure to predict a long-term hearing handicap. Similarly, any transient pathology apparent at one test and resolved by the time of follow-up will appear as a false-positive although not necessarily indicative of a weakness in the test procedure. As a consequence, an unresolved issue ensues: should the presence of false-positives be considered a reflection of the accuracy with which ABR audiometry (or any other electrophysiologic test procedure) can accurately predict permanent hearing loss? It is our impression that ABR precisely monitors the status of the peripheral auditory system at the time of testing but cannot predict change from unforeseen transient auditory or neurologic pathology.

The effective management of each patient requires integration of information obtained from a variety of sources. This principle is also true from the standpoint of diagnostics in the young and uncooperative patient. The relationship between behavioral and electrophysiologic measures of auditory function will require greater attention in the future, particularly with respect to the effect of neurologic disorders impinging on the various portions of the central auditory pathway. Quite clearly it is possible to have a patient who is functionally deaf yet has an intact peripheral auditory apparatus and even normally functioning brain stem auditory pathways as reflected in the ABR. Improved correlations between electrophysiologic and behavioral data will undoubtedly require the inclusion of other electrophysiologic measures of auditory function, including the middle latency and cortical evoked potentials. Historically, these latter measures were the first to appear as viable candidates for objective evoked potential audiometry and were in large part rejected by most practitioners. Their reintegration into the overall test battery will be facilitated by an improved understanding of these responses and improved criteria for the recognition of abnormalities therein. Efforts to correlate abnormalities of behavioral measures with electrophysiologic abnormalities will undoubtedly necessitate expanding the behavioral test repertoire. It is to be hoped that the long-term outcome of these efforts will be an expanded battery of diagnostic measures better able to characterize abnormalities of suprathreshold function and therefore improve our understanding of human communication disorders.

Efforts at defining the etiology of neonatal hearing loss have been handicapped by the need to perform long-term follow-up before establishing the presence of significant hearing handicaps. The availability of the ABR and the immediacy of response interpretation opens up exciting possibilities in terms of precisely defining those conditions and agents responsible for the production of neonatal hearing loss. It is therefore anticipated that there will be increased activity among all hearing specialists involved in determining the pathogenesis and incidence of handicapping auditory disorders in infants.

REFERENCES

1. Berger, H. Uber das Elektrenkephalogram des Menschen. *Arch. Psychiatr. Nervenkr.* 27:527, 1929.
2. Caton, R. The electrical currents of the brain. *Br. Med. J.* 2:278, 1875.
3. Clark, W. A., Brown, R. M., Goldstein, M. H., Jr., Molnar, C. E., O'Brien, D. F., and Zieman, H. E. The average response computer (ARC): A digital device for computing averages and amplitude and time histograms of electrophysiological responses. *IRE Trans. Biomed. Electron* BME-8:46, 1961.
4. Coats, A. C., and Martin, J. L. Human auditory nerve action potentials and brainstem evoked responses. Effects of audiogram shape and lesion location. *Arch. Otolaryngol.* 103:605, 1977.
5. Davis, H. Principles of electric response audiometry. *Ann. Otol. Rhinol. Laryngol.* 85:1, 1976.
6. Davis, H., Davis, P. A., and Loomis, A. L. Electrical reactions of the human brain to auditory stimulation during sleep. *J. Neurophysiol.* 2:500, 1939.
7. Davis, H., and Hirsch, S. K. A slow brainstem response for low-frequency audiometry. *Audiology* 18:445, 1979.
8. Dawson, G. D. Cerebral responses to electrical stimulation of peripheral nerve in man. *J. Neurol. Neurosurg. Psychiatry* 10:134, 1947.
9. Despland, P. A., and Galambos, R. Use of auditory brainstem responses by premature and newborn infants. *Neuropaediatrie* 11:99, 1980.
10. Don, M., Eggermont, J. J., and Brackman, D. E. Reconstruction of the audiogram using brainstem responses and high pass noise masking. *Ann. Otol. Rhinol. Laryngol.* 56:1, 1979.
11. Emerson, R., et al. Effects of click polarity on brainstem auditory evoked potentials in normal subjects and patients: Unexpected sensitivity of wave V. *Ann. N.Y. Acad. Sci.: Evoked Potentials* 388:710, 1982.
12. Galambos, R., and Despland, P. A. The auditory brainstem response (ABR) evaluates risk factors for hearing loss in the newborn. *Pediatr. Res.* 14:159, 1980.
13. Galambos, R., and Hecox, K. E. Clinical

applications of the auditory brainstem response. *Otolaryngol. Clin. North Am.* 11: 709, 1978.

14. Galambos, R., Hicks, G., and Wilson, M. J. Hearing loss in graduates of a tertiary intensive care nursery. *Ear Hear.* 3:87, 1982.

15. Hausler, R., and Levine, R. A. Brainstem auditory evoked potentials are related to interneural time discrimination in patients with multiple sclerosis. *Brain Res.* 191:589, 1980.

16. Hecox, K. Electrophysiological Correlates of Human Auditory Development. In L. Cohen and P. Salapatek (Eds.), *Infant Perception: From Sensation to Cognition.* New York: Academic, 1975.

17. Hecox, K., and Moushegian, G. Brainstem auditory evoked potentials: I. Method and norms. *Arch. Otolaryngol.* In press, 1983.

18. Hecox, K., Squires, N. K., and Galambos, R. Brainstem auditory evoked responses in man. I. Effect of stimulus rise fall time and duration. *J. Acoust. Soc. Am.* 60:1187, 1976.

19. Jacobson, J. T., Morehouse, C. R., and Johnson, M. J. Strategies in infant auditory brainstem response assessment. *Ear Hear.* 3:263, 1982.

20. Jacobson, J. T., et al. Auditory Brainstem Response: A Contribution to Infant Assessment and Management. In G. T. Mencher and S. Gerber (Eds.), *Early Management of Hearing Loss.* New York: Grune & Stratton, 1981. P. 151.

21. Jerger, J., and Mauldin, L. Prediction of sensorineural hearing level from the brainstem evoked response. *Arch. Otolaryngol.* 104:456, 1978.

22. Jewett, D. L. Volume-conducted potentials in response to auditory stimuli as detected by averaging in the cat. *Electroencephalogr. Clin. Neurophysiol.* 28:609, 1970.

23. Jewett, D. L., and Romano, M. N. Neonatal development of auditory system potentials averaged from the scalp of the rat and cat. *Brain Res.* 36:101, 1972.

24. Jewett, D. L., Romano, M. N., and Williston, J. S. Human auditory evoked potentials: Possible brainstem components detected on the scalp. *Science* 167:1517, 1970.

25. Jewett, D. L., and Williston, J. S. Auditory-evoked far fields averaged from the scalp of humans. *Brain* 94:681, 1971.

26. Josey, A. F., Jackson, C. G., and Glasscock, M. E. Brainstem evoked response audiometry in confirmed eighth nerve tumors. *Am. J. Otolaryngol.* 106:285, 1980.

27. Kevanishivili, Z., and Aphonchenko, V. Frequency composition of brain-stem auditory evoked potentials. *Scand. Audiol.* 8:51, 1979.

28. Lev, A., and Sohmer, H. Sources of averaged neural responses recorded in animal and human subjects during cochlear audiometry. *Arch. Klin. Exp. Ohren. Nasen. Kehlkopfheilkd* 201:79, 1972.

29. Loomis, A., Harvey, E., and Hobard, G. Disturbances of patterns in sleep. *J. Neurophysiol.* 1:413, 1938.

30. Maudlin, L., and Jerger, J. Auditory brainstem evoked responses to bone-conducted signals. *Arch. Otolaryngol.* 105:656, 1979.

31. Picton, T. W., Hillyard, S. A., Krausz, H. I., and Galambos, R. Human auditory evoked potentials. I: Evaluation of components. *Electroencephalogr. Clin. Neurophysiol.* 36: 179, 1974.

32. Picton, T. W., et al. Evoked potential audiometry. *J. Otolaryngol.* 6:90, 1977.

33. Picton, T. W., et al. Brainstem evoked potentials to tone pips in notched noise. *J. Otolaryngol.* 8:289, 1979.

34. Salamy, A., and McKean, C. M. Postnatal development of human brainstem potentials during the first year of life. *Electroencephalogr. Clin. Neurophysiol.* 40:418, 1976.

35. Schulman-Galambos, C., and Galambos, R. Brainstem auditory-evoked responses in premature infants. *J. Speech Hear. Res.* 18: 456, 1975.

36. Selters, W. A., and Brackmann, D. Acoustic tumor detection with brainstem electric response audiometry. *Arch. Otolaryngol.* 103: 181, 1977.

37. Sohmer, H., and Feinmesser, M. Cochlear action potentials recorded from the external ear in man. *Ann. Otol. Rhinol. Laryngol.* 76:427, 1967.

38. Stapells, D. R., and Picton, T. W. Technical aspects of brainstem-evoked potential audiometry using tones. *Ear Hear.* 2:20, 1981.

39. Starr, A., and Achor, L. J. Auditory brainstem responses in neurological disease. *Arch. Neurol.* 32:761, 1975.

40. Starr, A., et al. Development of auditory function in newborn infants revealed by auditory brainstem potentials. *Pediatrics* 60:831, 1977.

41. Stockard, J. E., and Westmoreland, B. F. Technical considerations in the recording and interpretation of the brainstem auditory evoked potential for neonatal neurologic diagnosis. *Am. J. EEG Technol.* 21:31, 1981.

42. Stockard, J. E., et al. Brainstem auditory-evoked responses: Normal variation as a function of stimulus and subject characteristics. *Arch. Neurol.* 36:823, 1979.

43. Stockard, J. J., Stockard, J. E., and Sharbrough, F. W. Brainstem Auditory Evoked Potentials in Neurology: Methodology, Interpretation, Clinical Application. In M. J. Aminoff (Eds.), *Electrodiagnosis in Clinical*

Neurology. New York: Churchill Livingstone, 1980.

44. Suzuki, T., Hirai, Y., and Horiuchi, K. Auditory brainstem responses to pure tone stimuli. *Scand. Audiol.* 6:51, 1977.

45. Terkildsen, K., Osterhammel, P., and Huis In't Veld, F. Recording Procedures for Brainstem Potentials. In R. F. Naunton and C. Fernandez (Eds.), *Evoked Electrical Activity in the Auditory Nervous System.* New York: Academic, 1977.

46. Thornton, A. R. D. The measurement of surface recorded electrocochleographic responses. *Scand. Audiol.* 4:51, 1975.

6

Laboratory Diagnosis of Otologic Diseases

Joseph D. White, Jr.

Laboratory tests add a dimension of accuracy to the art and science of medical diagnosis. In some situations, laboratory tests are needed to confirm a suspected diagnosis; in others, they are used as health screening procedures. Sometimes the laboratory test itself serves to provide a quantitative result, a qualitative result, or a morphologic finding. The quantitative studies provide results in numbers. The qualitative studies record a physical effect such as a change in color or a clumping of particles. The morphologic studies identify a given entity such as a bacterium, a fungus, a cell, or a parasite.

It is to be cautioned that laboratory tests do not and cannot take the place of a thorough history and physical examination. However, on occasion, after such a methodical evaluation, the physician either may be totally puzzled by the patient's complaints, symptoms, and lack of concrete evidence to support a diagnosis or may not have a definite diagnosis in mind but may have a good idea about the underlying mechanisms involved in the disorder. Although laboratory tests usually help clarify these situations, the more general circumstance is that the physician has established a clear impression of the patient's problem(s) and uses the laboratory test results to confirm the diagnosis.

There should be no doubt that the use of laboratory tests in clinical medicine has greatly increased the accuracy of otologic diagnosis. All members of the medical care team, including audiologists, have a continuing need to know the general nature, the meaning, and the significance of clinical laboratory tests. Although the responsible otolaryngologist or otologist must be knowledgeable about the administration and interpretation of clinical laboratory tests, the audiologist needs a broad appreciation and understanding of the clinical laboratory as a major tool for the diagnosis and treatment of disease.

This chapter is organized into two sections. The first deals with specific diseases affecting the external, middle, and inner ear, respectively. Within each of these areas, diseases will be categorized as traumatic, infectious, neoplastic, congenital, or idiopathic in origin. At the end of each category are the medical laboratory tests believed to be most appropriate. The second section presents a glossary of the medical laboratory tests that have been detailed in the first section. It is the author's hope that this chapter will be a frequently used reference source for the audiologist in the investigation of specific problem(s). It is also hoped that the description of the otologic diseases together with the delineation of the appropriate medical laboratory tests will give the audiologist a finer appreciation in the understanding of each disease entity and a feeling of satisfaction as a member of the medical team concerned with the overall care and treatment of the patient.

DISEASES OF EXTERNAL EAR
Traumatic Lesions of the Pinna
Hematoma. A hematoma is a collection of blood between the cartilage of the pinna and its nutritive connective tissue covering (perichondrium). The pinna reveals loss of its normal contour, and marked redness may be present in addition to tenderness.
Medical laboratory test: culture and sensitivity (via sterile needle aspiration).

Frostbite. Frostbite is damage to the tissues of the pinna caused by extreme cold. Portions of the pinna appear white and feel solid to touch.
Medical laboratory test: culture and sensitivity (via sterile needle aspiration).

Keloid. A keloid is excessive scar tissue formation following trauma or surgery to the pinna. It is a shiny, firm mass found on the lobule often caused by ear piercing. It occurs most commonly in blacks.
Medical laboratory test: culture and sensitivity (via sterile needle aspiration).

Inclusion Cyst. An inclusion cyst is a lesion found on the pinna. It often follows incision or trauma and occurs as a result of implantation of skin cells into the underlying subcutaneous tissue. Lesions are firm and tense when palpated.
Medical laboratory test: culture and sensitivity (via sterile needle aspiration).

Infectious Lesions of the Pinna
Cellulitis. Cellulitis is an inflammatory condition affecting the pinna. It is characterized by redness, warmth to touch, tenderness, and tenseness on palpation.
Medical laboratory tests: complete blood count and culture and sensitivity (via sterile needle aspiration) if fluid collection is present.

Subperichondral Abscess. A hematoma, if not cared for properly, and especially in the presence of a contaminated wound, may become an abscess collection.
Medical laboratory tests: complete blood count and culture and sensitivity (via sterile needle aspiration) if fluid collection is present.

Herpes Zoster Oticus. These painful vesicular lesions, also known as Ramsay Hunt syndrome, involve portions of the pinna. They are caused by the reactivation of a herpes virus (chickenpox), and are usually unilateral. A few cranial nerves may be involved.
Medical laboratory tests: complete blood count.

Neoplastic Tumors and Lesions of the Pinna
Senile Keratosis. Senile keratosis, which is benign, appears as yellow, brown, or black lesions, usually less than 1 cm in diameter and caused by sun exposure. It is believed to be a precancerous lesion.
Medical laboratory tests: biopsy.

Seborrheic Keratosis. These yellow, brown, gray, or black lesions, which are benign, are usually elevated on the skin and quite greasy. They are characterized by many pits and fissures. These are the most common skin tumors of the elderly.
Medical laboratory tests: Biopsy (if clinically suspicious).

Nevi. Nevi, both benign and malignant, are proliferative lesions of the skin and, occasionally, the mucosa. These lesions can be either raised or flat and present with variation in color. The majority are benign but degeneration into a malignancy can occur (see Malignant Melanoma).
Medical laboratory tests: biopsy (if clinically suspicious).

Chondrodermatitis Nodularis Chronica Helicis. These grayish, firm, nodular lesions are benign. They are pea-shaped and occur in the free edge of the pinna. They are exquisitely tender with male predominance.

Medical laboratory tests: biopsy (if clinically suspicious).

Squamous Cell Carcinoma. Squamous cell carcinoma is the most common malignant tumor of the pinna. It is characterized by thickening of the skin with scaling, development of a painless pale outgrowth, and finally formation of an ulcer with a raised edge. A good possibility for metastasis (tumor spread to other locations) exists.

Medical laboratory tests: biopsy and metastatic workup (if indicated).

Basal Cell Carcinoma. Basal cell carcinoma is a slow-growing skin cancer (malignant) that develops as an ingrowth. It is initially seen as a flat, painless, slightly raised lesion followed by the development of a rolled edge with a penetrating ulcer that bleeds readily ("rodent ulcer"). There is little possibility for metastasis.

Medical laboratory tests: biopsy and metastatic workup (if indicated).

Malignant Melanoma. Malignant melanoma is a rare but extremely aggressive tumor that may develop from melanocytes (skin pigment cells) within small, rounded pigmented tumors (nevi; previously discussed), or from the melanocyte itself as separate from the nevus. The lesion becomes progressively more pigmented and may ulcerate and bleed. Satellite lesions around the suspicious area make the diagnosis more probable.

Medical laboratory tests: biopsy and metastatic workup (if indicated).

Congenital Lesions of the Pinna
Pinna Malformations. The patient may exhibit microtia (small ear), macrotia (large ear), cleft or trifid pinnae, absent ear lobes, or the complete absence of the pinna. The clinician should regard unusual ear configuration as a possible clue to hidden defects of more importance (e.g., middle ear abnormalities).

Preauricular Cysts and Fistulas. Faulty embryologic closure along tissue planes causes these congenital abnormalities. They may be unilateral or bilateral and present as pit-like depressions in front of the pinna with, in many cases, discharge of foul-smelling material.

Medical laboratory tests: complete blood count and culture and sensitivity. Both tests should be ordered if infection is present.

Hemangiomas. Hemangiomas consist of localized vascular dilatations and often involve adjacent facial areas. They are usually subclassified into two types: (1) capillary hemangioma, which is characterized by clusters of many small capillaries, and (2) cavernous hemangioma, which is characterized by abnormally large blood vessel channels.

Arteriovenous Fistula. An arteriovenous fistula is an abnormal direct communication between an artery and a vein. It usually appears in infancy and enlarges in the first few years of life. The pinna is warm to touch and may pulsate. Eventually the entire pinna may become involved.

Idiopathic Lesions of the Pinna
Dermatitis. Dermatitis is a nonspecific skin condition that may be characterized by dryness, itching, crusting, or weeping. It has been associated with many systemic conditions including anemia, vitamin deficiencies, and endocrine disorders.

Medical laboratory tests: complete blood count.

Relapsing Polychondritis. Relapsing polychondritis is an episodic, inflammatory disease of connective tissue and various cartilages in the body including those of ears, larynx, nasal septum, and trachea. It is believed to be an autoimmune disease (i.e., the body rejecting a portion of itself).

Medical laboratory tests: tests for collagen vascular disease (connective tissue disorders).

Traumatic Diseases of the External
Auditory Canal
Abrasions and Lacerations. Abrasions and lacerations commonly occur in the external auditory canal and can be caused by the patient or by the physician while trying to

extract a foreign body or cerumen. Deep lacerations may become infected if not treated appropriately.

Medical laboratory test: culture and sensitivity if pus is present.

Foreign Bodies. A wide variety of items can be found in the ear canal, the most common being vegetable matter and insects. These, after long-standing, may set up an underlying infection of the ear canal. They require removal by an otolaryngologist.

Medical laboratory test: culture and sensitivity if pus is present.

Infectious Diseases of the External Auditory Canal

Bullous Myringitis. Bullous myringitis is a condition affecting the external auditory canal and, in particular, the tympanic membrane. Viral etiology is proposed. Generalized inflammation is present in addition to multiple blebs, which are red and inflamed. There may be an associated sensorineural hearing loss.

External Otitis. External otitis is an inflammatory condition within the external auditory canal and is one of the most common conditions treated by both the general practitioner and the otolaryngologist. It can be caused by both fungi (molds) and bacteria. The patient may have ear pain, discharge from the external auditory canal, tenderness on movement of the tragus, and occasionally fever and cellulitis.

Medical laboratory tests: complete blood count (in severe infections), culture and sensitivity, fasting blood glucose (for recurrent episodes), and glucose tolerance test.

Malignant External Otitis. Malignant external otitis is a severe inflammation caused by a bacterial agent involving the external auditory canal. It occurs usually in elderly diabetic patients and is associated with a high mortality. The infection may spread through the eardrum to the middle ear space and mastoid system, or it may spread into adjacent preauricular tissue and involve a few of the cranial nerves on the involved side.

Medical laboratory tests: complete blood count, culture and sensitivity, fasting blood glucose, glucose tolerance test, and blood cultures.

Furunculosis. Furuncles are painful, raised, reddened lesions resembling pimples. They occur in the outer third of the external auditory canal. They may be quite painful in the fitting of an ear mold, and may require incision and drainage.

Medical laboratory test: culture and sensitivity (via sterile needle aspiration).

Herpes Zoster Oticus. See Herpes Zoster Oticus under Infectious Lesions of the Pinna. This disease can affect the ear canal.

Neoplastic Tumors and Diseases of the External Auditory Canal

Papilloma. Papilloma is a benign warty growth in the external auditory canal that must be distinguished from a middle ear polyp or a malignancy.

Medical laboratory test: biopsy.

Keratosis Obturans. Keratosis obturans (benign) is, literally, a "skin ball" tumor caused by faulty migration of the surface skin outward in the external auditory canal. There is subsequent mixing of the skin mass with cerumen.

Medical laboratory test: biopsy.

Exostosis. Exostosis is a benign, smooth, rounded nodule of extremely hard bone covered with skin. It is usually multiple and occurs near the tympanic membrane.

Osteoma. Osteoma is a benign, smooth nodule of somewhat spongy bone covered with skin. It is usually single and occurs in the bony cartilaginous junction within the canal.

Basal Cell Carcinoma. See Basal Cell Carcinoma under Neoplastic Tumors and Lesions of the Pinna.

Squamous Cell Carcinoma. See Squamous Cell Carcinoma (Malignant) under Neoplastic Tumors and Lesions of the Pinna.

Both basal cell carcinoma and squamous cell carcinoma are associated with poor prognoses because the diagnosis is often delayed. These patients may have ear canal mass, pain, and ear drainage, which may be bloody.

Medical laboratory tests: biopsy and metastatic workup (if indicated).

Congenital Diseases of the External Auditory Canal

Atresia. Atresia is usually a unilateral condition, which can be either membranous or bony. Membranous atresia is characterized by a dense soft tissue plug between the external auditory canal and middle ear space. Bony atresia is characterized by a wall of bone separating the ear canal from the middle ear space.

Idiopathic Diseases of the External Auditory Canal

Dermatitis. See Dermatitis under Idiopathic Lesions of the Pinna.

DISEASES OF THE MIDDLE EAR

Trauma of the Middle Ear

Tympanic Membrane or Ossicular Damage. These injuries can occur with both sharp and blunt trauma, explosions, or burns.

Medical laboratory test: culture and sensitivity if persistent infection is evident in presence of perforated tympanic membrane.

Temporal Bone Injury. There are two types of temporal bone fractures: longitudinal and transverse. Longitudinal is more common. These fractures often tear the tympanic membrane and disrupt the ossicles. A cerebrospinal fluid leak may occur. Facial paralysis on the side of injury may also occur. Transverse is less common and is usually associated with severe head injury. Inner ear structures are markedly affected. Damage to the facial nerve and the vestibulocochlear nerve can occur as well.

Medical laboratory tests: culture and sensitivity if persistent infection is present with perforated tympanic membrane and cerebrospinal fluid identification tests in presence of clear fluid discharge from ear or nose.

Infectious Diseases of the Middle Ear

Acute Suppurative Otitis Media. See Chapter 8. Briefly, acute suppurative otitis media is an acute bacterial infection of the middle ear space characterized by the presence of pus. A history of previous recurrent serous otitis media is common.

Acute Mastoiditis. Acute mastoiditis is an extension of acute suppurative otitis media rarely seen today because of the use of antibiotics. Complications of this condition include acute suppurative labyrinthitis (see Chap. 8), facial nerve paralysis, meningitis, and brain abscess.

Medical laboratory tests: complete blood count and culture and sensitivity (either from tympanic membrane perforation or from a myringotomy site); in addition: lumbar puncture (spinal tap) and blood cultures.

Neoplastic Tumors and Diseases of the Middle Ear

Polyps. These benign lesions typically present as an external auditory canal tumor protruding through a defect in the tympanic membrane. They may be attached to important middle ear structures (e.g., stapes).

Medical laboratory test: biopsy with extreme caution only if deemed necessary to perform preoperatively.

Cholesteatoma. Cholesteatoma, which is benign, may be either congenital or acquired. The end result is the same—a slowly enlarging collection of skin tissue that can cause perforation of the tympanic membrane. If this lesion is allowed to grow further, facial nerve injury, damage to the labyrinth, or both may occur.

Medical laboratory test: biopsy if cholesteatoma is readily seen via perforation in the tympanic membrane.

Osteomas. These benign, firm, bony growths rarely invade the middle ear and mastoid systems. Osteomas usually do not produce symptoms.

Glomus Tumors. Glomus tumors, which are benign, are formed from embryologic nervous system tissue and may be associated with the jugular bulb (glomus jugulare tumors) or with the middle ear (glomus tympanicum tumors). Both of these lesions may be visualized through the tympanic membrane as a reddish blue mass. The patient may experience pulsatile tinnitus in the affected ear. Numerous cranial nerves on the side of the lesion may be affected (cranial nerves IX, X, XI, and XII).

Medical laboratory test: biopsy is done in the operating room at the time of the operative procedure.

Squamous Cell Carcinoma. Squamous cell carcinoma is the most common middle ear malignancy. The patient may experience otorrhea (usually bloody), pain, decreased hearing, and possibly aural polyps. Facial nerve weakness or paralysis on the side of the lesion indicates serious pathology.
Medical laboratory test: biopsy.

Congenital Diseases of the Middle Ear
Ossicular Anomalies. Examples of ossicular anomalies are congenital fixation of the stapes footplate, absence of portions of the ossicles, and fusion of the ossicles to themselves or to adjacent temporal bone.

Vascular Anomalies. Vascular anomalies include a persistent stapedial artery (an artery that supplies the stapes in embryonic life and degenerates thereafter), anomalous internal carotid artery, or anomalies of the internal jugular vein.

Facial Nerve Anomalies: Anomalies of the Bony Partitions Separating the Middle Ear Space from Adjacent Areas. This condition may allow, for example, a portion of the brain to herniate through the roof of the middle ear space and allow for intermittent cerebrospinal fluid leakage or the spread of infection into the central nervous system, which may result in recurrent meningitis.
Medical laboratory tests: cerebrospinal fluid identification and tests for meningitis if clinically believed to be present (see Trauma of the Middle Ear and Temporal Bone Injury).

Idiopathic Diseases of the Middle Ear
Otosclerosis (Otospongiosis). See Chapter 9 for a discussion of otosclerosis.

DISEASES OF THE INNER EAR AND INTERNAL AUDITORY CANAL
Trauma of the Inner Ear and Internal Auditory Canal
Fractures. (see Temporal Bone Injury under Trauma of the Middle Ear.

Presbycusis. Presbycusis is a progressive sensorineural hearing loss that usually starts at about age 60. Audiogram can have flat, sloping, or rapidly falling contour. A proportionate decrease in the audiometric speech discrimination score accompanies the hearing loss (see Chap. 14).

Noise-induced Hearing Loss. Noise-induced hearing loss is evidenced on audiogram as a sensorineural hearing loss that is most severe at 4000 Hz. It may be accompanied by a decrease in discrimination score. Usually the patient will give a history of noise exposure such as an explosion or gunfire (see Chap. 12).

Infectious Diseases of the Inner Ear and Internal Auditory Canal
The labyrinth can be affected by both bacterial and viral agents. These agents can enter the labyrinth from the middle ear or mastoid system, after surgery of the middle ear, from fractures of the temporal bone, or as an extension of meningitis through well-formed pathways.

Bacterial Labyrinthitis. There is a wide variation in the ways that this bacterial entity can present. There may be labyrinthitis confined to a small area of the labyrinth (such as the horizontal semicircular canal), which may produce vertigo, or there may be frank pus in the labyrinth, which usually causes complete sensorineural hearing loss and severe vertigo.
Medical laboratory tests: complete blood count, blood culture, and culture and sensitivity if pus can be obtained from the middle ear space.

Syphilitic Labyrinthitis. Syphilitic labyrinthitis is a rare but quite serious form of bacterial labyrinthitis. It may be either congenital or acquired. The congenital form usually produces more severe sensorineural hearing loss.
Medical laboratory tests: VDRL and fluorescent treponemal antibody absorption (FTA-ABS) test.

Viral Labyrinthitis. A number of viral agents have been implicated in labyrinthitis such as mumps, measles, influenza, and viruses causing the common cold. All can cause sensorineural hearing loss and vertigo.

Medical laboratory tests: complete blood count and viral titers (if indicated).

Neoplastic Tumors and Diseases of the Inner Ear and Internal Auditory Canal
Acoustic Neuroma. Acoustic neuroma is a benign tumor that arises in the internal auditory canal or just outside the internal auditory canal from the nerve sheath of a vestibular nerve. This tumor, as it slowly enlarges, can compress the vestibular nerves, which causes vertigo. The patient complains, in the early part of the tumor's growth, of unsteadiness. If compression of the cochlear nerve occurs, there is evidence of a sensorineural hearing loss with very poor discrimination. Tinnitus may also be present. The facial nerve may be affected, but usually late in the course of the disease (see Chap. 15).

Medical laboratory test: lumbar puncture.

Meningioma. Meningioma is a benign tumor arising from lining cells of the braincase. It presents in a similar fashion to an acoustic neuroma, discussed previously.

Medical laboratory test: lumbar puncture.

Congenital Diseases of the Inner Ear and Internal Auditory Canal
Congenital ear defects fall into two broad categories: those present at birth or that develop shortly after birth and those in which there is a gradual, genetically programmed deterioration in hearing later in life. It is impossible in this chapter to discuss all of the different causes of congenital hearing loss. Only the major categories are listed. The reader is encouraged to review Chapter 13 should more detailed information on this subject be desired.

Prenatal Factors. The following prenatal factors are associated with hearing loss: (1) congenital rubella, (2) maternal ototoxicity, (3) cytomegalovirus, (4) toxoplasmosis, and (5) maternal syphilis.

Medical laboratory tests: viral titers, VDRL, and fluorescent treponemal antibody absorption (FTA-ABS) test.

Neonatal Risk Factors. The following neonatal risk factors are associated with hearing loss: (1) hypoxia (decreased oxygen to the fetus), (2) elevated serum bilirubin (occurs in erythroblastosis fetalis, a condition resulting from blood incompatibility between fetal and maternal circulation), (3) low birth weight, (4) serious infections (such as meningitis, encephalitis), and (5) evidence of congenital deformities of the head and neck.

Medical laboratory tests for hypoxia and elevated serum bilirubin: arterial blood gas and serum bilirubin level. *For low birth weight, infections, and congenital deformities:* complete blood count, blood cultures, and lumbar puncture.

Genetic Syndromes. Most genetic syndromes are transmitted by a recessive pattern. The reader should at least be familiar with the following syndromes (D = dominant mode of genetic transmission; R = recessive mode of genetic transmission):

1. Waardenburg's syndrome (D)
2. Klippel-Feil syndrome (D)
3. Marfan's syndrome (D)
4. Alport's syndrome (D)
5. Pendred's syndrome (R)
6. Usher syndrome (R)
7. Jervell and Lange-Nielsen syndrome (R)
8. Möbius' syndrome (R)

Medical laboratory tests: urinalysis, complete blood count, electrocardiogram, thyroid function tests, and karyotype (buccal smear).

Idiopathic Diseases of the Inner Ear and Internal Auditory Canal
Otosclerosis (Osteospongiosis). See Chapter 9 for a discussion of otosclerosis. This disease entity can also affect the inner ear resulting in progressive sensorineural hearing loss and vertigo and tinnitus.

Meniere's Disease. Meniere's disease is characterized by the sudden onset of tinnitus, vertigo, and fluctuating sensorineural hearing loss. The patient is usually without symptoms between attacks (see Chap. 11).

Medical laboratory tests: thyroid function tests and glycerol test.

Multiple Sclerosis. Multiple sclerosis is characterized by unsteadiness, frank vertigo, or both, and a fluctuating sensorineural hearing loss. It is usually associated with visual disturbances as well. The disease is of unknown etiology and is characterized by exacerbations and remissions.

Medical laboratory test: lumbar puncture (for protein content and other specialized laboratory determinations).

GLOSSARY OF MEDICAL LABORATORY TESTS

arterial blood gas   Designed to determine, among other things, the oxygen content of the blood. It is also an indirect way of assessing the capacity of the lungs and kidneys to rid the body of waste products.

bilirubin level   Bilirubin is a pigment formed in the breakdown of the red blood cells. Normally this pigment is altered by the liver and then stored in the gallbladder as bile. If there is malfunction of the liver or gallbladder or if there is the sudden massive breakdown of red blood cells (such as in erythroblastosis fetalis), the serum (blood) level of bilirubin will be elevated.

biopsy   Examination of tissue specimens removed from the patient. Biopsies may be performed on many kinds of tissue from almost any area. They can be classified as incisional when only a portion of the lesion to be biopsied is removed, or excisional when the entire sample is removed for evaluation. Biopsy is most often done to differentiate benign from malignant lesions.

blood culture   Identifies a bacteria producing a bloodstream infection (bacteremia). The blood is removed from the patient's vein and placed immediately into a growth medium so that the bacteria will be able to survive and grow well.

cerebrospinal fluid (CSF) identification   Identifies clear fluid leaking from the nose or ears as CSF. Also called *spinal fluid,* CSF fills the cavities within the brain and the central canal of the spinal cord. It is believed that its function is to protect the brain and spinal cord from compression injuries. It also may play a role in supplying the brain and spinal cord with oxygen and other nutrients. Usually CSF is obtained by lumbar puncture (see lumbar puncture). Occasionally with trauma or with erosive disease affecting the temporal bone, CSF may leak (appearing as clear fluid) from the nose or the ear. CSF is odorless, colorless, and contains glucose (sugar).

collagen vascular disease, tests for   Collagen vas-
cular diseases (also called connective tissue disorders) include rheumatoid arthritis, relapsing polychondritis, and systemic lupus erythematosus (SLE). The tests to evaluate these conditions include rheumatoid factor (RF), erythrocyte sedimentation rate (ESR), and antinuclear antibody (ANA).

complete blood count (CBC)   Refers to the red cell count, white cell count, and the white cell differential count. A CBC may be ordered either to help with a particular problem or to follow the results of treatment.

1. *red cell count*   The red cells contain hemoglobin, which is the essential oxygen carrier in the blood. An increase in red cells may indicate a concentration of the blood (such as in severe dehydration or in diseases in which too many red cells are produced). A decrease in the red blood cell count may occur from hemorrhage or from various forms of anemia.

2. *white cell count*   White cells are important in the defense of the body against invading microorganisms. An increase in the white blood cell count is usually seen in infections. It can, however, be seen in other medical conditions, some of which are quite serious, such as leukemia. A decrease in the white cell count may be seen in overwhelming infections, drug and chemical toxicity, as well as in several other medical entities.

3. *white cell differential count*   There are several types of white blood cells that can be distinguished microscopically. It is often helpful and important to know if the percentage of these cells has changed. The *neutrophils* are increased in most bacterial infections. The *eosinophils* are seen in allergic conditions and those in which parasites are involved. The *basophils* again may be seen in allergic conditions as well as other specific disease entities. The *lymphocytes* may be increased in viral infections and in a few bacterial infections. The *monocytes* may be increased during recovery from severe infections.

culture and sensitivity

1. *culture*   Identifies causative organisms. Specimens for culture are taken at the bedside or in the office and sent to the laboratory where the material is inoculated into growth media.

2. *sensitivity*   Determines which antibiotics are most effective against a particular strain of bacteria causing a patient's illness.

electrocardiogram   A recording of the changes

in electrical potential of the heart that are transmitted through the limbs and chest wall. This recording is useful in diagnosing cardiac rhythm disturbances and in diagnosing and following a heart attack.

fasting blood glucose Determines disorders of glucose (blood sugar) metabolism. An increase in blood glucose is seen in severe diabetes, chronic liver ailments, and in overactivity of the endocrine glands. In mild diabetes, there may be a normal fasting blood glucose and a more sensitive test may be needed (see glucose tolerance test).

fluorescent treponemal antibody absorption (FTA-ABS) test Measures the ability of a patient's serum to coat the bacteria responsible for causing syphilis. This is the most specific and sensitive of all the serologic tests for syphilis.

glucose tolerance test Discovers disorders of glucose metabolism that have not become severe enough to change the blood glucose levels in the fasting state. In this test, the fasting patient is given a large amount of glucose either intravenously or orally. At regular intervals, the blood glucose levels are measured to determine how long it takes for the body to handle the additional glucose. There is evidence of an abnormality in glucose metabolism if the glucose remains in the blood for an excessive period of time.

glycerol test Improves the diagnostic accuracy in patients suspected of having Meniere's disease. The glycerol acts as a diuretic (increases urine output). The patient ingests 6 oz of a mixture of 50% glucose and water. Pure-tone thresholds and discrimination scores are measured before and 3 hours after the ingestion of this mixture. In Meniere's disease, a temporary improvement in hearing occurs after this mixture is given. The test is considered positive when there is a pure-tone shift of more than 15 dB in at least one frequency (250–4000 Hz) and/or improvement in the speech discrimination score of at least 12%.

karyotype A very specialized test whereby the chromosome characteristics of an individual cell (usually taken from the buccal mucosa inside the mouth) can be examined for possible abnormalities under the microscope.

lumbar puncture Usually obtains cerebrospinal fluid (see cerebrospinal fluid identification). Fluid is withdrawn after passing a needle between two vertebrae of the lower back into the fluid bathing the spinal cord. At the time of the puncture, the physician can measure just how much pressure the spinal fluid is under. In addition, the fluid can be sent to the laboratory for chemical analysis (i.e., glucose content, protein content, white cell content).

metastatic workup Diagnostic tests (bone scans, CAT scans, liver-spleen scans) to detect the metastasis of tumors. Certain malignant tumors have the ability to metastasize (spread) to both close and distant sites. Depending on the probability of spread to specific sites, certain diagnostic tests can be performed. In addition, certain laboratory tests can be ordered that may give clues as to whether metastatic disease is present.

thyroid function tests A battery of blood tests to evaluate the function of the thyroid gland. In addition, these tests can be helpful in evaluating the other endocrine organs involved with the production of thyroid hormone (i.e., pituitary gland).

urinalysis An analysis of the urine. This simple test indicates if there is any blood or blood derivatives in the urine, if there is glucose (sugar) or protein in the urine, and, among other things, if there are cells (i.e., red cells, white cells) in the urine. In addition, certain drug determinations can be performed on the urine.

viral titers A special battery of tests to detect the presence of viral agents in the serum (blood) of a patient.

VDRL A blood test for syphilis that is positive in a variety of other diseases in which syphilis plays no part. Thus, the FTA-ABS test (previously discussed) is still the most specific and sensitive test for syphilis.

SUGGESTED READING

Levinson, S. A., and MacFate, R. P. *Clinical Laboratory Diagnosis* (7th ed.). Philadelphia: Lea & Febiger, 1969.

Northern, J. L., and Downs, M. P. *Hearing in Children* (3rd ed.). Baltimore: Williams & Wilkins, 1984.

Paparella, M. M., and Shumrick, D. A. *Otolaryngology*. Philadelphia: Saunders, 1980.

Widmann, F. K. *Clincial Interpretation of Laboratory Results*. Philadelphia: Davis, 1973.

Wood, R. P., and Northern, J. L. *Manual of Otolaryngology*. Baltimore: Williams & Wilkins, 1979.

7

Radiology in Otologic Diagnosis

Jeffrey S. Rose

The German physicist Wilhelm Conrad Röntgen discovered a unique form of radiant energy in 1895, which had the ability to penetrate solid matter. He named the newly observed emanations "x"-rays, and almost immediately they began to assume an important and expansive role in medical practice. Revolutionary recent developments in manipulating, refining, and computerizing data generated by the interactions of the x-rays with human tissues has led to more recent radiologic technology that has particular utility in otologic diagnosis. Indeed, the detection of a hearing abnormality, which, in the judgment of the clinician, may be caused by a structural lesion, demands the application of one or several appropriate radiologic modalities if a correct diagnosis and efficacious treatment plan are to be accomplished.

The x-rays that Röntgen discovered are a form of electromagnetic radiation similar to visible light but with much shorter wavelengths and higher energies*; these wavelength and energy characteristics allow x-rays to penetrate substances they encounter, to an extent dependent on the physical density and atomic number of the material they must traverse. A photosensitized film placed in the path of the radiation after it has passed through an object is differentially exposed to the degree that x-rays have been unimpeded in their travel. A conceptual understanding of the creation of routine radiographic images is not only prerequisite for understanding the more complex radiologic modalities used to investigate abnormalities affecting the ear, but facilitates the selection of radiologic examinations that (1) are most effective at detecting a presumed abnormality, (2) are least invasive (e.g., involve little intrinsic morbidity), (3) are most cost-effective, and (4) are least likely to expose patients to potentially damaging amounts of ionizing radiation.

STANDARD RADIOGRAPHY

Standard radiographs are obtained when x-rays are generated in the roentgen ray tube and focused on a photographic film,

---

* Visible light, 400–700 nm; x-rays, 0.5–5.0 nm (1 nm $= 10^{-9}$ meters).

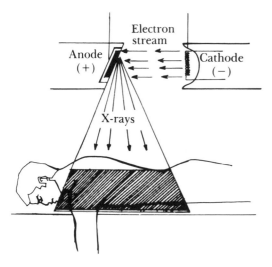

A

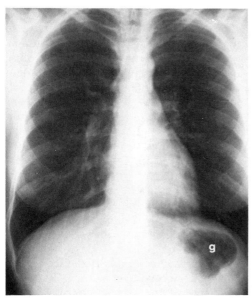

B

Figure 7-1. A. *Roentgen ray tube and patient position for PA chest film. Current applied across the coil at the cathode causes electrons to be "boiled off," and a voltage difference between the anode and this cathode attracts the negatively charged electrons toward a tungsten target in the anode. On striking the target the electrons cause the generation of x-rays in a beam, which then traverse the patient (from back to front) to expose an x-ray film (crosshatching). B. The exposed film results in a representation of the patient based on the impedance of the x-rays on their way to the film. The bones (ribs, clavicles, scapulae, and spine) are dense structures that absorb the x-rays and pre-*

with the patient positioned between the two (Fig. 7-1A).

On their path to the photosensitive plate, the rays encounter the body tissues and are absorbed or attenuated depending on the density of the structures confronted. For example, the lungs, which contain mostly air, only minimally impede x-ray transmission and allow relatively large amounts of energy to reach the film. The resulting high exposure yields a dark area on the processed image. In contrast, the bones, with their dense calcium component, absorb more of the radiation than they allow to reach the photographic film and appear as white areas on the film (Fig. 7-1B). In between these extremes of transmission are two other radiographic densities that may be determined visually: "water," which represents the soft tissues (nerves, muscles, connective tissue, and blood vessels), and "fat," which represents areas of lipid materials in the soft tissues. These areas allow slightly more x-rays to the film than the other soft tissues, but less than occurs with air-containing structures. These four densities, bone, soft tissue, fat, and air, bear the same relationship to each other in all of the techniques in the following discussion.

The tissue-specific absorption of the rays allows the production of a two-dimensional roentgenogram, but a perceptual problem occurs because patients are three-dimensional. All structures in the path of the beam are imaged, and multiple densities overlying a single point appear on the film as a conglomerate shadow. Several projections or positions must therefore be used to comprehend the anatomy (Fig. 7-2).

A projection is generally named based on the patient's position relative to the incident beam. A frontal projection is a view of the patient as seen from the front, whereas a lateral projection is a side view

vent film exposure, and therefore appear white, whereas the lungs transmit x-rays and cause dark areas on the image. The gas bubble in the stomach (g) also demonstrates transmission properties of air. The heart and subdiaphragmatic soft tissues represent an intermediate density between bone and air; fat is not seen on this radiograph.

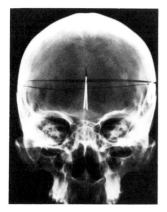

A

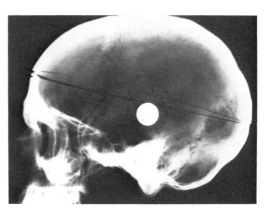

B

Figure 7-2. Importance of projection in radiography. A. In this dried skull preparation (note the air where the skull has been circularly cut and where small holes have been drilled), a lateral roentgenogram has been taken, and a coin is projected over the midportion of the squamous temporal bone. It cannot be predicted from this view if the coin is on the right calvaria, left calvaria, or somewhere between in the cranial vault. B. The same specimen is seen in a frontal projection, and the coin is clearly seen "end on" adjacent to the left calvaria and has been successfully "localized" with two views. Now, however, two metal pins are seen in the midline used to hold the top of the calvaria to the remainder of the skull. These pins are located far anteriorly and posteriorly, and the anterior pin can be seen on the lateral view (arrows) on careful scrutiny; the posterior one is obscured by the dense bone overlying it.

of the patient. A frontal projection can be obtained by passing the x-rays from the anterior surface of the body toward a film at the posterior surface, in which case an anteroposterior (AP) frontal projection is obtained, or by passing the beam from the posterior surface toward a film on the anterior surface of the patient, in which case a posteroanterior (PA) frontal projection is obtained. The subtle differences in the appearance of films obtained in the AP versus PA projections are beyond the scope of this chapter, but what should be kept in mind is that regardless of the beam trajectory, the final roentgenogram is always viewed as though the patient were facing the clinician; that is the right side of the film represents the left side of the patient. Similarly, a lateral film can be made by

passing the rays from the right side toward a film on the left or conversely. For lateral films, no convention is established for viewing the roentgenogram, but one should be aware that a left lateral projection is accomplished with the left side of the patient closest to the film.

Other projections are obtained with varying degrees of beam obliquity along any conceivable axis and are understandably limitless; the more useful of such projections often bear the name of the investigator who originated them, and these views must be described in reference to the anatomy they best display.

Traditional views that are most useful in evaluating otologic abnormalities include frontal, lateral, and Towne's views of the skull (Figs. 7-3 to 7-5). Supplemental positions for better evaluation of the internal auditory canal and the mastoid process are often obtained but need not be described here.

Despite these multiple projections, interpreting otologic films can be difficult. Expansion of the internal auditory canal, which indicates an acoustic neuroma (Fig. 7-6A), or other destructive lesions of the temporal bone, such as infection, neoplasm, or trauma (Figs. 7-6B and C), are usually detected. For these abnormalities, standard radiographs are sufficient screening examinations. Exposure to radiation is negligible and cost is at a minimum with these studies. More subtle abnormalities involving the auditory apparatus may not be ascertained with standard radiography, and if preliminary films are normal in the face of

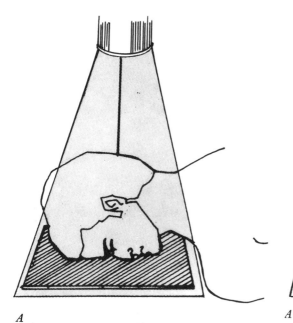

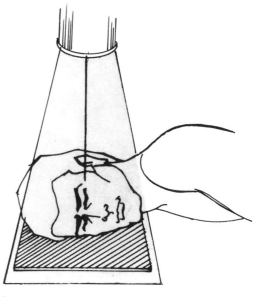

A

A

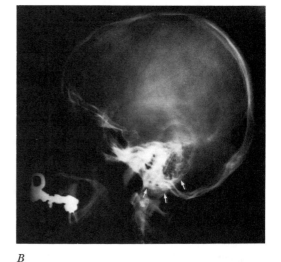

B

B

Figure 7-3. The frontal projection. A. The patient position for a frontal roentgenogram of the skull. The x-ray tube is posterior to the patient, and the film is beneath the patient's face (cross-hatching). Because the x-rays travel from posterior to anterior through the patient, the resultant radiograph will be a PA frontal film. B. The resulting radiograph projects the petrous bones within the orbits, and is often useful in

Figure 7-4. The lateral projection. A. The lateral film is obtained with the patient lying on the film as shown with the beam of x-rays directed at the middle of the skull. The side of the patient closest to the film determines whether the resultant radiograph is a right lateral or left lateral film. B. The lateral skull radiograph shows the overlapping density of the petrous bones and is not often revealing unless tomography is performed (see Fig. 7-8B). It does demonstrate the mastoid tips and air cells well (arrows).

otologic diagnosis. A close-in view of this region would be necessary to delineate the ear anatomy in detail.

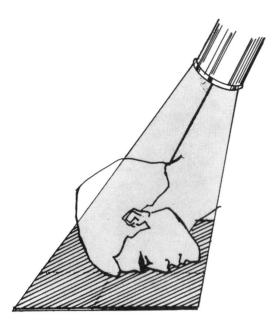

A

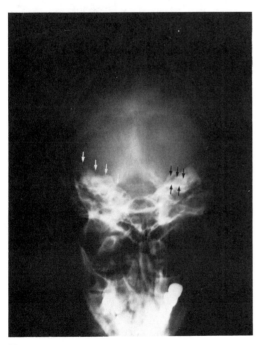

B

Figure 7-5. *Towne's projection of the skull. A.
The position for a Towne's view is similar to
that for a PA frontal position, except that the
x-ray beam is angled such that it traverses the
patient from the lower back of the head toward
the upper forehead (compare with Fig. 7-3A).
B. This Towne's view skull roentgenogram projects the petrous pyramids (white arrows) above
the facial structures and is a very useful stan-*

strong clinical suspicion, additional steps
must be taken to reach a diagnosis. When
the audiologic and otologic examinations
suggest a congenital abnormality of the
temporal bone, a vascular lesion affecting
the ear, or a neural deficit characteristic of
the cerebellopontile angle mass, higher resolution conventional tomography, computerized tomography, or angiography may be
indicated without preliminary plain radiography.

POLYTOMOGRAPHY

Conventional tomography (also called laminagraphy) is a method devised to deal
with the overlapping densities seen on a
regular radiograph. The same x-ray source
and film are used, but in laminagraphy
both the x-ray tube and the film are moved
in opposite directions during the exposure
(Fig. 7-7). In this manner, only a single
plane through the patient is in focus on
the films; objects above or below that plane
are blurred and the eye perceives more
crisp detail in the plane of interest. The
thickness of these slices may be varied from
less than one millimeter to more than several centimeters, and adjacent planes may
be imaged by changing the distance from
the patient to the tube a calculated amount.
The tomogram technique does not alleviate the need for multiple projections to aid
in interpretation; some structures are best
seen in a frontal projection, whereas others
can be studied only in a lateral projection
(Fig. 7-8).

For many years, petrous bone tomography has been the high-resolution x-ray modality of choice in looking for subtle structural lesions affecting hearing. It has had
most utility in detailing congenital anomalies of the ear (Fig. 7-9) as well as in detecting early inflammatory or neoplastic
involvement of the temporal bone (Fig.
7-10), in revealing trauma to the auditory
canal or ossicles (Fig. 7-11), and in diagnosing the subtle changes of otosclerosis and

*dard view for otologic diagnosis. The internal
auditory canals are often well seen (black arrows), and more detailed anatomy is visible on
close-up views.*

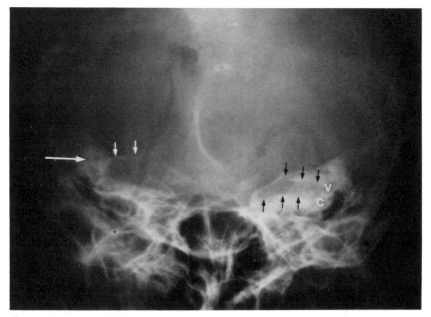

A

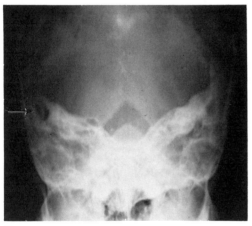

B

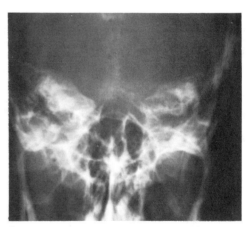

C

Figure 7-6. Lesions evident on standard radiographs. A. Expansion of the internal auditory canal. This close-up view of a Towne's projection reveals normal left auditory structures including the superior and inferior margins of the internal auditory canal (black arrows), the cochlea (c), and the vestibule (v). On the right, however, the internal auditory canal is expanded, its roof and medial margins thinned and indistinct (short white arrows); the vestibuli and superior semicircular canal (long arrow) are unremarkable. The findings in the internal auditory canal on the right are typical of an expansile intracanalicular or juxtacanalicular neoplasm, most often an acoustic neuroma, which was the final diagnosis in this case.
B. Abnormal petrous bone lucency. This Towne's view demonstratees an abnormal

"hole" in the lateral portion of the right petrous bone (arrow), which is not present on the left. Other projections would be necessary to localize this lesion precisely, but a bone-destroying lesion in this position is often due to a cholesteatoma, which was discovered in this patient with chronic middle ear disease. C. Diffuse petrous bone demineralization and apical bone destruction. This Towne's view was obtained in the patient whose case is presented in Fig. 7-16. The right petrous bone is normal, but the left is "washed" out in density, and its medial aspect demonstrates erosion and asymmetry when compared to the other side. These changes were due to an adjacent glomus jugulare tumor, but acute infection and metastatic neoplasms were also considered in the differential diagnosis.

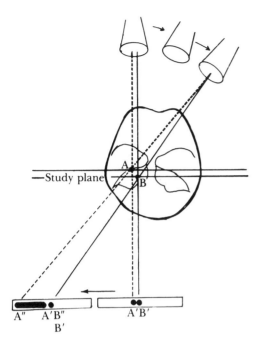

—Study plane

A″ A′B″   A′B′
     B′

Figure 7-7. Tomographic technique. In conventional linear tomography the x-ray tube and the film move in opposite directions during the exposure. The object of interest (B) and other objects in the same plane of focus will remain sharp and clear on the film because they maintain a constant position relative to the moving tube and film, whereas objects above or below the plane of focus (A) will be blurred because of their motion relative to the arc of the x-ray beam. The unfocused objects are readily ignored by the eye, and the plane of study is more clearly seen. (Redrawn from L. F. Squire, Fundamentals of Radiology, *Cambridge, Mass.: Harvard University Press, 1975. P. 23.)*

Meniere's disease. Although tomography generally has a higher diagnostic yield than radiography, it involves considerably more time and expense and a much higher patient radiation dose. It should not be ordered as a screening test, but rather should be reserved for problem cases or presurgical evaluation. It may not always be necessary to perform petrous tomography; if a vascular lesion is detected on physical examination, angiography may be more useful, and when audiologic studies indicate a lesion in neural pathways geographically removed from the temporal bone, laminagraphy is certainly not indicated.

COMPUTED TOMOGRAPHY

The most revolutionary new technique in radiology, perhaps since the discovery of x-rays, has been the development of computerized axial tomography, or CT scanning. This modality uses a small, mobile micro x-ray tube mounted in a circular gantry. Detector crystals are aligned in a circle directly opposite the tube (Fig. 7-12A). The rays that the tube emits are finely collimated (thin and contained), such that the beam thickness can be as little as 2 mm. As the patient lies within the gantry (Fig. 7-12B), the tube is activated and moved along the gantry circumference. X-rays pass through the patient in differing degrees determined by the tissues penetrated, and each of the detectors opposite the beam at any instant reads the transmitted amount of radiation for that position and sends this information to a computer. The motion of the tube continues through a 360-degree rotation, at which point all of the detectors have received their "tissue specific" units of x-ray exposure. The information gathered by the detectors and accumulated in the computer is then reconstructed using complex algorithms, such that the average density of the scanned object in each of thousands of tiny volumes or "voxels" is calculated. The density information is then displayed on a monitor, where the visual data representation may be modified by the radiologist so that an optimal image is achieved.

CT is a computer reconstruction of absorption density measurements obtained with the use of minidose x-rays. The image appears as a slice of predetermined thickness in a projection dependent on the patient's placement within the gantry. The axial projection is most frequently obtained, and by convention it is displayed so the slice is viewed from below; that is, looking upward from the patient's feet. The posterior portion of the patient is down, anterior up, and the right side of the patient appears on the left side of the image (Fig. 7-12C).

The major advantage of CT is that very minor differences in density are sensed and displayed. Although the general rules for the pictorial appearance of tissues in standard radiography apply, rather than there

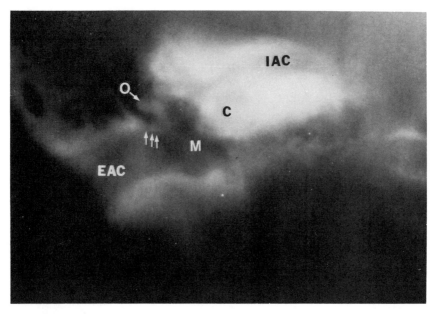

A

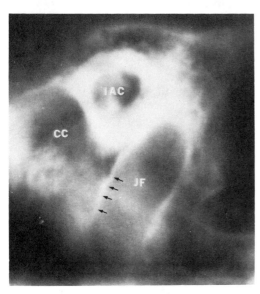

B

Figure 7-8. Petrous tomograms. A. This single section from a frontal tomographic study of the right petrous bone demonstrates the external auditory canal (EAC), the scutum (the bony projection to which the tympanic membrane is attached superiorly; white arrows), the middle ear cavity (M), and the incus and malleus ossicles superiorly (O). Also discernible, but out of focus because they are not directly in the plane of study, are the cochlea (C) and a portion of the internal auditory canal (IAC). B. The lateral tomogram of the right ear is often useful in evaluating the region of the jugular bulb, and this section demonstrates the sharp crest of bone (arrows) that separates the carotid canal (CC) from the jugular fossa (JF). This structure is not visible on frontal tomograms and illustrates the necessity of multiple projections even when tomography is employed to increase anatomic clarity. The jugular crest may be eroded by tumors in the region, particularly in the case of glomus jugulare tumors (see Fig. 7-16). A cross section of the internal auditory canal is also apparent (IAC).

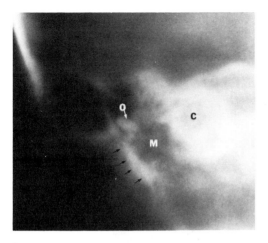

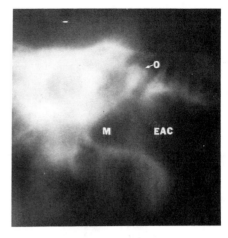

A

B

Figure 7-9. Congenital anomaly on frontal tomography. A. External ear anomaly. The abnormal right ear of this child may be compared with the normal opposite side (B). The middle ear cavity (M) and the incus and malleus (O) are seen, as is the cochlea (C), but there is a bony atretic plate where the tympanic membrane should be (arrows), and the external auditory canal is absent. B. Normal ear. This frontal tomogram of the left ear is in the same plane of focus as the film of the abnormal right side and clearly demonstrates a well-formed external auditory canal (EAC), healthy-appearing middle ear ossicles (O), and no bony plate in the region of the tympanic membrane that separates the middle ear (M) from the external auditory meatus.

being only four or five apparent densities, there are literally hundreds. Blood vessels may be individually detected (see next section), different soft tissue densities within the brain can be seen, and even different states of a single substance (e.g., clotted vs fresh blood) can be discerned. It is available for studying the brain and the ear with impressive advantages over conventional tomography. The contrast between the bone and soft tissue, which is the limiting factor in plane tomography, is of far less importance with CT; small tumors in the cerebellopontile angle that have not affected the temporal bone can be detected; and perhaps most importantly, brain lesions causing otologic problems (e.g., stroke, central nervous system tumor, infection) can be exposed and localized.

CT remains a costly but essential tool in otologic diagnosis. It is noninvasive, less hazardous from a radiation standpoint than polytomography, and of superior diagnostic yield in most instances. Its limitation is in the fact that the reconstructed CT images have not yet achieved the spatial resolution of plain radiography or conventional tomography; that is, the ability to distinguish one anatomic structure separated from another by a very small distance is slightly inferior. For this reason it may still be desirable to evaluate congenital ear problems or temporal bone trauma with routine petrous bone tomography. As technology improves, CT may eventually surpass the more established radiologic techniques altogether (Fig. 7-13).

CONTRAST-ENHANCED RADIOGRAPHIC METHODS

In an attempt to better define structures seen on conventional radiographs, various substances have been injected into different body spaces to opacify them, or to make them sufficiently different in their x-ray absorption characteristics from surrounding soft tissues to render them visible. In most cases the materials used have been iodinated compounds that absorb x-rays well, and provide a density greater than that of bone. The opposite extreme on the contrast scale, air, is occasionally used for studies of the spinal cord and cisternal ventricular spaces in the brain. The advent of CT, which can usually delineate the same struc-

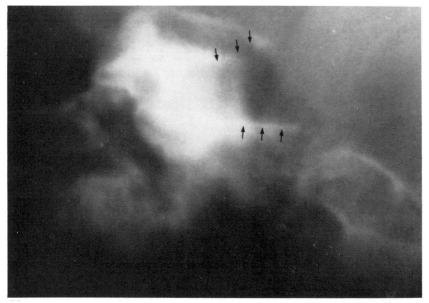

A

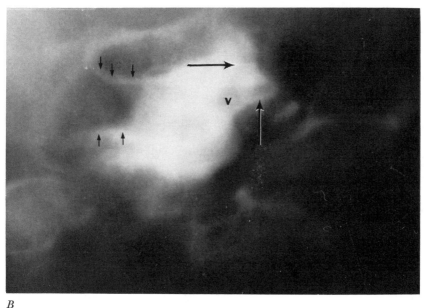

B

Figure 7-10. Acoustic neuroma on frontal to-mography. A. This frontal tomogram demonstrates changes similar to those seen on the plain film in Fig. 7-6A, but with greater clarity. The medial portion of the right internal auditory canal is expanded (arrows), and its superior margin is absent. The erosion and expansion are due to an acoustic neuroma growing within the canal. B. The normal left side in this patient illustrates the expected sharp, smooth borders of the internal auditory canal (arrows). Also note the vestibule (v) and superior and horizontal semicircular canals (long arrows) seen to advantage in this plane.

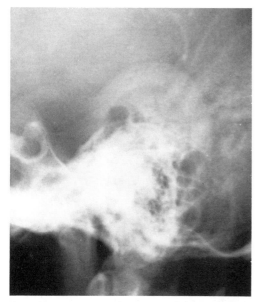

A

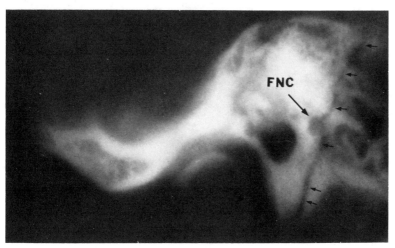

B

Figure 7-11. Petrous bone fracture on lateral tomography. A. This plain film was obtained on a patient with symptoms of facial nerve damage after head trauma in an automobile accident. There is no apparent fracture line. B.

The lateral tomogram of the same patient clearly reveals a fracture extending from the inferior portion of the mastoid process through the facial nerve canal (FNC) and upward to the top of the petrous bone (arrows).

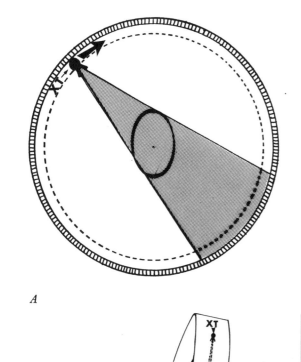

A

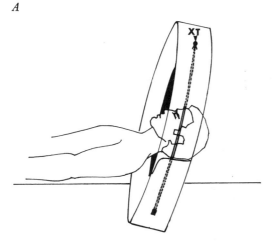

B

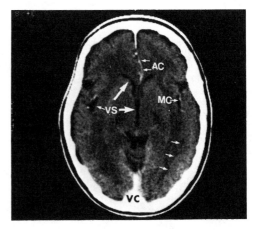

C

Figure 7-12. Computed axial tomography. A. Cross-section view of the computed tomographic scanner gantry. The patient's head is represented in the center of the gantry, as if one were looking at the axle of a wheel. Around the periphery of the gantry are the detector elements, and just inside these is the x-ray tube (XT), which is emitting a finely collimated beam. The tube will travel along the dotted line for 360 degrees, thereby exposing all of the detectors, which will store data relating to their relative exposures for computer processing. B. Side view of patient in scanner gantry. This drawing illustrates the patient's position in the gantry, and displays the collimated fan beam in relation to the head. The "radiograph" that results from this position is a section in the axial projection, a thin slice that will be viewed from the perspective of the patient's feet. C.

Axial CT scan of the head. This is an image obtained with CT in a patient positioned as in B. The image is viewed from the patient's feet looking "upward" at the section, so that the patient's posterior skull is down, forehead is up, and the right side of the head is to the left of the image. The patient has been given intravenous contrast material to allow the anterior (AC) and middle (MC) cerebral arteries to be seen as well as the confluence of the venous sinuses posteriorly (VC). The ventricular and subarachnoid spaces (VS) are well seen, and the subtle density differences between gray and white matter in the brain (small arrows) can be appreciated. (A is redrawn from E. E. Christensen, T. S. Curry, III, and J. E. Dowdy, An Introduction to the Physics of Diagnostic Radiology *(2nd ed.), Philadelphia: Lea & Febiger, 1978. P. 334.)*

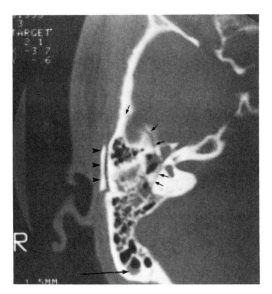

A

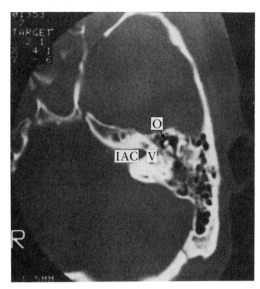

B

Figure 7-13. Temporal bone fracture on computed tomography. A. This CT section through the right temporal bone demonstrates several areas of traumatic damage to the ear. A fine fragment of bone has been dislodged from the calvaria (arrowheads), and a fracture line extends anteriorly through the middle ear and posteriorly into the mastoid air cells (arrows). Compare this image to the patient's normal side (B), and note the disruption of the ossicles and the soft tissue (blood) in the middle ear cavity, which should contain only air. Blood is also present in a posterior mastoid air cell on the right (long arrow). B. The left side of the patient clearly demonstrates the normal temporal bone aerated middle ear cavity and ossicles (O). The internal auditory canal (IAC) and vestibule (v) are also nicely visualized.

tures without air, has greatly diminished the need for pneumoencephalography.

Until they are removed from the blood and excreted in the urine by the kidneys, iodinated contrast media perfuse different organs in relatively low concentrations. This form of contrast administration is useful in CT scanning because it provides enough vascular enhancement to be detected by this very sensitive modality. When certain lesions of the brain are present, they may alter the blood-brain barrier such that the contrast may leak from the blood into the lesion and produce a blush in an area that might otherwise appear normal. A contrast-enhanced scan is routinely done when a neoplastic, inflammatory, or vascu-

lar lesion is suspected as the cause of a neurologic problem (Fig. 7-14). It should be remembered that the contrast material is safe in most instances, but it may cause renal failure in dehydrated patients or those with underlying renal disease and is a rare cause of death from allergic reaction.

The peripheral intravenous administration of contrast media does not provide sufficient density to be detected by standard x-ray techniques, unless the iodinated material is somehow trapped in the veins near the injection site. What has been useful in instances when visualization of fine vascular detail is necessary is rapid filming with standard x-ray technique while contrast is forcefully infused. This technique is referred to as *angiography* and requires the passage of catheters into the arteries or veins that are to be injected. In most instances the femoral artery or vein is entered percutaneously, and the catheter is threaded up the aorta or inferior vena cava and positioned in the vessel to be studied. This is an invasive procedure and has a small but significant incidence of complications including stroke, thrombosis or bleeding from the vessel punctured, allergy, and death. The risk of a serious complication is less than 1 in 100, but careful consideration of the indications for angiography should always be made before subjecting patients to the potential hazards.

As a general rule, angiography in pa-

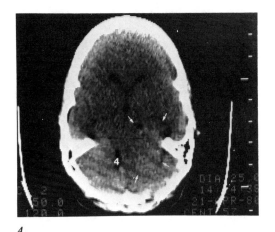

A

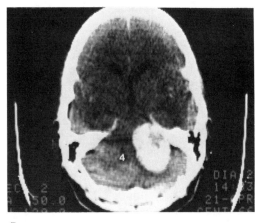

B

Figure 7-14. Nonenhanced and contrast-enhanced CT scan of an acoustic neuroma. A. This precontrast axial CT scan of the head was obtained in a patient with a left hearing loss and ataxia. In the posterior fossa near the apex of the temporal bone, there is a suggestion of a mass (arrows) that is displacing the nor- mally midline fourth ventricle (4) to the right. B. After intravenous contrast administration, the mass brightly "enhances" and is seen to be adjacent to the petrous pyramid on the left. This was an acoustic neuroma that had arisen from the eighth cranial nerve and was growing in the cerebellopontile angle.

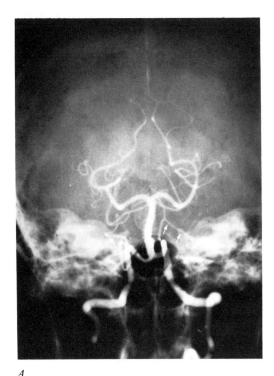

A

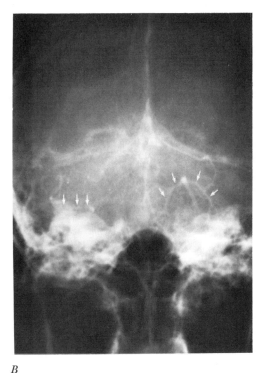

B

Figure 7-15. Angiography of an acoustic neu- roma. A. Arterial phase. Soon after the injec- tion of contrast media into the left vertebral artery, the arteries of the posterior fossa are seen (some contrast media has "refluxed" into the right vertebral artery). Comparing the right and left arterial tree in this Towne projection, it is apparent that the left posterior inferior cerebellar artery is taking an abnormal asym- metric course in the region of the internal audi- tory canal (arrows). B. Venous phase. Later in the injection, the contrast media has flowed from the arteries into the veins, and it is ap- parent that the petrosal veins on the left are displaced upward and bowed (arrows) and no longer closely applied to the temporal bone, as are their compatriots on the right (arrows).

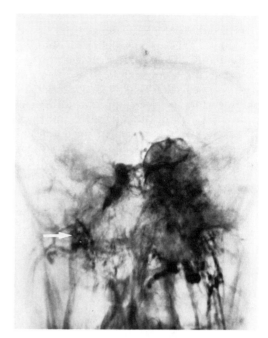

Figure 7-16. Glomus jugulare tumor. This arterial phase angiogram in a Towne projection has been photographically manipulated to "subtract" overlying bone density, and the contrast medium in the blood vessels appears black. This patient has a large left glomus jugulare tumor, also called a chemodectoma, which is represented by the mass of tangled abnormal blood vessels at the skull base extending up into the petrous bone. This mass had eroded the petrous apex and generally demineralized the temporal bone (see Fig. 7-6C). A smaller jugulare tumor is present on the right (arrow), as is the case in nearly 15% of such lesions.

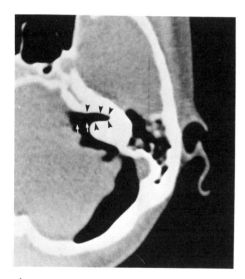

A

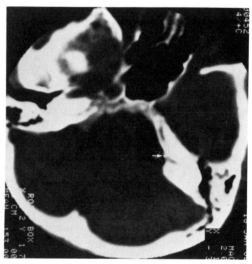

B

Figure 7-17. Air cisternography with computed tomography. A. Normal air cisternogram. The cisternal spaces in this patient have been filled with air to evaluate the internal auditory canal (arrowheads). The small nerve bundle extending from the brain stem into the canal is seen with air on either side (arrows), and there is no soft tissue in the cerebellopontile angle. The scan is viewed as in routine axial tomography, although the patient was positioned with his left side up in the gantry to keep the air in the region of interest. B. Small intracanalicular tumor. This patient also has air in the cisternal spaces, but rather than an air-filled internal auditory canal, which would be normal, there is a small soft tissue density (box) at the entry to the inner ear. This was a tiny acoustic neuroma that had caused hearing loss but was undetectable by other radiologic modalities.

tients with otologic abnormalities is ordered after CT to better define an observed abnormality. The invasive procedure may delineate the blood supply to a lesion and disclose its effect on neighboring arteries and veins; factors that are important to the surgeon in planning an operative approach (Fig. 7-15). More frequently, an abnormality is identified as vascular during a physical examination or on an enhanced CT scan, and angiography is used to secure precise diagnosis (e.g., malignancy, aneurysm, glomus tumor (Fig. 7-16). Because angiography is invasive, expensive, and involves significant radiation exposure, it should be ordered judiciously.

Another contrast medium used to diagnose otologic abnormalities is metrizamide, an iodinated water-soluble material. Metrizamide is injected into the subarachnoid space in the spine, and the patient is manipulated by rotation so it eventually enters the cisternal spaces within the brain. This increased contrast in the cerebellopontile angle cistern, combined with CT or conventional tomography, may reveal minute lesions that have not yet displaced the cerebellum or brain stem or involved the temporal bone. As with vascular contrast media, metrizamide is not without some adverse effects: headache, nausea, and vomiting are common. Air may often be used in small amounts to accomplish the same study without the adverse effects of metrizamide (Fig. 7-17). Such procedures are rarely necessary, but may be called for in patients whose less invasive studies are normal despite substantial clinical symptoms, or in patients with presumed traumatic cerebrospinal fluid otorrhea to define the site of the leak.

NUCLEAR MEDICINE

A final imaging modality of occasional use in the diagnosis of ear problems involves the administration of radioisotope-labeled substances that can subsequently be seen by a scintillation or gamma camera. A Technetium 99 m-DTPA (diethylene triamine pentaacetic acid) is often used in brain scanning; it is administered intravenously and, like radiographic contrast material, may leak through the blood-brain barrier into a lesion, thereby revealing its presence. Tumors of the brain and cerebellopontile angle have been demonstrated in this fashion, as have vascular lesions and cerebral infarctions. Detail and resolution are poor, and this method of detection has been largely replaced by CT.

An additional radioisotope technique involves injection of material into the cerebrospinal fluid of the spine, as with metrizamide cisternography, with imaging to reveal a site of CSF otorrhea. Again, however, the resolution is suboptimal, but in this case the nuclear medicine method may be reasonably used to screen patients for the metrizamide CT study, because the latter examination is tedious and not without the risk of iodinated contrast medial administration.

SUGGESTED READING

Christensen, E. E., Curry, T. S., III, and Dowdey, J. E. *An Introduction to the Physics of Diagnostic Radiology* (2nd ed.). Philadelphia: Lea & Febiger, 1978.

Guinto, F. C., and Himadi, G. M. Tomographic anatomy of the ear. *Radiol. Clin. North Am.* 713:405, 1974.

Meschan, I. *An Atlas of Anatomy Basic to Radiology*. Philadelphia: Saunders, 1975.

Paul, L. W., and Juhl, J. H. *The Essentials of Roentgen Interpretation* (3rd ed.). Hagerstown, Md.: Harper & Row, 1972.

Samuel, E., and Lloyd, G. A. S. *Clinical Radiology of the Ear, Nose and Throat*. Philadelphia: Saunders, 1978.

Squire, L. F. *Fundamentals of Radiology*. Cambridge, Mass.: Harvard University Press, 1975.

Tavaras, J. M., and Wood, E. H. *Diagnostic Neuroradiology* (2nd ed.). Baltimore: Williams & Wilkins, 1977.

Zizmore, J., and Noyek, A. M. *An Atlas of Otolaryngologic Radiology*. Philadelphia: Saunders, 1978.

II

Medical Aspects of Hearing Loss

8

Otitis Media

Nigel R. T. Pashley

Otitis media is the most common problem (other than upper respiratory infection) for which a child is seen by a physician. Otitis media is suspected in the differential diagnosis of fevers, implicated in the development of bacterial meningitis or other life-threatening infections, the common basis for prescribing antibiotics and decongestant medications, and the basis for the most commonly performed operation of infancy and childhood—a myringotomy with or without the insertion of tympanostomy tubes.

Recently, it has been recognized that the disease has many forms that may overlap or even progress or regress into each other, but which nevertheless are almost certainly a pathologic continuum.

Otitis media is an inflammation of the middle ear space. The inflammation occurs most commonly as a result of an infection, at which stage pus is present behind the eardrum. The eardrum may rupture during this period of time, in which case purulent otorrhea (a discharge through a nonintact eardrum) occurs (Fig. 8-1). An acute infective process is termed *acute purulent otitis media* (APOM). An inflammation without infection in evidence is always accompanied by the production of liquid that accumulates in the middle ear space and dampens or restricts movement of the tympanic membrane, resulting in hearing loss. When liquid is present (fluid is an incorrect term as a fluid may be a liquid or a gas), this is termed otitis media with effusion (OME; Fig. 8-2). The effusion of liquid may be thin (serous), probably resulting from transudation of serum into the middle ear space, or thick and mucoid (mucoid or secretory otitis).

The presence of OME may be punctuated by APOM, in which the liquid becomes infected and a purulent effusion is therefore possible as a part of the spectrum. OME may occur in three types based on progression and time.

1. Acute, from 0 to 5 weeks
2. Subacute, from 6 to 11 weeks
3. Chronic (COME), from 12 weeks onward

The tympanic membrane photographs were taken by Robert J. Keim, M.D., Oklahoma City, Oklahoma.

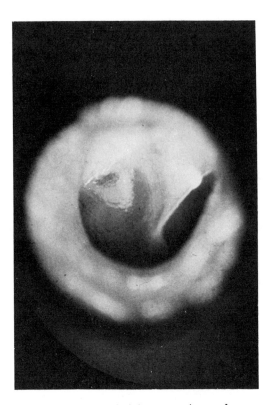

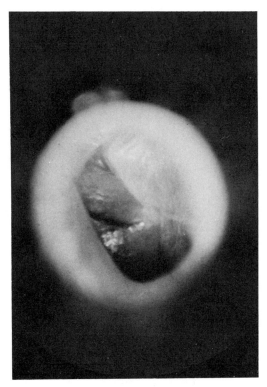

Figure 8-1. A normal right tympanic membrane. Posteriorly through the translucent drum the incus and stapedius tendon are seen.

Figure 8-2. A left tympanic membrane with acute OME. The drum is retracted—the short process of the malleus is more prominent and the long process foreshortened in appearance. Inferiorly the drum is sucked inward and pneumatic otoscopy reveals an immobile tympanum from liquid in the middle ear space.

The effusion must be present constantly, and it is recognized from studies of middle ear mucosa that changes occur progressively in the lining with time, that is, COME is less likely to resolve to normal spontaneously. Unfortunately, the type of effusion does not always behave on time and so serous, mucoid, or seromucous effusions are seen in all types of OME.

COME may progress through three stages.

1. Initiation: entering the 12th week of effusion
2. Full expression: effusion present; this stage may be stable for a prolonged period or progress
3. Degeneration: the tympanic membrane "degenerates" and tympanosclerosis, retraction, or both may start to be in evidence

Chronic otitis media is a precise term for inflammation persisting beyond the expected course. Common usage has dictated that when a perforation exists in the tympanic membrane from whatever cause (infection or trauma), it is also called chronic otitis, although inflammation may have long since left (Fig. 8-3). Unfortunately, chronic otitis has been loosely used by some authors to include chronic otitis media with effusion.

EPIDEMIOLOGY

Many of the factors overlap and interact in the epidemiology of this disease. Factors that may be of importance include age, race and socioeconomic status, sex, genetic facts, and the season or climate.

Age

The highest incidence of APOM occurs in early childhood, and a progressive decline

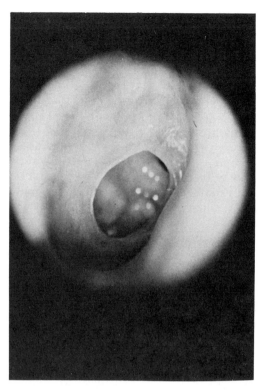

Figure 8-3. A right tympanic membrane with a chronic perforation anteriorly. The margins of the perforation are rolled and smooth, and there is no discharge. The middle ear mucosin is smooth and salmon pink. Chronic otitis media is the term applied to this process even though no active inflammation is present.

Although the skull base shape may be implicated in eustachian tube function, socioeconomic, dietary, climatic (the change from igloo, high-humidity nomadic living to centrally heated, low-humidity living in Eskimos), and the exposure to "white man's" diseases also play a part. If these factors are simplified by using a class system, children in low socioeconomic classes have a six times greater incidence of otitis media than children in high socioeconomic classes.

Sex

Most studies show a greater preponderance of males; and because reports exist that show a greater susceptibility to infection in boys, this preponderance may be artificial.

Genetic

Otitis media is observed to run in families but no studies have proved this. A history of otitis media in parents or siblings is common in children with otitis media.

Season and Climate

APOM occurs in increased incidence during cold winter months—December to February—and the incidence falls in warm months—June to September—in the northern hemisphere.

in incidence is seen after age 6. The child with attacks of APOM occurring before age 2 years is most likely to go on to be in one of two groups: the OME group, or the recurrent APOM group.

Suggested reasons for the heightened incidence in children include greater susceptibility to infection with young age, the possible importance of breast and cow's milk feeding (no statistical significant difference), less competent eustachian tube function in young children, more abundant nasopharyngeal lymphoid tissue, and the postural factor (bottle feeding in bed seems to be consistently related to OME persistence).

Race and Socioeconomic

Some races, notably native American Indians and Eskimos, have been noted to have a much higher incidence of otitis media.

PATHOGENESIS

The eustachian tube may be the key to otitis media. Impaired function occurs in the development of most cases of otitis media, and restoration of the air contained in the middle ear space, either by resolution of the problem or by insertion of a tympanostomy tube, results in the return of the lining of the middle ear to normal. The functions of the eustachian tube are (1) ventilation of the middle ear space, (2) protection of the ear, and (3) clearance of the middle ear space.

Compromise of the renewal of air in the middle ear space from the nasopharynx via the eustachian tube initiates a complex inflammatory response that includes effusion of liquid, compromise of the mucociliary transport mechanism, and metaplasia of the middle ear lining, tending to lead to persistence of the problem.

An alteration in eustachian tube function and a rise in incidence of otitis media are seen in diseases in which anatomic changes are present in the eustachian tube. In infants with cleft palate, the equilibration of air pressure differences between the nasopharynx and middle ear space is compromised, and a functional obstruction exists owing to increased compliance of the lower end of the eustachian tube. This may be due to decreased function of the tensor muscle of velum palatini and other muscles of the levator sling. There may be other muscles implicated in function such as the medial pterygoid. Otitis media decreases in incidence after palate repair but does not approach that of normal children.

Children with Down's syndrome and other children with cranial base anomalies also have a high incidence of otitis media, possibly because of alterations in the eustachian tube anatomy or muscular hypotonia or alterations in muscular insertions.

Allergies tend to lead to mucosal changes in the nasopharynx and eustachian tube and may also be implicated in eustachian tube dysfunction. Adenoid hypertrophy, tumors of the nasopharynx, and barotrauma lead to swelling in the middle ear mucosa or eustachian tube mucosa. Other contributory factors are radiotherapy to the nasopharynx, nasal obstruction from a deviated nasal septum, and recurrent nasopharyngitis causing persistent infection and edema in the region.

Chronicity of otitis is specifically related to the following three factors:

1. Acquired bacterial resistance to antibiotics
2. Anatomic predisposition to persistent disease
3. Irreversible changes present in the middle ear or mastoid with which it communicates

Most chronic otitis media (other than the rare congenital trapping of skin during development of the middle ear or the ear trauma group) is the result of an initial APOM episode. Recent studies suggest that most OME also results from an attack of APOM, and the suggestion has been studied that prompt antibiotic treatment early in APOM cuts short the child's antibody response to the bacterial agent and may actually predispose the child to OME. On the other hand, prompt antibiotic treatment of APOM has led to an almost complete irradication of suppurative coalescent mastoiditis and its potentially lethal sequelae of lateral sinus thrombosis, purulent bacterial meningitis, subdural and brain abscesses, all of which were frighteningly common in the preantibiotic and early postantibiotic era. These rare complications have become more difficult for training otolaryngologists to recognize because of their rarity, although occasionally in a compromised host or in a child with a mastoiditis from skin growing into the mastoid cavity (cholesteatoma), occasionally a severe complication is seen.

In the case of coalescent mastoiditis, there is an inexorable progress of infection leading to demineralization of bone and tissue necrosis. Quite often there is an anatomic block between the middle ear space and the mastoid, which predisposes the patient to this occurrence. If an anatomic block is not present, the tympanic membrane can rupture. The reader is referred to the following discussion of APOM for a further understanding of the pathogenesis of this disease.

ACUTE PURULENT OTITIS MEDIA

When a bacterial infection is present within the middle ear space, four progressive stages of inflammation exist.

1. Hyperemia. Congestion of vessels along the long process of the malleus and the posterosuperior region of the tympanic membrane is followed by gradual hyperemia of the entire drum head. Hearing may be normal but there is discomfort. There is little pus or exudate in the middle ear space.
2. Exudation. A gradual increase in liquid (serum, fibrin, and bacteria in the middle ear space) occurs. The tympanic membrane is thickened, red, and often bulging with obscured landmarks. Pain, fever, and hearing loss are present. Prompt antibiotic therapy at this stage cuts short the progress.

3. Suppuration. A slow tympanic membrane rupture occurs with discharge of pus through a small perforation that does not enlarge. In necrotizing otitis media (often associated with the infectious diseases such as measles or chickenpox), there is necrosis and enlargement of the perforation with continued foul-smelling discharge, quite often accompanying necrosis of ossicles (particularly the incus). At the start of drainage from the exudative-suppurating ear, there is a defervescence of fever and a reduction, if not abolition, of pain.
4. Resolution. Once the abscess (pus within a closed cavity such as the middle ear space) is drained, resolution of the infection occurs. The perforation should close spontaneously and hyperemia diminish. The drum may remain thickened and liquid remains in the middle ear space.

Clearance of the liquid varies although there is good evidence that in treated APOM (cut short in the stage of exudation by antibiotics), the effusion (liquid) may remain in 40% of children 1 month and in 10% of children up to 3 months after the infection. The liquid may be a suitable medium for other infections, and a pattern of persistent liquid with intermittent infection may be established. This cyclical recurrent APOM can be satisfactorily cut short by either of the following two methods:

1. Prophylactic antibiotics, which do not increase the rapidity of eustachian tube clearance of liquid and therefore do nothing for the hearing loss associated with the liquid
2. Placement of a tympanostomy tube, which prevents recurrent infection and promptly resolves hearing loss from effusion.

When a dry perforation is present (either a spontaneous or hole from the insertion of a tube), the onset of exudation from infection is heralded by prompt purulent drainage. (The exudative stage is "eliminated" and suppuration occurs directly.)

MORBIDITY OF OTITIS MEDIA

APOM causes the morbidity of any acute infection, disruption of the family unit while the child is sick, and financial stress. Hearing loss will exist in the presence of an exudate but will resolve over several weeks to months. Recurrent APOM, if frequent, may well have an additive effect in that hearing is less than optimal for a period of time after each infection. A predisposition to chronic otitis media also exists in recurrent APOM.

OME predisposes the patient to recurrent APOM as well as causes a low level of conductive hearing loss. The major question of whether a mild to moderate conductive hearing loss from fluid directly causes a delay in speech development has surprisingly been difficult to prove statistically, although the evidence indicates that it does. Recurrent APOM and OME predisposes the patient to degenerative tympanic problems such as tympanosclerosis and retraction (Fig. 8-4), and thereby (or even directly) to chronic otitis media.

Hemophilus influenzae is the most commonly encountered organism in otitis media in children less than the age of 5 and may be seen in older children. (Fifteen percent of *Hemophilus influenzae* is resistant to the antibiotic ampicillin.) Other organisms, as one might expect, are the common respiratory pathogens, pneumococcus and beta-hemolytic streptococcus. Less commonly, *Staphylococcus aureus* or the gram-negative organisms, *Klebsiella pneumoniae* and *Pseudomonas* are found. Acute necrotizing otitis is often caused by the beta-hemolytic streptococcus or staphylococcus infection associated with a systemic illness that is often infectious in nature.

Occasionally, mini "epidemics" of otitis media occur in association with viral upper respiratory infections or bullous myringitis (in which painful blebs occur on the tympanic membrane or adjacent canal wall). The middle ear is usually not involved, and the causative agents are the influenza virus and *Mycoplasma pneumoniae*. Bullous myringitis is self-limiting and resolves within a few days.

Chronic otitis media is a potentially dangerous situation with irreversible com-

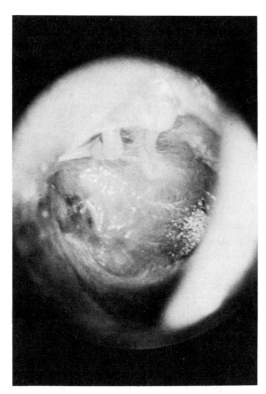

Figure 8-4. A right tympanic membrane with degenerative disease (retraction). The tympanum is thinned, retracted, and stuck around the incus posteriorly. The stapedius tendon appears in broad relief, and the drum is pulled into the round window niche inferoposteriorly. This condition of the drum is termed atelectasis.

plications including suppurative coalescent mastoiditis, suppurative labyrinthitis, facial paresis, cholesteatoma, cholesterol granuloma, ossicular sclerosis or destruction, meningitis, and sensorineural hearing loss. Brain abscess, subdural abscess, lateral sinus, and sigmoid sinus thrombosis are all possible but are fortunately rare. Long-term cochlea hydrops and sensorineural loss have been shown to be increased in incidence in chronic otitis media.

Treatment
A flow-directional diagram is shown in Figure 8-5. Appropriate antibiotics are suggested based on the commonest known bacteria for different age groups. The known incidence of occurrence of each step in the cascade of progressive disease is described. In Figure 8-5, one can see that myringot-

omy or tympanocentesis is used to confirm the presence of effusion and also to obtain liquid for culture when there is persistent purulent otitis. Myringotomy is not curative as the therapeutic mode in OME because the lining changes observed in the middle ear need time and aeration to resolve to normal.

When a complication of APOM (such as meningitis or facial paresis) exists, a myringotomy, tympanocentesis, or both is often performed as a first-line approach to obtain pus for culture and gram stain and to start the patient on the most appropriate antimicrobial agent and provide drainage for what is basically an abscess.

Often further surgical treatment (e.g., complete mastoidectomy) may be required.

It has become the responsibility of the health care provider to document that there is no delay in speech development in a child in whom a hearing loss, even if it is mild, is present. This has been historically neglected and is particularly prone to happen when multiple antimicrobial courses are used. As can be seen by the flow chart, a considerable time can elapse with a hearing loss present, unless a careful check on the number of attacks is documented. A hearing loss is always present in otitis media with effusion and transiently with acute APOM, and it is simply not allowable to treat a child and not follow him carefully when otitis media is identified.

Tympanostomy tubes (Fig. 8-6) are indicated in

1. Recurrent APOM (more than three attacks of otitis media in the preceding 6 months)
2. Chronic or persistent otitis media with effusion
3. Degenerative changes in the tympanic membrane (particularly pocketing and excessive retraction)

OTHER TREATMENTS FOR OTITIS MEDIA
Adenoidectomy With or Without Tonsillectomy
Adenoidectomy and tonsillectomy unfortunately are commonly performed to prevent recurrent episodes of otitis media, but

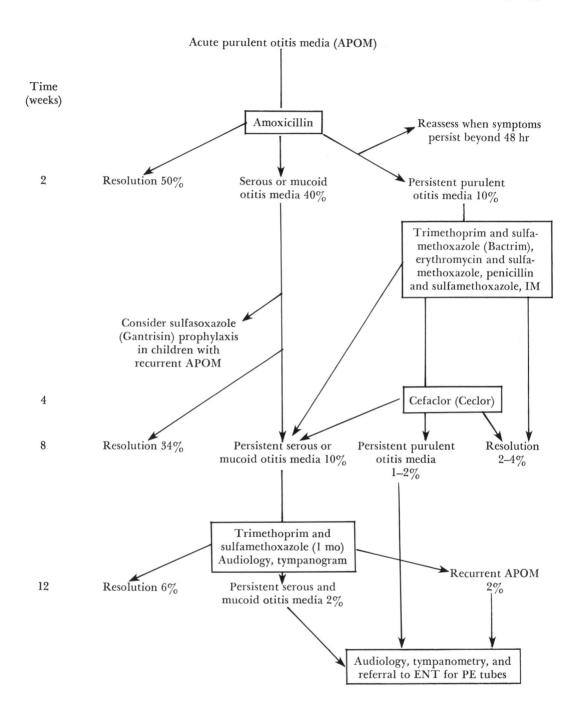

Figure 8-5. Flow diagram for the management of otitis media.

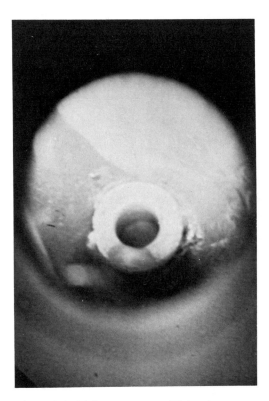

Figure 8-6. A left tympanum with tympanostomy tube anteroinferior to the long process of the malleus. The tube is dry and will gradually be pushed laterally by tympanic membrane growth behind it.

there are few prospective studies that can show their efficacy.

When children are carefully selected and if there is a temporal relationship between attacks of tonsillitis and otitis media, then a tonsillectomy is likely to assist in preventing this disease. If all children with otitis media with effusion have an adenoidectomy performed without there being nasal symptoms or signs, then in approximately 20% the effusion is cured. These data are unfortunately confusing in that most practitioners do not perform an adenoidectomy routinely unless there are nasal signs of obstruction, recurrent nasopharyngitis, or persistent otorrhea with a tympanostomy tube already in place. Studies are still progressing to better determine the role of adenoidectomy as there certainly are children who have otitis media caused by the

reflux of secretions from the nasopharynx into the eustachian tube. The problem is to identify these children.

Myringotomy for Acute Otitis Media
Myringotomy has been studied in coordination with antimicrobial agents based on the theory that myringotomy may assist in resolving the disease. Most studies show that myringotomy does not hasten or improve the efficacy of antimicrobial agents alone.

Polyvalent Pneumococcal Vaccines
Studies have been done but no conclusions are evident as to the efficacy of vaccines in preventing pneumococcal otitis media. Present results are discouraging and it would appear that in general vaccines are not capable of preventing otitis media.

Decongestant or Antihistamine Medications
Both for APOM and in the treatment of persistent OME, decongestants alone, antihistamines alone, and decongestant antihistamine combinations have been found to be ineffective. There is some data to suggest that some decongestants or antihistamines may lead to persistence of the effusion in OME.

Steroid Medications
Steroid preparations have been used nasally and systemically to attempt to treat OME. There are both encouraging and negative studies and literature and so the answer is not clear if steroids will resolve otitis media with effusion.

SUGGESTED READING
Diagnosis and management of the child with persistent middle ear effusion: Proceedings of a symposium. *Pediatric Infect. Dis.* (Suppl.) 1:5, 1982.

Schwartz, R. H., et al. Acute otitis media: Towards a more precise definition. *Clin. Pediatr.* 20:550, 1981.

Paparella, M. M. Current treatment of otitis media based on pathogenesis studies. *Laryngoscope* 92:292, 1982.

Paradise, J. L. Otitis media in infants and children. *Pediatrics* 65:917, 1980.

9

Otosclerosis

Eugene L. Derlacki

Otosclerosis might be termed the stable lesion of the labyrinthine capsule and of the stapedial footplate. It is initially a primary spongifying disease beginning in the endochondral layer of the capsular bone. The most common site of predilection is the area just anterior to the oval window.

There is universal agreement that an otosclerotic lesion in and around the footplate of the stapes results in impaired stapedial mobility, and thereby produces the characteristic gradually progressive conductive hearing loss. However, the concept of a sensorineural hearing loss caused by otospongiotic or otosclerotic involvement of the cochlear capsule, with or without stapes ankylosis, is not so universally accepted.

PATHOLOGY

The focal pathology of the otosclerotic lesion is actually in an unpredictable state of change varying from an active vascular otospongiosis to a healed, quiescent, and mature sclerotic bone within the dense bony labyrinthine capsule. This disease occurs anywhere within the otic capsule and to any degree.

The localized focus may be irregularly arranged in lamellae of new bone containing many vascular spaces with osteoblasts and osteoclasts. This immature bone stains more deeply with hematoxylin-eosin stain when viewed on microscope slides, sometimes bluer or redder, than the surrounding normal capsule. In its more mature form the bone is denser with only a few narrow vascular spaces and very few cells. Both "active" immature areas of vascular spongy bone and the more dense mature histologic structure may be present in one otosclerotic focus.

Stapedial fixation is considered *nonobliterative* if the entire footplate can be separated and removed at the annular margin, and *obliterative* if any marginal segment cannot be freed for removal. The site and extent of involvement of the stapes footplate by otosclerosis causing fixation is classified as follows: (1) anterior, (2) diffuse and thin, (3) diffuse and thick, (4) bipolar, and (5) posterior. In addition, otosclerotic

Research sponsored by the American Hearing Research Foundation.

111

stapes ankylosis can be caused by fibrous fixation with or without compression of the footplate by otosclerotic narrowing of the oval window [3].

ETIOLOGY

Despite extensive light microscopic studies, experimental work, and clinical observations, the etiology and pathogenesis of otosclerosis is quite obscure. To the clinician who has seen many otosclerotic patients, certain factors of probable pathogenetic significance are frequently repeated in patient histories. A positive family history for otosclerosis is often noted. Otologic surgeons with lengthy experience can cite numerous families with two, and even three, generations of family members with surgically proven stapedial otosclerosis. Both Shambaugh [13] and Schuknecht [12] are impressed by the same statement that described the probable mode of inheritance as a "monohybrid autosomal dominant inheritance with a penetrance of the pathologic gene of between 25 to 40 percent." Tato, de Lozzio, and Valencia [16] reported finding trisomy and tetrasomy of chromosome 13 as well as mosaicisms with 46/47/48 chromosomes in a study of 10 patients with otosclerosis and 4 normalhearing relatives of such patients. Carhart and Derlacki [2] conducted a pilot study on chromosomal patterns in 13 otosclerotic patients representing 3 families but could not confirm that even patients with familial otosclerosis are characterized by chromosomal aberrations.

Racial and sex incidence are other interesting and self-evident factors in otosclerotic patient populations. In the United States, otosclerosis is almost exclusively an affliction of the white population. Most clinicians are in agreement with the 2 : 1 female-male ratio of incidence noted by many observers, as well as in the often-quoted studies of histologic otosclerosis by Guild [6].

Initial awareness of the hearing loss or an accelerated progression of an existing loss during or following pregnancy is a fairly common observation when taking histories from women with otosclerosis. This impression, however, does not permit us to give a very factual risk figure to any woman with otosclerosis for informed family planning. Shambaugh [13], after a careful study of 475 mothers who had undergone fenestration surgery, emphatically states that "actually, the risk of increased hearing loss from any one pregnancy in a woman with stapedial otosclerosis is thus about 1 chance in 4."

NATURAL HISTORY

The onset and course of the otosclerotic bone lesion as it affects hearing has been studied preoperatively and postoperatively in many surgical patients with many years of serial hearing tests. The reported age of onset of the conductive hearing loss from stapedial otosclerotic fixation varies greatly from midchildhood to as late as the seventh decade of life. The most common age of onset is in the third and fourth decades. Once the conductive hearing loss has been reported by the patient, it is often thought to be unilateral, but hearing tests will usually reveal a significant loss in one ear and an incipient conductive loss in the so-called normal ear.

Bilateral conductive otosclerotic hearing loss is the rule, but unilateral involvement reportedly occurs in 10 to 15% of cases. In bilateral involvement, symmetry in degree of the conductive hearing loss may be consistent throughout the progression to complete stapes ankylosis. However, linear progression in hearing loss may occur in one ear, and the other may plateau at a stage of partial stapedial fixation indefinitely. The most predictable fact about an individual otosclerotic focus as it affects stapedial motility is its unpredictability.

The mechanism of the early immobilization of the stapes by otosclerosis may be fibrous fixation, or the enlarging focus at the anterior end of the oval window forces the footplate into posterior impaction. When the otosclerotic lesion inexorably progresses, firm bony ankylosis by involvement of the anterior annular ligament may produce just as great a conductive air-bone gap as that caused by lesions totally obliterating the oval window. Maximum air-bone gaps rarely exceed 50 dB in complete functional fixation of the stapes, whatever the extent of the otosclerotic lesion in the oval window.

The pathologic findings in stapedial otosclerosis and their relationship to the conductive hearing loss are universally accepted because there is good correlation between the audiometric results and the polytome radiographic findings, gross otomicroscopic surgical observations, and histopathologic studies. However, otologic clinicians and histopathologists disagree about whether otosclerosis damages the inner ear and causes progressive sensorineural hearing loss in cases of stapedial otosclerosis. The concept of pure sensorineural hearing loss caused by involvement of the cochlear capsule by so-called cochlear otosclerosis is a matter of controversy. Schuknecht [12] states that "this idea cannot be accepted on the basis of histologic studies." Shambaugh [13] is completely committed to the concept of cochlear otosclerosis, with and without stapedial involvement, and feels that "the mechanism of the sensorineural loss of otosclerosis has not been so clearly explained."

DIAGNOSIS
The results of the otologic history, examination, and hearing tests usually provide an easy diagnosis of a bilateral conductive hearing loss from otosclerosis. The typical history is one of an insidious onset of a gradually progressive hearing loss, usually bilateral, which begins in early to middle adult life without any specific etiologic information other than a family history of progressive hearing loss or even of surgically proven otosclerosis. Variable tinnitus may precede, coincide with, or develop after the discovery of the hearing loss, but it is not an invariable symptom. In the absence of prior or coexisting ear disease, the tympanic membranes are normal. At times there is a reddish glow of the posteroinferior promontory visible through the transparent membranes. The latter finding is termed a *positive Schwartze sign.*

There are numerous false-positive indications in both the history and examination that may make the diagnosis less certain. A patient may report a sudden onset of the hearing loss, often unilateral and associated with trauma or with an acute ear infection. Careful examination should rule out any middle ear fluid as a residual of acute otitis media. Polytomography and tympanometry can confirm either a diagnosis of stapedial ankylosis by otosclerosis or traumatic ossicular discontinuity. Congenital ossicular anomalies with normal tympanic membranes may also be diagnostic problems, particularly in unilateral cases. These anomalies include well-documented conditions such as the fixed malleus syndrome or congenital stapes ankylosis.

The otoscopic examination is hindered when the tympanic membrane is scarred, retracted, or tympanosclerotic. If the history indicates repeated ear infections in childhood, but the onset of progressive conductive hearing impairment occurs many years later, otosclerosis may be the primary diagnosis.

Properly performed audiometry should provide reliable air- and bone-conduction thresholds, as well as speech reception thresholds and speech discrimination scores, all consistent in establishing a conductive hearing loss. However, it is our regular routine to check our audiometric tests with masked tuning fork testing. If there is a discrepancy between the audiometric test results and the tuning fork tests, or between audiometry and the otologic examination, then polytomography, acoustic impedance measurements, or even exploratory tympanotomy may help provide the explanation.

Audiometric test relationships between the pure-tone bone and air thresholds, as well as the Rinne test with tuning forks at 256, 512, and 1024 Hz, will establish the degree of otosclerotic stapes fixation. The bone-conduction audiogram and the Schwabach tuning fork test help establish and confirm the presence or absence of an accompanying sensorineural hearing loss. However, in making the final assessment of sensorineural function, the experienced clinician must keep in mind the mechanical effect of stapes ankylosis on bone-conducted hearing. Although the average mechanical effect of stapes fixation causes approximately 10 dB poorer bone responses, stapes fixation can produce shifts of as much as 25 to 30 dB in depressing the bone-conduction thresholds. The final proof of the excessive mechanical notch depression in bone thresholds is the air-conduction threshold achieved by so-called overclosure of the preoperative air-bone gap through completely successful stapes surgery.

The degrees of stapes fixation may be classified as *beginning, partial,* and *complete.* A beginning stapes fixation would be revealed by an equal or positive 256 Hz Rinne, which would be equivalent to a 20 to 25 dB air-bone gap at that frequency. Partial fixation would be demonstrated by an equal or barely negative 512 Rinne, and an overall air-bone gap of 30 dB for the speech frequencies. When the 256, 512, and 1024 Hz tuning forks are all negative, complete stapes ankylosis is present. The degree of stapes fixation has no influence on speech discrimination scores.

There is no correlation between the degree of otosclerotic stapedial fixation and the extent of a coexistent sensorineural hearing loss, whether the latter is due to cochlear otosclerosis or another cause. In even severe threshold depression from cochlear otosclerosis, speech discrimination remains relatively intact. However, when a maximum conductive component is combined with a moderate to severe sensorineural hearing loss, the total hearing loss may be profound and at the limits of standard testing equipment. In such cases, the use of speech discrimination tests with amplification to limits well beyond regular equipment ranges may demonstrate that the discrimination function is surprisingly intact. Removal of the conductive component by successful stapes surgery may restore the hearing level to a degree that permits successful amplification with even an ear-level hearing aid in ears with good speech discrimination potential.

SURGICAL TREATMENT
Case Selection for Stapes Surgery
Because successful stapes operations can improve the hearing threshold to a maintained postoperative level within 10 dB of the preoperative bone-conduction threshold or may equal or far exceed it, most decisions should be made by the patient after he knows the meaning of the hearing improvement he may reasonably expect to achieve. This decision must always be tempered by just as much emphasis on risks as on the rewards of successful stapes surgery. The principal risk is the 1 to 2% chance of sustaining an increased hearing loss, which is usually an irretrievable cochlear loss. Transient postoperative facial nerve paresis is possible, but complete paralysis requiring a long period of recovery with or without surgical intervention is rare. Postoperative disequilibrium is rarely so severe as to be disabling or to require labyrinthine ablation for relief. However, positional unsteadiness may affect patients whose livelihood depends on perfect balance, for example, an athlete or a construction worker. If the otologist, the clinical audiologist, or both have determined that the patient's hearing loss constitutes a disability of sufficient magnitude to require active rehabilitative efforts, the excellent performance of hearing aids in otosclerotic patients should be discussed with adequate emphasis and not dismissed with a cursory mention. In fact, it is customary in our practice to perform a hearing aid evaluation, which often results in a recommendation that the patient try a binaural hearing aid fitting in his initial experience with amplification.

Discussion of management with a patient with sufficient bilateral stapedial fixation and good cochlear function poses no problem, because this is the ideal candidate for amplification or for stapes surgery. The more sensorineural hearing loss in excess of 25 dB the more other considerations influence decisions concerning the desirability of surgery. Yet the otologic surgeon must remember that he has no more right to deny an individual patient to seek a potential surgical improvement in hearing from a 90 dB level to a 45 dB level with adequate discrimination ability than he has to encourage the "ideal" candidate to undergo surgery.

The ear selected for surgery should be the ear with the poorer hearing threshold, provided discrimination is equal. If the thresholds are approximately equal, patient factors may decide the ear to be operated. Sometimes audiometrically equal ears may be surprisingly unequal in response to amplification. The poorer hearing aid ear should be selected for surgery.

The advisability of surgery in a purely unilateral otosclerosis is justifiable only when the cochlear function will permit achieving a better than 25 dB level, and no greater than a 10 to 15 dB difference in thresholds. A greater disparity in hearing levels will seldom result in the hoped-for binaural hearing. Surgery on the second ear should be delayed for at least 1 year in adults, but several years after a maintained first-ear success should elapse in teenagers or very young adults.

Surgery for Otosclerosis
There is no point in reviewing the historical development of stapes surgery because it has been covered in detail in numerous articles and books. Currently stapedectomy is the universal primary approach to stapes surgery. The main technical variations have to do with differences in footplate removal, the type of oval window cover, and the favorite incudovestibular-connecting prosthesis.

Once the incudostapedial surgical anatomy has been adequately exposed, the surgeon must make a decision concerning the chorda tympani nerve. The least permanent taste disturbance results from minimum manipulation. Cutting the nerve causes only moderate patient distress. Stretching and excessive manipulation causes far more postoperative taste disturbance.

The mucous membrane covering the stapes footplate and the sloping sides of the oval window niche are handled in two ways. Some surgeons incise the mucosa either longitudinally or transversely and reflect the two sides to permit footplate removal. They then replace the mucosa and cover it with their grafting material. Others strip the mucosa widely and denude the oval window niche, feeling that they will get more rapid and secure graft attachment.

When the footplate is thin with only anterior or anteroposterior otosclerotic involvement, many surgeons will perforate or transect the footplate prior to fracture removal of the superstructure. Then the anterior and posterior halves are removed. The thick but well-defined "biscuit" footplate may be easily removed by outfracture

with a wide spud after widening the inferior or superior annular groove with a knife curette. The dense obliterative footplate can be saucerized with the motor-driven burr or knife curettes, prior to either total removal or establishing a small central opening into the vestibule to receive some type of piston prosthesis.

In 1978 Smyth and Hassard [15] initiated a still continuing debate on the merits of the small fenestra stapedectomy in allegedly minimizing "the inevitable loss of high tone response which complicates all types of stapedectomy and which is very significantly greater following total removal of the footplate." The small fenestra technique gained support from Perkins' [10] very preliminary report on 11 laser stapedectomies in 1979, and again in 1981 by McGee [8] in a study of 280 cases analyzed over a 7-year period. Austin [1] in 1980 and Farrior [5] and Robinson [11] in 1981 presented very convincing statistical evidence supporting those surgeons who prefer total footplate removal. This controversy is not over and the footplate fenestration will be a major technical issue in the next several years.

An important point to remember once the stapes superstructure has been removed is to routinely palpate the malleus handle and incus long process to make certain that they are mobile.

Covering the vestibular window can be done with Gelfoam, or with tissue grafts such as vein, fat, fascia, loose areolar tissue, periosteum, or perichondrium. My associates and I prefer fascia from the temporalis muscle.

There is an even greater number of connective prostheses. Stainless steel or tantalum wire, with or without an attached Gelfoam, fat, or connective tissue plug, have all had their advocates. Stainless steel wire with attached steel or Teflon pistons have been popular. Piston prostheses of complete Teflon or complete steel are also currently being used.

Complications Following Stapes Surgery
Other than persistent and often unpleasant taste disturbances or dry mouth symptoms from chorda tympani nerve trauma or section (particularly when bilateral),

Case _7023_ **Age** _54_ **Date** _11-17-69_

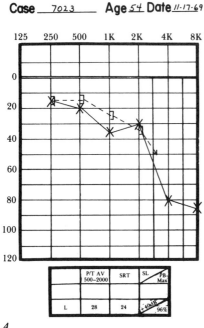

	P/T AV 500–2000	SRT	SL	PB-Max
L	28	24	+40dB	96%

A

Case _7023_ **Age** _66_ **Date** _6-15-81_

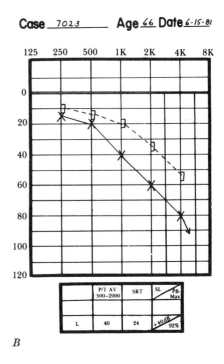

	P/T AV 500–2000	SRT	SL	PB-Max
L	40	24	+40dB	92%

B

the most frequent serious complications are those resulting in conductive hearing recession or all degrees of cochlear loss. Persistent incapacitating vertigo is a rare complication.

Conductive hearing loss following a stapedectomy may be the remaining deficit because of a primary failure to close the air-bone gap, or it may be a conductive recession after an initial completely successful closure. In both circumstances similar soft tissue reactions and prosthesis problems may be at fault. Strong postoperative fibrous tissue bands may partially bind the incus to the promontory or dislocate a prosthesis to a marginal position during the immediate healing period. However, an eccentric displacement of the distal prosthesis can happen as a slow migration as long as a year or two after surgery, which results in an audiometric test pattern that is pathognomonic of a distal wire prosthesis displacement. Such a marginal eccentric dislocation of the distal end of the prosthesis results in a high frequency air-bone gap, usually greatest at 2K, and less pronounced at 4K and 1K (Fig. 9-1). Revision surgery confirms the validity of this diagnostic audiologic finding and re-

Figure 9-1. A. Five-year postoperative audiogram after left Gelfoam wire stapedectomy. B. Seventeen-year postoperative audiogram of left ear demonstrating 1, 2, and 4K air-bone gap pathognomonic of distal wire loop displacement.

sults in a worthwhile hearing improvement. McGee [9], on the other hand, presented a group of 43 patients who developed a postoperative syndrome of loss in auditory acuity, speech discrimination, and sound distortion from a "loose wire syndrome." Apparently the syndrome was caused by inadequate crimping of the proximal wire loop at its incus attachment or to notching, reduction, or both in the diameter of the long process of the incus.

A sudden onset of recurrent conductive hearing loss should raise the suspicion that a gradual incus tip amputation has taken place. Revision surgery has also demonstrated that the vestibular membrane has apparently contracted and maintained an attachment only to the shaft of a correctly centered wire prosthesis. This attachment has been seen principally when using prefabricated wire prostheses over a compressed Gelfoam splint or the prefabricated wire–Gelfoam prosthesis. The experienced

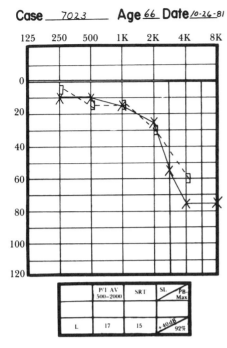

Case ___7023___   Age _66_ Date _10-26-81_

	P/I AV 500-2000	SRT	Sl.	PB-Max
L	17	15	+40dB	92%

Figure 9-2. Four-month postoperative audiogram of left ear after revision surgery correcting wire displacement with the use of fascia graft and Robinson stainless steel piston prosthesis.

otologic surgeon is aware of the various causes of postoperative conductive hearing losses and is able to deal with the surgical problem successfully during revision surgery (Fig. 9-2).

A more important cause of recurrent conductive hearing loss is the regrowth of massive otosclerosis after primary stapedectomy in a patient with a massive obliterative lesion of the oval window. It usually takes place within several months after surgery regardless of the variable techniques advocated by innovative surgeons. The risk of sensorineural damage rises dramatically in attempting revision surgery in these cases.

Sensorineural hearing loss after stapedectomy can also be an immediate or delayed phenomenon. If one discounts the surgical catastrophe from the occasional massive floating footplate and overly aggressive attempts to retrieve it (which has been an iatrogenic cause for immediate severe cochlear trauma and hearing loss), postoperative sensorineural hearing loss

can be a diagnostic problem. Schuknecht [12] has written extensively on the finding of reparative granuloma as a large tissue mass in the oval window, which may be so large as to even fill the posterosuperior mesotympanum, and which he finds responsible for cochlear loss or unsteadiness occurring between the seventh to the fifteenth postoperative days. He has found this complication in approximately 1 out of 100 cases. Retrospectively, my associates and I have found that reparative granulomas were much less frequent and occurred only in cases in which we had used Gelfoam as an oval window splint.

In my experience, perilymph leak through an oval window membrane fistula has been a more common early complication causing vertigo and a sensorineural hearing loss. Harrison and associates [7] have reported extensively on diagnosis, surgical findings, and surgical repair of perilymph fistulas. It may be extremely difficult to differentiate the clinical picture of perilymph fistula from that of endolymphatic hydrops (Meniere's disease), which may occur in the stapedectomized ear. A rapid response to medical management of endolymphatic hydrops has often saved a patient from surgical exploration for a fistula.

The most enigmatic and frustrating postoperative complication is that of so-called delayed sudden sensorineural hearing loss, which may result in permanent profound loss, and tympanotomy reveals a normal prosthesis-vestibular membrane relationship with no fistula. I am excluding the cases in which polyethylene tube strut is forced into the vestibule by barotrauma. Whether the unexplained sudden sensorineural deafness is exactly the same syndrome seen in the general unoperated nonotosclerotic population is a matter of conjecture.

One of the most carefully accurate assessments of the results of primary stapedectomy in properly selected cases appears in Schuknecht's book [12]: "It is my impression that competent surgeons can expect to achieve an initial air-bone gap of 10 dB or better in 80 to 90 percent of their cases and that a sensorineural hearing loss with a loss of speech discrimination of 30 percent or more can be expected in 1 to 3 percent. It is quite clear from my own observations and from the reports of others that neither the thresholds nor the air-bone gaps will be maintained at the early postoperative level in all patients."

COCHLEAR OTOSCLEROSIS— DIAGNOSIS AND TREATMENT

The closing remarks on cochlear otosclerosis are presented more or less as an epilogue since the concept of such otic capsular involvement is still controversial. I have watched this concept during its formative years and participated in the early polytomographic studies of the patients in our group practice. This early interest produced a study reported in 1965 by Derlacki and Valvassori [4] in which our otologic and radiologic findings in the presumptive entity of labyrinthine (cochlear) otosclerosis were described. We stated that a sensorineural hearing loss that antedated, developed coincidentally with, or ensued after a recognizable otosclerotic stapes ankylosis was no diagnostic problem. The following were the unweighted criteria of so-called primary or pure labyrinthine (cochlear) otosclerosis sensorineural hearing loss presented in our article:

1. Insidious onset from late childhood to middle adult life
2. No other specific etiologic history
3. Progressive, or becomes stable after having been slowly progressive
4. A family history of clinical otosclerosis, or, less helpful, a family history of prepresbycusis, progressive hearing loss
5. Positive Schwartze sign
6. Variable audiometric configuration, with frequent bilateral symmetry in the patient, but only occasional symmetry within a family

Shambaugh's last report [14] reviewed the results of 10 years' experience in fluoride treatment of cochlear otosclerosis. The most important conclusion was stated as follows: "Moderate dosage NaF, 40 to 60 mg daily with calcium supplement, is generally (in 80% of cases) but not always effective in promoting recalcification and inactivation of an actively expanding demineralized focus of otospongiosis with stabilization of a progressing sensorineural hearing loss. To prevent reactivation of the focus a maintenance dose of 20 mg daily is advised."

My own reaction at present is still the same as it was in my 1965 paper [4], "In the final analysis, labyrinthine (cochlear) otosclerosis as a clinical entity must find its decisive evaluation in the histopathologic documentation."

REFERENCES

1. Austin, D. F. Stapedectomy with Tissue Seal. In J. B. Snow, Jr. (Ed.), *Controversy in Otolaryngology.* Philadelphia: Saunders, 1980.
2. Carhart, R., and Derlacki, E. L. Chromosomal patterns in familial otosclerosis. *Arch. Otolaryngol.* 91:376, 1970.
3. Derlacki, E. L., and Anson, B. J. Histology of fifty-six surgically excised stapes in relation to otomicroscopic observations. *Laryngoscope* 78:1337, 1968.
4. Derlacki, E. L., and Valvassori, G. Clinical and radiological diagnosis of labyrinthine otosclerosis. *Laryngoscope* 75:1293, 1965.
5. Farrior, B. Contraindications to the small hole stapedectomy. *Ann. Otol. Rhinol. Laryngol.* 90:636, 1981.
6. Guild, S. R. Histologic otosclerosis. *Ann. Otol. Rhinol. Laryngol.* 53:246, 1944.
7. Harrison, W. H., et al. The perilymph fistula problem. *Laryngoscope* 70:1000, 1970.
8. McGee, T. M. Comparison of small fenestra and total stapedectomy. *Ann. Otol. Rhinol. Laryngol.* 90:633, 1981.
9. McGee, T. M. The loose wire syndrome. *Laryngoscope* 91:1478, 1981.
10. Perkins, R. C. Laser stapedecotomy for otosclerosis. *Laryngoscope* 90:228, 1980.
11. Robinson, M. Total footplate extraction in stapedectomy. *Ann. Otol. Rhinol. Laryngol.* 91:630, 1981.
12. Schuknecht, H. F. *Stapedectomy.* Boston: Little, Brown, 1971.
13. Shambaugh, G. E., Jr. *Surgery of the Ear* (2d ed.). Philadelphia: Saunders, 1967.
14. Shambaugh, G. E., Jr., and Causse, J., Jr. Ten years' experience with fluoride in otosclerotic (otospongiotic) patients. *Ann. Otol. Rhinol. Laryngol.* 83:635, 1974.
15. Smyth, G. D. L., and Hassard, T. H. Eighteen years experience in stapedectomy. *Ann. Otol. Rhinol. Laryngol.* [Suppl. 49] 87:3, 1978.
16. Tato, J. M., de Lozzio, C. B., and Valencia, J. I. Chromosomal study in otosclerosis. *Acta Otolaryngol.* 56:265, 1963.

10

Ototoxicity

LaVonne Bergstrom
Patricia L. Thompson

Advances in medicine have not been without compromises, and chemotherapy is no exception. Almost any available drug, effective for treatment of a certain ailment, has the potential to compromise the human system. It is well known that the inner ear is susceptible to damage by a variety of pharmaceutical agents. Chemotherapy is, however, an integral part of modern health care, and drugs known to be ototoxic for some 30 years are still being used and will be for some time to come. Management then becomes a fine-line decision, weighing the potential benefit to the patient against the risks of adverse side effects.

Ototoxicity is the result of the action of certain chemicals that damage the cochlear or vestibular portion of the inner ear, causing hearing loss, with or without vertigo, nausea, or gait instability. These symptoms may be temporary or permanent.

Ototoxicity is usually regarded as an inner ear disorder acquired in adulthood. However, a congenital hearing loss may be ototoxic in origin, because of the administration to a pregnant woman of an ototoxic drug that crossed the placental barrier and damaged fetal ear structures [31]. Ototoxic drugs are also administered to neonates and infants with some risk of ototoxicity. In pursuing a differential diagnosis of inner ear disease with suspected congenital or early onset, it is important to obtain a history regarding drug use during prenatal and postnatal life.

The incidence of ototoxicity, either on an overall basis or for most specific drugs, has not been accurately determined. Most incidence figures for ototoxicity have been derived from anecdotal accounts of patients who experienced toxicity, from drug trials in normal patients, or from treatment trials in which the focus was primarily on drug efficacy. In recent years, prospective studies of patients receiving aminoglycoside antibiotics have been designed to achieve a more comprehensive evaluation of the ototoxicity of these drugs in human beings. These studies have focused on the need for standardizing protocols for clinical research, using objective methods of testing inner ear function and refining our knowledge of the various risk factors associated with ototoxicity.

RISK FACTORS

Increased Drug Serum Level

Ototoxic drugs reach the inner ear primarily through the bloodstream, and it is believed that the higher the concentration of the drug in the serum, the higher the risk of damage to inner ear structures. An increased dosage or increased length of administration time of the drug presumably results in increased serum levels, and ototoxicity is thus said to be dose-related. From the therapeutic standpoint, the aminoglycoside antibiotics must achieve a certain minimum serum concentration level to act effectively on the offending bacteria. The narrow range between these therapeutic and toxic serum levels presents a real dilemma to the physician using these drugs, as he or she faces risks in both underdosing and overdosing the patient. Physicians use guidelines for the amount, duration, and method of administering these drugs, although there is a wide variation in the dosages affecting toxicity among individual cases reported in the literature [17]. Attempts to define precisely the levels of unsafe doses or course durations have been frustrating. Some of the recent clinical studies [3, 14, 37, 38, 51, 69, 74] have shown contradictory findings regarding statistically significant correlations between ototoxicity and increased daily dosages, increased course durations, and even total accumulated dosages. Considerable variation has been noted from subject to subject in dose-serum level ratios [46, 60]. Because of these uncertainties, many clinicians have advocated monitoring the serum concentration level of the drug as a more reliable predictor of ototoxicity. However, as data have accumulated, it has become apparent that the association between serum level and ototoxicity is a complex one, depending on such variables as whether peak or trough serum levels are measured, what assay method is used, or whether renal function is normal. It is not known precisely what constitutes a toxic serum concentration and how often or how long it needs to remain to become toxic. Ototoxic cases have been documented in which serum levels were well within the presumed safe range [14, 38, 69, 74].

Decreased Renal Function

The kidney is primarily responsible for filtering ototoxic drugs from the bloodstream and excreting them from the body. Based on knowledge of normal renal function, a drug is administered in doses and at time intervals designed to prevent its unnecessary accumulation in the bloodstream. In the presence of either acute or chronic renal dysfunction, the accumulation of drug levels in the bloodstream and thus the cochlea is less predictable. The immediate and accurate monitoring of alterations in renal function to adjust dosage is problematic because of the many variables involved. The aminoglycoside antibiotics are also nephrotoxic; that is, they can damage the proximal tubular epithelium of the kidneys. The renal impairment is usually reversible but can last several weeks, during which the excretion of the ototoxic drug will be slowed. Abundant clinical and experimental data indicate that the incidence of ototoxicity in patients who have received aminoglycosides at a time of diminished renal function is increased.

Concomitant Treatment With More Than One Ototoxic Drug

The use of more than one ototoxic drug simultaneously or the administration of consecutive courses of ototoxic drugs has become a worrisome problem in recent years. Clinical reports and experimental work [6, 28, 33] indicate that concurrent use of the ototoxic diuretics and aminoglycosides, even at otherwise safe dosages, may carry an increased risk of ototoxicity.

Other Risk Factors

Since some early reports, increased age has been considered a possible risk factor in ototoxicity, but more recent studies have not confirmed this [14, 37, 38]. Other risk factors, such as heredity [29, 54] and concurrent noise exposure [11, 27], have been proposed as well, but have yet to be substantiated by further evidence.

Special Patient Conditions

Patients with certain conditions deserve special consideration, not because they are at high risk to develop ototoxicity, but because an otototoxic reaction could be especially disastrous to them. It is not known whether a patient with preexisting hearing loss from any cause is more susceptible to damage by an ototoxic drug. However, if a reaction does occur and is additive to the hearing loss already present, the resulting loss could be severe. A patient with severe visual impairment or blindness would be devastated by either cochlear or vestibular damage: hearing is his only means of communication and his mobility would be severely affected by vestibular loss. Other persons who are especially dependent on intact hearing or vestibular function for their livelihoods need cautious observation during ototoxic drug therapy.

AMINOGLYCOSIDE ANTIBIOTICS

The aminoglycoside antibiotics constitute a family of drugs that have a common chemical structure, therapeutic use, and ototoxic and nephrotoxic potential. The drugs represent an important era in medicine, the development of better drugs for the treatment of infections with gram-negative and acid-fast bacteria. They are an essential part of the therapeutic regimen of many often life-threatening infectious diseases, and in many instances they are the only drugs of choice. They are also the most worrisome of all the ototoxic drugs and are infamous for their potential in damaging the inner ear.

General Clinical Characteristics

These drugs as a group have common toxic manifestations. When hearing loss occurs, it is sensorineural. It is usually characterized as bilaterally symmetric, although asymmetric and even unilateral cases have been frequently documented. The occurrence of asymmetry is somewhat of an enigma (as in mumps), as it would seem logical that hearing loss from a systemic cause be symmetric. Hearing loss is initially evident in the high-frequency range; if it progresses or is more severe, all audiometric frequencies may become affected. In a hearing loss involving all frequencies, the characteristic high-frequency slope configuration is usually evident. When the midfrequency, or speech-frequency, range is affected, auditory discrimination ability

is also impaired. In fact, discrimination is often disproportionately poorer than the degree of sensitivity loss. The degree of hearing loss can vary from mild to severe to even total deafness. It is typically permanent, although some cases of reversible hearing loss have been reported. The primary site of lesion is believed to be in the cochlear end-organ structures. Accordingly, characteristic cochlear findings are reported on special audiologic tests: positive short increment sensitivity index (SISI) scores, minimal tone decay, recruitment shown by loudness balancing techniques or by reduced acoustic reflex threshold levels, and type II Bekesy tracings.

The onset of hearing loss is often preceded by tinnitus, usually of a high-pitched or ringing quality. Whether it precedes or coincides with the onset of hearing loss, it is usually present. Further, it often begins intermittently, then becomes constant.

If vestibular damage occurs, the patient may or may not experience true vertigo. Quite often, the complaint is of light-headedness or giddiness. The patient may have a sensation of disequilibrium and may exhibit ataxia, an unsteady walk, and a broad-based gait. Vestibular symptoms can be quite debilitating during the first few weeks. On the other hand, symptoms can be so mild as to cause only a slight sensation or discomfort on rapid head turns or positional changes. On clinical examination, spontaneous nystagmus is usually not seen. The Romberg test may be abnormal. When vestibular function is evaluated with electronystagmography, the bithermal caloric studies are usually the most informative of the battery of tests. A depressed or absent response to caloric stimulation is seen, usually bilaterally. The damage to vestibular epithelium is believed to be permanent, as with cochlear insult, although the clinical symptoms usually resolve within a few months. This resolution is attributed to central compensatory mechanisms and depends on intact deep proprioceptive and visual senses. However, if these senses are also impaired, the patient may be permanently incapacitated.

These characteristics apply generally to the toxic effects of the aminoglycosides. The individual drugs differ in severity of toxicity and site of damage, as well as clinical usage.

Streptomycin. Streptomycin* was the first aminoglycoside to be isolated, in 1943, and within a few years it was reported as having ototoxic effects on the inner ear. Streptomycin was the successful result of a search for an antituberculous agent, and it is still used systemically and on a long-term basis primarily against tuberculous infections such as pulmonary tuberculosis and tuberculous meningitis. Unfortunately, streptomycin has been used casually and intermittently for a variety of clinical disorders. At one time it was marketed in combination with penicillin, a preparation that was very popular among many physicians. Streptomycin is associated with vestibular damage and, much less frequently, with hearing loss. Symptoms usually appear concurrently with drug use. When hearing loss does occur, it is usually preceded by vestibular symptoms. The degree of hearing loss caused by streptomycin varies considerably. Archieri [1] has indicated the incidence of ototoxicity with streptomycin use to be 3.6%.

Dihydrostreptomycin was introduced as an antituberculous agent shortly after streptomycin in the hope that it would not be ototoxic. However, it proved to be more hazardous than its predecessor: it usually damaged the auditory system, with a characteristic delay of onset of up to 6 months. As it proved to be less effective therapeutically than streptomycin, it gradually came into disuse.

Neomycin. Neomycin, introduced in 1949, has the widest antibacterial spectrum of any antibiotic. Unfortunately, it was soon found to have such severe ototoxicity when injected that it is not now recommended for parenteral use, except in life-threatening situations when it is the only drug of choice. Archieri [1] has reported the incidence of ototoxicity from neomycin to be 8%. Its current popular use is as a sterilizing agent. It is given orally as a preoperative bowel sterilizer; in solution for wound

* Although most aminoglycoside antibiotics have a common suffix, other drugs end in -mycin that do not belong to this group and do not possess ototoxic properties.

and cavity irrigations (peritoneal cavity, pleural cavity, and orthopedic wounds are the most frequent sites of instillation); it is even administered in aerosol form for inhalation.

Cases of ototoxicity have been reported by all routes of administration. Neomycin primarily damages the auditory system and rarely the vestibular portion. The onset of symptomatic hearing loss can be concurrent with administration of the drug or can be delayed up to several months, a characteristic that makes its use particularly hazardous. Once evident, the hearing loss typically progresses over a rapid or long course to severe or total deafness.

CASE REPORT: Figure 10-1 depicts a hearing loss attributed to neomycin solution instilled in the peritoneal cavity during a renal transplant operation on an 18-year-old woman (total dose estimated to be 0.5 gm). Although her hearing was not tested until approximately 1 year later, she dates the onset of hearing loss to the immediate posttransplant period, which is also well-documented by hospital notes. Over an 8-year follow-up period there has been no change in hearing status. She has not complained of vestibular symptoms. Electronystagmography, obtained several years after onset, revealed normal and symmetric responses to bithermal calorics. Seven years after the onset of hearing loss she sought advice regarding amplification. Although she initially rejected the suggestion of a hearing aid, communicative problems with family and friends were causing considerable stress. She now wears a behind-the-ear contralateral routing of signals (CROS) right-to-left hearing aid with a left "open" earpiece, on a part-time basis with help in limited situations.

CASE REPORT: Figure 10-2 represents neomycin ototoxicity effecting a different clinical response. Neomycin was given as treatment for peritonitis in a young boy with renal failure. It was instilled into the peritoneum, through the dialysate, while he was undergoing peritoneal dialysis (total dose estimated to be more than 50 mg). He first noted hearing loss approximately 4 months after treatment, which was soon confirmed by audiometry (7/1/66). On follow-up testing (7/19/66; 9/9/66) the hearing loss appeared to be progressive. Further testing revealed a marked deterioration in discrimination (9/20/66); prior to this test neomycin had again been used in an intraperitoneal wound irrigation. Over the following 3-month period the hearing loss apparently progressed to near

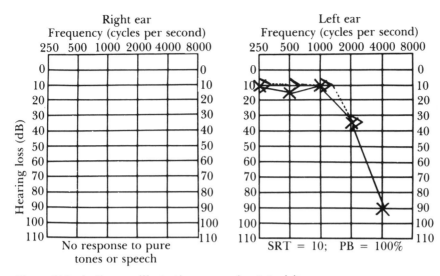

Figure 10-1. Audiogram illustrating neomycin ototoxicity.

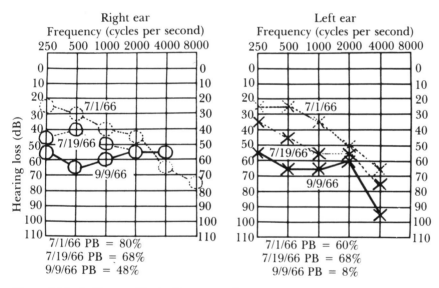

Figure 10-2. Audiogram illustrating neomycin ototoxicity. (From L. Bergstrom et al., Hearing loss in renal disease: Clinical and pathological studies. Ann. Otol. Rhinol. Laryngol. 82:555, 1973.)

totality. (Audiometry not available for this period.) He had never reported any vestibular symptoms; electronystagmography had revealed normal findings.

These two cases were chosen to illustrate the variety that can be seen in clinical response to neomycin ototoxicity. The doses causing ototoxicity were of different magnitudes; onset and configuration of the hearing losses also differed. Neither case exhibited vestibular damage.

Framycetin. Framycetin was isolated in 1953 and soon noted to have characteristic ototoxic properties. However, it was later discovered to be chemically identical to, and thus indistinguishable from, neomycin.

Kanamycin (Kantrex). Kanamycin was isolated in 1957 and is typically used as an injectable antibiotic for bacterial organisms. Although its ototoxicity is less severe than neomycin, it also preferentially damages the cochlea rather than the ves-

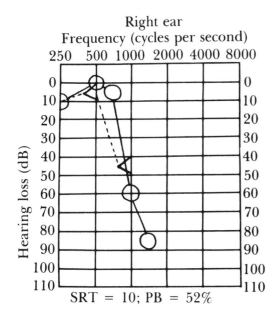

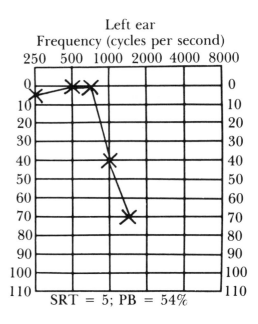

Right ear
Frequency (cycles per second)

SRT = 10; PB = 52%

Left ear
Frequency (cycles per second)

SRT = 5; PB = 54%

Figure 10-3. Audiogram illustrating kanamycin ototoxicity.

tibular end-organs. However, it does appear to damage the vestibular system more often than does neomycin. Archieri [1] has reported the incidence of ototoxicity as 4.9%, from a review of more than 1000 treated patients. Usually the onset of hearing loss accompanies the administration of the drug and progresses quite rapidly to a stable level. Kanamycin does not show the delay of onset characteristic of neomycin.

CASE REPORT: Figure 10-3 illustrates a hearing loss from kanamycin, which has been stable over 6 years of follow-up testing. The patient has been bothered by constant, bilateral, high-pitched tinnitus since onset. She has worn binaural behind-the-ear hearing aids (vented earmolds) full-time, with good benefit. However, she does feel she has developed lipreading skills and depends on supplementing audition with visual clues. She communicates quite efficiently, yet indicates her hearing loss causes her much stress and embarrassment, and she still does not psychologically accept it.

CASE REPORT: Figure 10-4 demonstrates ototoxic hearing loss in a 15-year-old patient exposed to both kanamycin and neomycin. This hearing loss was detected by audiometry 1 month after the exposure to drugs, although she was subjectively unaware of hearing loss at the time.

Her hearing was previously documented to be normal. Results of audiologic testing indicate cochlear pathology. This patient initially did not complain of dizziness but walked with an unsteady and broad-based gait. There was no spontaneous or gaze nystagmus; however, bithermal caloric responses were significantly reduced bilaterally. By 1 year, audiometry and electronystagmography showed no change, although clinically, vestibular problems were resolved within 6 months. At present, she does not feel her unilateral hearing loss creates a problem for her and has preferred not to investigate hearing aid use.

Gentamicin (Garamycin). Although clinical experience and experimental research with gentamicin has been over a short period, it appears to be significantly less toxic than either neomycin or kanamycin. Archieri [1] reports the incidence of "significant ototoxicity" to be 2.3%, from a review of more than 1000 patients administered the drug. Archieri's figures indicate that gentamicin is less ototoxic than streptomycin; however, others have rated gentamicin as being more hazardous than streptomy-

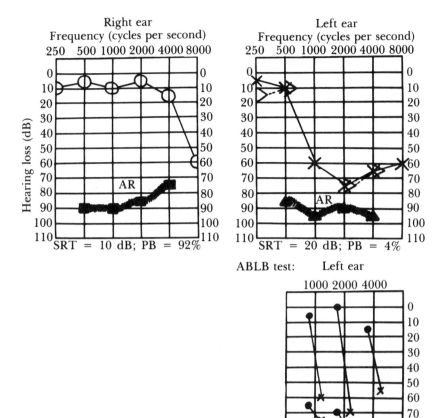

Figure 10-4. Audiologic studies of ototoxicity in patient exposed to kanamycin and neomycin. (■, ▲ = acoustic reflex thresholds.)

cin. Gentamicin is a broad-spectrum antibiotic [14, 74] and has gained considerable popularity for systemic use. Vestibular toxicity occurs about twice as frequently as does cochlear damage; thus, the comparative occurrence of hearing loss does not appear to be rare. When hearing loss does occur, it is usually preceded by the onset of vestibular symptoms. The degree of hearing loss is usually mild or moderate. It is not yet clear whether onset of clinical symptoms occurs with any regularity after the drug has been discontinued.

CASE REPORT: A 33-year-old man had an intermittent lengthy course of gentamicin, administered for a chronic wound infection. The course of gentamicin covered a 3-month period during which he had periodic audiometric monitoring. During the first 2 months, he was free of symptoms and hearing was normal. In the last month he began to complain of intermittent true objective vertigo, which became severe and constant over the next 4 weeks. His dizziness was so severe that he could not arise from bed. Bilateral, intermittent, ringing tinnitus also accompanied the onset. Although he did not complain of hearing loss, he stated his ears "felt funny." Figure 10-5 presents audiometry done at this time. Electronystagmography revealed absent caloric responses bilaterally. He died from his infection 2 weeks later. The hearing loss did not appear to progress (subjective observation), but he still had severe constant vertigo.

Other Aminoglycosides. New aminoglycoside derivatives such as tobramycin and Amikacin have been released for clinical

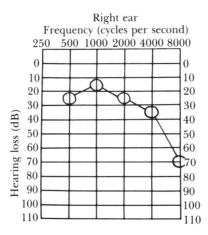

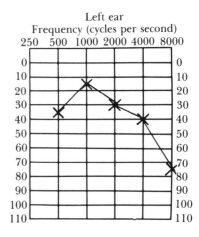

Figure 10-5. Audiogram illustrating gentamicin ototoxicity. Tested at bedside; low-frequency thresholds probably affected by ambient noise.

use to broaden antibacterial activity against strains resistant to gentamicin. The ototoxicity of tobramycin was first demonstrated in experimental animals using excessive dosages [5, 42] and subsequently in clinical examinations [63]. Amikacin ototoxicity has been demonstrated in a number of good clinical studies [3, 37, 40, 62]. Vancomycin (Vancocin) is also a member of the aminoglycoside family, but is much less ototoxic than the others. Reported cases of ototoxicity have resulted from its systemic use in high doses and usually in patients with severe renal failure [41]. Hearing loss appears to be the predominant symptom. Polymyxin B was used parenterally after its ototoxicity was discovered. It is used now as an ototopical antibiotic, and has other topical use. Ototoxicity from this application has not been conclusively demonstrated.

POTENT DIURETICS

Ethacrynic acid (Edecrin) and furosemide (frusemide, Lasix) are powerful diuretic agents given to patients with refractory edema. They are used commonly in patients with pulmonary edema or edema from renal failure; the diuresis brought about by the drug relieves fluid overload. Other, less potent diuretics have not been implicated in ototoxicity. Ethacrynic acid and furosemide are normally ototoxic only in very high doses [47, 61, 73]. They are usually administered either orally or intravenously. Ethacrynic acid appears to have significantly greater toxicity than fu-

rosemide; however, their clinical manifestations are similar when toxicity is evident. Hearing loss is usually the most dramatic and severe side effect, although vestibular symptoms quite often accompany hearing loss. The onset is usually sudden, often within minutes of intravenous administration. Unlike the aminoglycosides, diuretic ototoxicity has been characterized as reversible, with recovery usually occurring within 24 hours. However, there have been instances of incomplete recovery or permanent hearing loss [53]. In contrast to the configuration of hearing loss from other drugs, which is usually a high-frequency slope, the diuretic-induced hearing loss often shows greater involvement in the low- to mid-frequency ranges. Discrimination ability is characteristically poor.

CASE REPORT: Figure 10-6 depicts audiologic studies in a patient with suspected furosemide ototoxicity. A young, male, renal transplant patient was administered a minimal dose of furosemide (40 mg). He had fairly poor kidney function at the time. The following morning he awakened with a feeling of disequilibrium and was unsteady on his feet when he attempted to rise from bed. He did not have true vertigo. He then noted a left-sided ringing tinnitus and a plugged feeling in his left ear. He had not experienced similar symptoms previously, nor had he been given furosemide or other ototoxic drugs as far as we can determine. His hearing was previously documented as normal. Audiometry showed a moderate to severe sensorineural

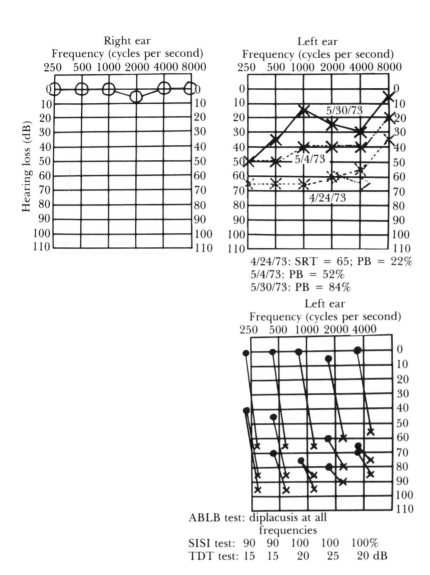

4/24/73: SRT = 65; PB = 22%
5/4/73: PB = 52%
5/30/73: PB = 84%

ABLB test: diplacusis at all
frequencies
SISI test: 90   90   100   100   100%
TDT test: 15   15   20   25   20 dB

Figure 10-6. Audiologic studies of hearing loss in a case of suspected furosemide ototoxicity.

hearing loss in the left ear, which was unchanged the following week (4/24/73). During this period he had received four additional daily doses of furosemide, 40 mg each. The drug was then discontinued. Electronystagmography initially revealed some spontaneous nystagmus, increasing in the left lateral position. There was a borderline left unilateral weakness to calorics. Over the next month of weekly interval testing his hearing showed a gradual recovery to a mild loss (5/30/73). By this time he had no vestibular symptoms. After 1 year, hearing tests showed no further improvement in hearing. Repeat electronystagmography at 1 year showed normal symmetric responses to calorics. The positional recordings did indicate adaptation to previous vestibular damage. This case may represent an idiosyncratic response to furosemide because the dose was minute in comparison to doses regularly, and apparently, safely used, even in the presence of significant kidney failure.

OTHER OTOTOXIC DRUGS

Acetylsalicylic acid (salicylate, aspirin, aspirin compounds), the oldest known ototoxic drug, has been in use since 1899. It is prescribed for its analgesic properties. Salicylates typically do not have an ototoxic effect unless the patient is on unusually high daily doses, such as used in treatment for arthritis [49]. Ototoxicity may also be a complication from overdoses of aspirin [59, 66]. Toxicity is evident as hearing loss, and vestibular symptoms are rarely, if ever, present. Although sensorineural, the hearing loss is characteristically seen as a temporary threshold shift, reversible if medication is discontinued or if the dosage is reduced. Hearing loss appears in the high frequencies, is bilaterally symmetric, and commonly preceded by tinnitus. In fact, tinnitus is often used as a guideline in establishing dose levels in chronic treatment: the patient is given as much as he can tolerate, at a dosage level just less than that which will elicit tinnitus. The ototoxicity of salicylates is rarely considered worrisome, no doubt because the hearing loss is reversible; however, some cases of permanent deafness have been reported [2, 26].

In describing the ototoxic properties of quinine and chloroquine phosphate, it is common to group them with the salicylates. Indeed, salicylates, quinine, and chloroquine phosphate have similar ototoxic characteristics. It should be noted, however, that many cases of congenital permanent hearing loss have been reported with the use of quinine or chloroquine phosphate during pregnancy. Quinine and chloroquine phosphate are known primarily as antimalarials. However, quinine has also been used as an abortifacient and to "cut" heroin. Chloroquine phosphate has also been found useful in treatment of various collagen diseases.

Aural defects are listed among other deformations in offspring of pregnant women who have ingested thalidomide. Aural malformation can occur as an isolated phenomenon or in combination with other defects. Depending on the time of gestation during which thalidomide was taken, ear disorders can be variable: malformed pinnae, outer and middle ear aplasias, or inner ear aplasias involving either the cochlear or vestibular organs [8, 32]. This drug has been removed from the market.

Erythromycin, belonging to the macrolide group of antibiotics, is usually used in treating gram-positive infections, especially group A beta-hemolytic streptococci, pneumococci, and staphylococci. A few cases of suspected ototoxicity have been reported [68]. Erythromycin ototoxicity seems associated only with high dosages (up to 4 gm/day), with oral or intravenous use, and is characterized by reversible sensorineural hearing loss without apparent vestibular problems.

Propoxyphene (Darvon), a widely used mild analgesic, has been reported to be associated with severe sensorineural deafness in two cases, one of chronic abuse [20] and one of acute accidental overdosage [43].

Cisplatin, a relatively new anticancer drug, has a number of severe side effects. Its ototoxicity has been reported in both experimental animals [35] and humans [52].

A few cases of hearing loss associated with potassium bromate poisoning have been reported [58].

Viomycin is a polypeptide that has been used for treatment in tuberculous infections and reportedly has ototoxic properties similar to streptomycin [9, 34].

Additional drugs implicated in ototoxicity or eighth nerve toxicity are arsenic, lead, and other such poisons [56]; propylthiouracil [64]; nitrogen mustard [2]; hexadimethrine bromide (Polybrene) [2]; chloramphenicol [2]; colistin (Coly-Mycin); and propylene glycol [48]. Relatively little is known of the ototoxic risk of these drugs. Their clinical manifestations have not been well defined; or only a few isolated cases have been reported; or the effect was noted after exposure to high levels of the toxic agent. There is some evidence against colistin [18] and propylene glycol [70] being ototoxic.

ETIOLOGY
Histopathology
Aminoglycoside histopathology has been studied extensively in experimental animals. The various techniques used and findings noted have recently been reviewed [23, 72]. Owing to the paucity of human temporal bone specimens, studies of inner ear changes caused by ototoxic drugs have been more limited [30, 50]. Epithelial structures in the cochlea and vestibule show the primary damage. In the cochlea, atrophy of stria vascularis, spiral ligament, the sensory hair cells, and occasionally, the supporting cells are seen. It is not known whether damage to stria vascularis precedes hair cell loss or vice versa, although stria

vascularis is believed to be involved in the mechanism by which damage occurs. The basal and middle coils are more commonly affected than the apical coil, correlating clinically with the high-frequency hearing loss typically seen. With increased severity, the apical turn—and accordingly, the low-middle frequencies—can be involved. The outer hair cells are more vulnerable to insult; with increasing damage, the inner hair cells and supporting cells will usually be affected. In the vestibular system, the cristae of the ampullae seem the most vulnerable to assault, with less frequent or severe damage to maculae in the utricle and saccule. In both cochlear and vestibular systems some degeneration of the ganglion cells has been seen; however, it is generally agreed that this finding represents secondary degeneration. One investigation of the brain stem [45] in ototoxicity revealed no primary pathology.

There is a characteristic pattern of change found in sensory cell degeneration. Early changes are seen in the nuclei of the hair cells, and in a deformation of the characteristic "W" pattern of the hairs. The hair cell may show increased lucency and vacuolization, and finally collapses. The cell walls shrink from the phalanges of Deiters' cells, leaving a gap with the consequent formation of the "phalangeal scar."

The sequence of hair cell changes is much the same regardless of the immediate cause of injury—as in aging, noise exposure, and ototoxicity [22]. It is not known at which point in the sequence of degenerative changes the hair cell becomes moribund.

The drugs that usually do not cause permanent damage to the inner ear—salicylates, diuretics, and antimalarials—have not shown consistent pathology. In one study [56], no morphologic lesions were found in experimental animals intoxicated with salicylates, although previously, mitochondrial alterations in epithelial structures were reported. Various morphologic findings have been reported with diuretics: from minimal [4, 12, 57] to changes more typical of aminoglycosides [44].

Electrophysiology

Electrophysiologic changes in experimental animals correlate with the histopathology. In antibiotic insult, the cochlear microphonic (CM) as well as eighth nerve action potential (AP) responses are depressed.

When diuretics have been used experimentally, transitory changes in the endocochlear potential (EP) have often been noted [4, 12, 55]. Within minutes of administering the drug, EP goes to a negative value, then recovers in a matter of a few hours. One study [44] showed transient changes in CM and AP with furosemide, but permanently depressed electrophysiologic response with ethacrynic acid.

Mechanisms of Ototoxicity

A number of theories of the mechanisms of ototoxicity have been investigated. The aminoglycosides destroy a bacterial organism through inhibition of metabolic or respiratory functions that are vital to the bacterial cell. Similarly, it has been proposed that these drugs inhibit oxidative or metabolic enzymes of the affected cells in the inner ear. These epithelial structures depend on an adequate blood flow with oxygen and nutrients; a toxic chemical may destroy the essential metabolic activities.

It has also been suggested that the ionic transport system of the inner ear, crucial to its function, undergoes breakdown. The offending antibiotic may in some way alter membrane permeability, which then interferes with the normal electrostatic medium in the inner ear fluids. The essential mechanism may be a breakdown of microhomeostatic processes that govern rate of formation, volume, and ionic composition of the inner ear fluids [22].

It has been speculated that the selective ototoxic and nephrotoxic properties of the aminoglycosides may provide a clue to the mechanism of ototoxicity, although this association has not been fully explained [16, 17].

The mechanism by which the ototoxic diuretics act in treatment of edema, or fluid overload, involves ion transport. There is some evidence that these drugs alter the ion transport system in the inner ear [7, 12]. Other undesirable side effects from the diuretics are fluid and electrolyte imbalances that result from a rapid diuresis. Attempts to explain the ototoxic action by these imbalances have not been entirely successful.

Analgesics (vasoconstrictors) are thought to have a similar ischemic effect, or interference in the blood supply, of the capillaries supplying the inner ear. This interference is believed to be a temporary effect and related to an especially high level of salicylate found in the bloodstream.

MANAGEMENT

Methods of alleviating or reversing the ototoxic effect have been studied. Ozothin in combination with an aminoglycoside was thought to reduce the potential ototoxicity of the latter, although further research could not substantiate this effect [24, 33]. Dialysis, used commonly in the treatment of renal failure and in drug overdoses, sparked some interest in its use in removing ototoxic drugs to alleviate toxicity, but this has not had widespread application [13, 19, 36].

Since the early 1970s, with greater therapeutic application of the aminoglycosides and widespread use of loop diuretics, it is likely that the overall number of patients receiving ototoxic drugs has increased and that more patients receive concurrent or repeated courses of ototoxic drugs. Positive steps have been made toward more judicious use of these drugs, to limit their overuse or misuse. Prospective clinical investigations of these drugs have become more rigorous, using well-defined and standardized criteria and objective testing of inner ear function, in an effort to define more precisely the incidence of a drug's ototoxicity, the critical parameters associated with toxicity, and comparative toxicity and efficacy. Guidelines have been published emphasizing important clinical parameters that should be monitored by the physician to achieve safer drug therapy [39].

Audiometric monitoring of patients receiving ototoxic drugs has been used inconsistently. Its use has been advocated to provide early evidence of decreased hearing, so that a drug can be discontinued in an effort to prevent further hearing loss. However, its usefulness has been questioned, as continued drug treatment is often indicated in life-threatening illness despite early evidence of ototoxicity. Further objections to the routine use of monitoring audiometry have been that it is too costly, time-consuming, and not feasible for many seriously ill patients. A further reason for its inconsistent use may be that there are no well-established guidelines to determine which patients need to be monitored, what procedures should be used, and how the resulting information should be interpreted.

Audiometry can serve two important functions for better management of the patient receiving ototoxic drugs: (1) prevention and reduction of severity of ototoxicity and (2) identification of drug-induced hearing loss for immediate and appropriate rehabilitative management.

An audiometric monitoring program has recently been described [67], using as specific procedures as possible, given the current knowledge of the most important parameters associated with ototoxicity. The essential features of this audiometric monitoring program are summarized as follows:

The audiometric monitoring program is applied only to patients receiving ototoxic drugs who are considered to be at high risk for hearing loss. Table 10-1 indicates the risk factors that are used to select patients for audiometric monitoring. If a patient meets any one of the six conditions, he is monitored during drug therapy.

The program uses bedside testing with a portable audiometer; this is least demanding of the patient and other supportive personnel. Table 10-2 outlines the protocol recommended for bedside testing. The procedure takes only a short time, yields only

Table 10-1. Selection of High-Risk Patients for Audiometric Monitoring During Ototoxic Drug Therapy

Ototoxic drug administered during decreased renal function

Ototoxic drug administered in increased daily doses or for extended duration

Assay showing high serum level (peak or trough) of ototoxic drug

Multiple ototoxic drugs administered concurrently or in consecutive courses (within 1 wk)

Special patient conditions such as preexisting hearing loss, severe visual impairment, or blindness

The following symptoms reported by patient: tinnitus, hearing loss, or dizziness

Table 10-2. Test Protocol for Audiometric Monitoring of Patients on Ototoxic Drug Therapy

Establish "baseline" hearing level as soon as possible

Obtain air-conduction thresholds bilaterally at 500, 1000, 2000, 4000, and 8000 Hz

If hearing loss is noted, obtain bone-conduction thresholds and consider referral for additional audiologic and otologic workup

Question patient for ear symptoms: tinnitus, hearing loss, and dizziness. Refer dizzy patient for electronystagmography

Record results in patient's hospital chart

Criteria for change: 15 dB at any test frequency

essential information, involves the smallest possible number of hospital personnel, is minimally demanding of the seriously ill patient, and is done at reasonable cost.

Air-conduction thresholds at the indicated frequencies are obtained during each test in the course of drug therapy. Tests are repeated every two to seven days, depending on the degree of risk of ototoxicity for the patient. Patients with a demonstrated decline in hearing or high serum levels are followed especially closely.

Patients who develop symptoms of vestibular damage during the course of audiometric monitoring are referred for whatever electronystagmographic evaluation can be undertaken according to the patient's condition.

The importance of follow-up (summarized in Table 10-3) is stressed, particularly since an emphasis of the audiometric monitoring program is to provide appropriate

Table 10-3. Follow-up Protocol for Audiometric Monitoring of Patients on Ototoxic Drug Therapy

Continue bedside testing to end of drug therapy

After drug therapy, perform audiometric tests at: 1 week, 1 month, and 3 months after therapy, then p.r.n.

Follow-up in infant may be necessary up to 3–4 years of age

Provide counseling and rehabilitative management as needed

management for the person with drug-induced hearing loss.

TESTING THE INFANT

The same criteria are used to select high-risk pediatric patients on ototoxic drugs for routine audiometric testing. Testing techniques are altered for the infant and preschool child. The main difficulty will be that of follow-up, as it may be necessary to follow the child up to the age of 3 or 4 years until standard audiometric testing can be completed. The primary physician can be helpful in supporting and encouraging follow-up of these youngsters.

A nonbehavioral method of testing for ototoxicity in infants, measurement of auditory brain stem response, has been described as an alternative to behavioral audiometry, especially in multihandicapped infants [15].

HIGH-FREQUENCY AUDIOMETRY

Many studies have been published suggesting various clinical applications of high-frequency audiometry (8000–18,000 Hz), including the monitoring of patients on ototoxic drugs. One study [25] in which seven patients on kanamycin were tested demonstrated that the use of this technique forewarned of hearing loss from 30 to 60 days before its detection by standard audiometry. However, the high-frequency system used in this study later fell into disrepute because of numerous equipment problems.

A number of clinicians [70] have since developed their own instrumentation systems to study the significance of high-frequency hearing in certain conditions. They report that high-frequency audiometry can detect ototoxicity earlier than conventional audiometric testing, although the time elapsed between drug therapy and hearing loss is apparently quite variable among patients.

At present, equipment and testing techniques make high-frequency threshold audiometry a viable endeavor. Its role in monitoring effects of ototoxic drug therapy is still in the research stage. Its clinical use will depend primarily on whether the preventive role of audiometric monitoring will play a more prominent role in ototoxic drug therapy.

If a patient develops ototoxicity, the otologist and audiologist play a primary role in counseling and rehabilitation. With vestibular toxicity, patients can be expected to compensate naturally within a few months, with no residual effects. If, however, proprioceptive or visual senses are not intact, compensation may be less complete. Permanent hearing loss, even of mild degree, is usually more disabling. If the hearing loss is severe, the handicap can be devastating. Because of its rapid onset, a person has no time to gradually develop compensatory mechanisms. Rehabilitation is often limited, at best. Hearing aid use should always be a consideration even if there is limited residual hearing. Whether or not a hearing aid is recommended, speech-reading training should also be considered in rehabilitating the patient. Above all, moral support and encouragement will help the patient take advantage of rehabilitative measures and learn to accept his handicap more easily. A patient in whom partial ototoxic hearing loss has been identified should certainly be counseled regarding hearing conservation practices.

REFERENCES

1. Archieri, G. M., et al. Clinical research experience with gentamicin. Incidence of adverse reactions. *Med. J. Aust.* (Suppl.) 1:30, 1970.
2. Ballantyne, J. Ototoxicity. In J. Ransome, H. Holden, and T. R. Bull (Eds.), *Recent Advances in Otolaryngology* (4th ed.). Edinburgh: Churchill Livingstone, 1973. Pp. 163–175.
3. Black, R. E., et al. Ototoxicity of amikacin. *Antimicrob. Agents Chemother.* 9:956, 1976.
4. Bosher, S. K., et al. The effects of ethacrynic acid upon the cochlear endolymph and stria vascularis. *Acta Otolaryngol.* 75:184, 1973.
5. Brummett, R. E., et al. Ototoxicity of tobramycin in guinea pigs. *Arch. Otolaryngol.* 94:59, 1971.
6. Brummett, R. E., et al. Quantitative relationships of the ototoxic interaction of kanamycin and ethacrynic acid. *Arch. Otolaryngol.* 105:240, 1979.
7. Cohn, E. S., et al. Ethacrynic acid effect on the composition of cochlear fluids. *Science* 171:910, 1971.
8. d'Avignon, M., and Barr, B. Ear abnormalities and cranial nerve palsies in thalidomide children. *Arch. Otolaryngol.* 80:136, 1964.
9. Daly, J. F., and Cohen, N. L. Viomycin ototoxicity in man: A cupulometric study. *Ann. Otol. Rhinol. Laryngol.* 74:521, 1965.
10. Davia, J. E., et al. Uremia, deafness and paralysis due to irrigating antibiotic solutions. *Arch. Intern. Med.* 125:135, 1970.
11. Dayal, V. S., et al. Combined effects of noise and kanamycin. *Ann. Otol. Rhinol. Laryngol.* 80:897, 1971.
12. Dilling, J. M., et al. Effect of ethacrynic acid on endolymphatic D C potential. *Arch. Otolaryngol.* 98:183, 1973.
13. Edwards, K. D. G., and Whyte, H. M. Streptomycin poisoning in renal failure. An indication for treatment with an artificial kidney. *Br. Med. J.* 1:752, 1959.
14. Fee, W. E., Jr., et al. Clinical evaluation of aminoglycoside toxicity. Tobramycin versus gentamicin, a preliminary report. *J. Antimicrob. Chemother.* 4(Suppl. A):31, 1978.
15. Finitzo-Hieber, T. Auditory Brainstem Response in Assessment of Infants Treated with Aminoglycoside Antibiotics. In S. A. Lerner, G. J. Matz, J. E. Hawkins, and E. F. Lanzl (Eds.), *Aminoglycoside Ototoxicity.* Boston: Little, Brown, 1981. Pp. 269–280.
16. Fisch, L. The Selective and Differential Vulnerability of the Auditory System. In G. E. W. Wolstenholme and J. Knight (Eds.), *Sensorineural Hearing Loss.* London: Churchill, 1970. Pp. 101–116.
17. Frost, J. O., et al. Kanamycin II ototoxicity. *Am. Rev. Respir. Dis.* 82:23, 1960.
18. Gabrielson, R. M. Colistimethate not ototoxic (letter to the editor). *N. Engl. J. Med.* 283:600, 1970.
19. Gombos, E. A., et al. Dialysis properties of newer antimicrobial agents. *Antimicrob. Agents Chemother.* 5:373, 1964.
20. Harell, M., et al. Total deafness with chronic propoxyphene abuse. *Laryngoscope* 88:1518, 1978.
21. Hawkins, J. E. Biochemical Aspects of Ototoxicity. In M. M. Paparella (Ed.), *Biochemical Mechanisms in Hearing and Deafness.* Springfield: Thomas, 1970. Pp. 323–339.
22. Hawkins, J. E. Comparative otopathology: Aging, noise and ototoxic drugs. *Adv. Otorhinolaryngol.* 20:125, 1973.
23. Hawkins, J. E., and Johnsson, L. G. Histopathology of Cochlear and Vestibular Ototoxicity in Laboratory Animals. In S. A. Lerner, G. J. Matz, J. E. Hawkins, and E. F. Lanzl (Eds.), *Aminoglycoside Ototox-*

icity. Boston: Little, Brown, 1981. Pp. 175–195.

24. Holz, E., et al. Decrease of ototoxicity of streptomycin sulfate. *Arch. Otolaryngol.* 87:359, 1968.

25. Jacobson, E. J., et al. Clinical findings in high-frequency thresholds during known ototoxic drug usage. *Journal of Auditory Research* 9:379, 1969.

26. Jarvis, J. F. A case of unilateral permanent deafness following acetylsalicylic acid. *J. Laryngol. Otol.* 80:318, 1966.

27. Jauhiainen, T., et al. Combined effect of noise and neomycin on the cochlea. *Acta Otolaryngol.* 73:387, 1972.

28. Johnson, A. H., and Hamilton, C. H. Kanamycin ototoxicity—Possible potentiation by other drugs. *South. Med. J.* 63:511, 1970.

29. Johnsonbaugh, R. E., et al. Familial occurrence of drug-induced hearing loss. *Am. J. Dis. Child.* 127:245, 1974.

30. Johnsson, L. G., et al. Aminoglycoside-Induced Inner Ear Pathology in Man, as Seen by Microdissection. In S. A. Lerner, G. J. Matz, J. E. Hawkins and E. F. Lanzl (Eds.), *Aminoglycoside Ototoxicity.* Boston: Little, Brown, 1981. Pp. 389–408.

31. Jones, H. C. Intrauterine ototoxicity. A case report and review of literature. *J. Natl. Med. Assoc.* 65:201, 1973.

32. Jorgensen, M. B., et al. Thalidomide-induced aplasia of the inner ear. *J. Laryngol. Otol.* 78:1095, 1964.

33. Kabins, S. A. Interactions among antibiotics and other drugs. *J.A.M.A.* 219:206, 1972.

34. Kanda, T., and Igarashi, M. Ultra-structural changes in vestibular sensory end organs after viomycin sulfate intoxication. *Acta Otolaryngol.* 68:474, 1969.

35. Komune, S., et al. Pathophysiology of the ototoxicity of cis-diamminedichloroplatinum. *Otolaryngol. Head Neck Surg.* 89:275, 1981.

36. Krumlovsky, F. A., et al. Dialysis in treatment of neomycin overdosage. *Ann. Intern. Med.* 76:443, 1972.

37. Lane, A. Z., et al. Ototoxicity and nephrotoxocity of amikacin: An overview of phase I and phase III experience in the United States. *Am. J. Med.* 62:911, 1977.

38. Law, W. K., et al. Comparative efficacy and toxicity of amikacin/carbenicillin versus gentamicin/carbenicillin in leukopenic patients: A randomized prospective trial. *Am. J. Med.* 62:959, 1977.

39. Lerner, S. A., and Matz, G. J. Suggestions for minitoring patients during treatment with aminoglycoside antibiotics. *Otolaryngol. Head Neck Surg.* 87:222, 1979.

40. Lerner, S. A., et al. Comparative clinical studies of ototoxicity and nephrotoxicity of amikacin and gentamicin. *Am. J. Med.* 62:919, 1977.

41. Lindholm, D. D., and Murray, J. S. Persistence of vancomycin in the blood during renal failure and its treatment by hemodialysis. *N. Engl. J. Med.* 274:1047, 1966.

42. Logan, T. B., et al. Tobramycin ototoxicity. *Arch. Otolaryngol.* 99:190, 1974.

43. Lupin, A. J., and Harley, C. H. Inner ear damage related to propoxyphene ingestion. *Can. Med. Assoc. J.* 114:596, 1976.

44. Mathog, R. H., et al. Ototoxicity of new and potent diuretics. *Arch. Otolaryngol.* 92:7, 1970.

45. McGee, T. M., and Olszewski, J. Streptomycin sulfate and dihydrostreptomycin toxicity. *Arch. Otolaryngol.* 75:295, 1962.

46. Meyer, R. D., et al. Amikacin therapy for serious gram-negative bacillary infections. *Ann. Intern. Med.* 83:790, 1975.

47. Morelli, O. H., et al. Acute effects of high doses of furosemide in patients with chronic renal failure. *Postgrad. Med. J.* (Suppl.) 47:29, 1971.

48. Morizono, T., and Johnstone, B. M. Ototoxicity of chloramphenicol ear drops with propylene glycol as solvent. *Med. J. Aust.* 2:634, 1975.

49. Myers, E. N., and Bernstein, J. M. Salicylate ototoxicity—A clinical and experimental study. *Arch. Otolaryngol.* 82:483, 1965.

50. Nadol, O. B. Histopathology of Human Aminoglycoside Ototoxicity. In S. A. Lerner, G. T. Matz, J. E. Hawkins, and E. F. Lanzl (Eds.), *Aminoglycoside Ototoxicity.* Boston: Little, Brown, 1981. Pp. 409–434.

51. Nordstrom, L., et al. Prospective study of the ototoxicity of gentamicin. *Acta Pathol. Microbiol. Immunol. Scand.* [B] (Suppl.) 241:58, 1973.

52. Piel, J. J., et al. Effect of cis-diamminedichloroplatinum (NSC-119875) on hearing function in man. *Cancer Chemother. Rep.* 58:871, 1974.

53. Pillay, V. K. G., et al. Transient and permanent deafness following treatment with ethacrynic acid in renal failure. *Lancet* 1:77, 1969.

54. Prazic, M., et al. Familial sensitivity to streptomycin. *J. Laryngol. Otol.* 78:1037, 1964.

55. Prazma, J., et al. Ototoxicity of the ethacrynic acid. *Arch. Otolaryngol.* 95:448, 1972.

56. Quick, C. A. Chemical and Drug Effects on Inner Ear. In M. M. Paparella and D. A. Shumrick (Eds.), *Otolaryngology II: Ear.* Philadelphia: Saunders, 1973. Pp. 391–406.

57. Quick, C. A., and Duvall, A. J. Early changes in the cochlear duct from ethacrynic acid. On electronmicroscopic evaluation. *Laryngosope* 80:954, 1970.

58. Quick, C. A., et al. Deafness and renal failure due to potassium bromate poisoning. *Arch. Otolaryngol.* 101:494, 1975.

59. Schreiner, G. E., et al. Specific therapy for salicylism. *N. Engl. J. Med.* 253:213, 1955.

60. Schuartz, F. D. Vestibular toxicity of gentamicin in the presence of renal disease (editorial). *Arch. Intern. Med.* 138:1612, 1978.

61. Schwartz, G. H., et al. Ototoxicity induced by furosemide. *N. Engl. J. Med.* 282:1413, 1970.

62. Smith, C. R., et al. Controlled comparison of amikacin and gentamicin. *N. Engl. J. Med.* 296:349, 1977.

63. Smith, C. R., et al. Double-blind comparison of the nephrotoxicity and auditory toxicity of gentamicin and tobramycin. *N. Engl. J. Med.* 302:1106, 1980.

64. Smith, K. E., and Spaulding, J. S. Ototoxic reaction to propylthiouracil. *Arch. Otolaryngol.* 96:368, 1972.

65. Stupp, H., et al. Kanamycin dosage and levels in ear and other organs. *Arch. Otolaryngol.* 86:515, 1967.

66. Suprapathana, L., et al. Salicylism revisited: Unusual problems in diagnosis and management. *Clin. Pediatr.* 9:658, 1970.

67. Thompson, P., and Northern, J. L. Audiometric Monitoring of Patients Treated with Ototoxic Drugs. In S. A. Lerner, G. J. Matz, J. E. Hawkins, and E. F. Lanzl (Eds.), *Aminoglycoside Ototoxicity.* Boston: Little, Brown, 1981. Pp. 237–245.

68. Thompson, P., et al. Erythromycin ototoxicity. *J. Otolaryngol.* 9:60, 1980.

69. Tjernstrom, O., et al. The ototoxicity of gentamicin. *Acta Pathol. Microbiol. Immunol. Scand* [B] (Suppl.) 241:73, 1973.

70. Vernon, J., et al. The ototoxic potential of propylene glycol in guinea pigs. *Arch. Otolaryngol.* 104:726, 1978.

71. Voldrich, L. The kinetics of streptomycin, kanamycin and neomycin in the inner ear. *Acta Otolaryngol.* 60:243, 1965.

72. Wersall, J. Structural Damage to the Organ of Corti and the Vestibular Epithelia Caused by Aminoglycoside Antibiotics in the Guinea Pig. In S. A. Lerner, G. J. Matz, J. E. Hawkins, and E. F. Lanzl (Eds.), *Aminoglycoside Ototoxicity.* Boston: Little, Brown, 1981. Pp. 197–214.

73. Wigand, M. E., and Heidland, A. Ototoxic side effects of high doses of fursemide in patients with uraemia. *Postgrad. Med. J.* (Suppl.) 47:54, 1971.

74. Winkel, O., et al. A prospective study of gentamicin ototoxicity. *Acta Otolaryngol.* 86:212, 1978.

11

Meniere's Disease

Jack L. Pulec

Although vertigo is usually considered to be the most prominent and disabling symptom of Meniere's disease, the hearing loss associated with this condition can produce a serious handicap. The diagnosis and treatment of patients with Meniere's disease present a challenge to the otologist. This symptom-complex first described by Meniere [5] in 1861 is a disease of the membranous inner ear characterized by deafness, vertigo, and usually tinnitus. Its pathologic correlate of hydropic distention of the endolymphatic system was demonstrated by Hallpike and Cairns [3] in 1938. Alfaro [1] in 1958 added fullness and pressure in the ear to the symptom-complex.

An intensive 5-year study by the author [10] has revealed that the signs and symptoms of Meniere's disease can be produced by a multitude of causes. A specific cause can be identified in 55% of all cases for which specific therapy is dictated, which is usually successful in controlling the condition. Those for whom no known specific cause can be identified will ultimately require surgical treatment because of their failure to respond to nonspecific medical therapy. It is incumbent on the otologist who first sees the patient with Meniere's disease to accomplish a thorough diagnostic examination to rule out conditions that mimic Meniere's disease and to establish a specific etiologic diagnosis. Appropriate medical or surgical treatment should not be delayed if a permanent hearing loss is to be avoided.

DIAGNOSTIC CRITERIA

The classic signs and symptoms of Meniere's disease include vertigo with hearing loss, tinnitus, and pressure in the involved ear. The name of the condition is correctly *Meniere's disease* [11], and all other terms (such as Meniere's syndrome, Meniere's symptom-complex, Meniere's disorder, or atypical Meniere's disease) should be discarded. If it is not Meniere's disease, it is some other condition (postural vertigo, inner ear concussion, toxic labyrinthitis, or acoustic neuroma) and should be so designated.

Hearing loss is sensorineural, fluctuating, and progressive. Early in the course of the disease, deafness is primarily for the low tones. Late in the disease, when fluctuation decreases, the hearing loss is usually for the high tones. Tinnitus, pressure, and hearing loss often gradually build up before an attack of rotary vertigo, often with nausea and vomiting. Spells of vertigo characteristically last from 30 minutes to 2 to 3 hours, after which time the patient usually makes a prompt recovery and regains otologic function. Nystagmus is common during and after the attack of vertigo. Some patients have constant instability between spells of vertigo, but this is a less common finding. Early in the disease, tests of hair cell dysfunction are positive. Late in the disease when deafness is severe, these signs of hair cell dysfunction may be lost. Late in the course of the disease, spells of vertigo may occur suddenly without warning and last for only a few minutes.

There are two subvarieties of the disorder: cochlear Meniere's disease and vestibular Meniere's disease. Cochlear Meniere's disease, or Meniere's disease without vertigo, is characterized solely by a fluctuating and progressive sensorineural deafness with all auditory test results typical of Meniere's disease. Many patients notice a fullness in the ear coincident with the sudden drop in hearing. Some patients subsequently develop the definitive dizzy spells and the qualifying *cochlear* is discarded.

Vestibular Meniere's disease, or Meniere's disease without deafness, is characterized solely by the definitive spells of vertigo. Vestibular Meniere's disease is difficult to diagnose, as there are no objective findings between spells. The symptom of pressure in the ear is helpful to differentiate the condition from vestibular neuronitis. The diagnosis may be accepted on exclusion of other diseases. Some subsequently develop the deafness and the qualifying *vestibular* is dropped. Meniere's disease may affect both ears in 24% of patients.

EXAMINATION

Every patient whose symptoms suggest Meniere's disease must be carefully evaluated to rule out acoustic neuromas and other lesions of the cerebellopontile angle, as well as to establish an etiologic diagnosis so that specific appropriate treatment can be instituted [6, 7, 8]. Every patient should have an audiogram for pure tone and speech, short increment sensitivity index (SISI), and Bekesy tests; electronystagmography with both positional and bithermal caloric stimulation; and petrous pyramid x-ray views including Towne's, Caldwell's, and Stenver's projections. In many cases in which the possibility of an acoustic neuroma is even remotely suggested, a polytome isophendylate (Pantopaque) study should be done to confirm the absence of a tumor. Each patient should also have a five-hour glucose tolerance test, a reactive fluorescent antibody absorption (FTA-ABS) test for syphilis, and thyroid studies, including T_4 free thyroxine and Murphy-Pattee methods. A lipoprotein phenotype test should be carried out. A careful history of allergy should be taken. Should it be significant, an allergic evaluation may be indicated.

Careful evaluation of these techniques has revealed a specific etiology in 55% of the patients with Meniere's disease. Each of the several differently caused conditions requires a different but specific treatment, which when given is usually successful.

ETIOLOGY
Allergy
Allergy, especially to foods, may produce a sensorineural hearing loss and the symptoms of Meniere's disease [10]. Craving for a certain food, a seasonal variation in symptoms, or other allergic manifestations such as asthma, postprandial bloating, or fatigue may suggest this diagnosis. Investigation of allergic causes is involved, time-consuming, and difficult. Cytotoxic food tests, challenge feeding tests, and provocative skin food tests as well as the more conventional tests help identify the offending allergens. Relief of aural symptoms can be expected by elimination of the allergens or by desensitization. Fourteen percent of the patients with Meniere's disease have been found to have an allergic diathesis and respond to allergic treatment alone. In an additional 12%, satisfactory control of symptoms is obtained by the less specific combined treatment of thyroid replacement, allergic treatment, and a high-protein, low-carbohydrate diet.

Congenital or Acquired Syphilis

Symptoms referable to the ear have been known to be caused by syphilis since ancient times. In 1964 Collart [2] showed that live spirochetes resistant to all forms of antibiotic therapy could coexist with their host in late syphilis. Karmody and Schuknecht [4] demonstrated the pathologic disorders caused by syphilis to be both endolymphatic hydrops and osteitis of the otic capsule. The ear symptoms are typical of Meniere's disease and often begin in the fifth decade of life, first in one ear and after a few years involving the second ear. Typical low-tone hearing loss with fluctuation, pressure, tinnitus, and progressively deteriorating speech discrimination occurs. Frequently, hearing loss is sudden and, if not treated promptly, is permanent. Caloric vestibular examination frequently indicates bilateral, markedly reduced vestibular responses. When hearing loss is severe and sudden, this condition represents a true medical emergency, and treatment is the prompt administration of steroids.

The diagnosis is confirmed by obtaining a reactive FTA-ABS test. Commonly the patient has a nonreactive VDRL test or other nonspecific tests for syphilis, and for that reason we have abandoned the use of these other tests and rely wholly on the reactive FTA-ABS test. More than one examination should be done to confirm a positive reaction.

Treatment involves hospitalization and the administration of penicillin, 20 million units intravenously daily for 7 days, to remove the risk of overlooking a treatable syphilitic condition. The patient is placed on prednisone, 10 mg four times a day, with appropriate amounts of an antacid to prevent ulcer formation. The steroid is maintained at this dosage level for 1 month, after which time it is slowly reduced to the lowest level that will maintain hearing. If no improvement in hearing is noted during the month of treatment, the steroid is discontinued and the inevitable permanent loss accepted. If the hearing level drops, the patient must take more medication immediately until hearing is restored before the dosage level is again gradually reduced to the maintenance level. In 6% of the patients, Meniere's disease has been found to have a syphilitic etiology. Smyth [10] has recently suggested the use of adrenocorticotropic hormone (ACTH), 40 units injected twice weekly, as a substitute for long-term steroid therapy.

Hypoadrenalism and Hypopituitarism

Inadequate function of the pituitary and adrenal glands has been suggested as a cause of Meniere's disease in the patient with bilateral involvement who often has a chronic fluctuating problem. A flat five-hour glucose tolerance curve also suggests this cause. The ACTH plasma cortisol stimulation test can be used for both conditions. This test involves the removal of two blood specimens for study, the second 30 minutes after the injection of the ACTH or ACTH substitute. A rise of less than 7 μg/100 ml indicates hypofunction of these glands. The differential diagnosis can be made by a more involved insulin stimulation test to measure growth hormone and lowered adrenocortical reserve [10]. Seven percent of the patients with Meniere's disease have been found to have abnormal tests indicating hypofunction of these glands, and hormone replacement therapy is indicated. Rarely is low blood pressure present in this group of patients.

Myxedema

Hypothyroidism is known to produce endolymphatic hydrops and accounts for 2% of the cases of Meniere's disease. The protein-bound iodine test, triiodothyronine resin uptake test, blood cholesterol determination, and basal metabolic rate examinations are subject to false responses and for this reason should be abandoned in favor of the thyroxine (T_4) free index test and the thyroxine (T_4) serum-bound test of Murphy-Pattee. Thyroid replacement therapy is effective in eliminating the symptoms of Meniere's disease in patients with hypothyroidism [10].

Stenosis of the Internal Auditory Canal

A condition has been identified in which the internal auditory canal is abnormally small and produces a compression of its contents with involvement of the ear or the facial nerve [10]. The usual symptoms are progressive hearing loss or instability, but a small number of patients exhibit the signs and symptoms of Meniere's disease with typical fluctuations of hearing, tinnitus, pressure, and episodic vertigo. Symptoms can be precipitated sometimes by placing the head in the dependent position. The condition is suggested by the findings of an internal auditory canal measuring 3 mm or less on plain x-ray views. It is confirmed by the polytome isophendylate study, which shows a characteristic constriction or nonfilling of the canal. Decompression of the internal auditory canal by use of the middle cranial fossa approach, without disturbing or sectioning any of the nerves, may result in recovery of normal function. This diagnosis is made in 3% of the patients with Meniere's disease.

Trauma
Physical or acoustic trauma precedes the onset of symptoms in 5% of the cases. The trauma may be a temporal bone fracture or a labyrinthine concussion. Exposure to loud noise has been clearly shown to initiate symptoms. The treatment is medical with vasodilator therapy, or surgical by means of the endolymphatic subarachnoid shunt, or a destructive procedure may be necessary.

Vascular
In 3% of patients with Meniere's disease, the cause seems to be solely vascular. Symptoms generally occur in patients with obvious other manifestations of vascular disease in association with congestive heart failure, hypertension, diabetes, and elevated blood fat. Correction of the primary problems and the use of vasodilators often control the symptoms of Meniere's disease.

Estrogen Insufficiency
Inadequate supply of estrogen can produce Meniere's disease. No test is currently available to detect the problem. Empiric use of estrogen replacement prevents the signs and symptoms of Meniere's disease in 2% of patients.

Viral
Although preliminary immunologic viral investigations suggest that those cases still classified as idiopathic are probably initiated by a viral infection, a clear-cut cause

and effect has been demonstrated in only 1% of patients.

CAUSES OF MENIERE'S DISEASE

Allergy	14%
Adrenal-pituitary insufficiency	7%
Congenital or acquired syphilis	6%
Hypothyroidism	2%
Vascular	3%
Estrogen insufficiency	2%
Combination of above	12%
Internal auditory canal stenosis	3%
Physical trauma	3%
Acoustic trauma	2%
Viral	1%
Idiopathic	45%

PSYCHOLOGICAL IMPLICATIONS
The literature abounds with references to the psychological aspects of Meniere's disease. Certainly the patient consulting a physician because of his problem may have some anxiety because he is living in constant fear of a violent attack of disabling vertigo with nausea and vomiting. Intensive and conclusive psychological evaluation has shown that there is no basis on which to incriminate any emotional or psychiatric factor in the etiology of this disease [10]. This is not to suggest that patients already suffering from a vertiginous problem are not affected by psychological changes. They in fact sometimes exhibit an exaggeration of symptoms during periods of stress. Two causes seem likely. (1) Stress and fatigue tend to reduce the effectiveness of the vestibular efferent system and its suppressing effect on a malfunctioning labyrinth. When suppression is reduced, the existing abnormal labyrinthine stimulation becomes evident. (2) Patients with Meniere's disease whose cause is allergic or metabolic and who are on the borderline of control may have inadequate adrenocortical output during these periods of stress with the subsequent exaggeration of symptoms.

AUDIOLOGIC FINDINGS
AND CHANGES
Audiologic results vary depending on the stage of the disease. Meniere's disease is most often characterized by a low-frequency

sensorineural hearing impairment often accompanied by recruitment. Relatively good speech discrimination scores of 82% or better are usual. The low-tone hearing loss may fluctuate greatly in some patients. Most have SISI scores of 100% and a type II Bekesy pattern.

After medical or surgical treatment, 50% of the patients remain the same as far as pure-tone hearing is concerned. Johnson [10] found improvement in pure tone, speech reception threshold (SRT), and speech discrimination after treatment, showing that a patient who has had the disorder for many years can often obtain significant improvement in hearing. One patient had a shift in speech discrimination scores from 14 to 92% after having had Meniere's disease for 27 years. Another patient who had experienced 7 years of hearing difficulty obtained improvement in discrimination from 54 to 88% after treatment for allergy. An endolymphatic subarachnoid shunt operation effected hearing improvement from 40 to 92% discrimination in one patient, even though symptoms had been present for 22 years.

In patients with active Meniere's disease, electrocochleography (ECoG) has demonstrated changes suggesting that the outer hair cells are affected first. Amplitude and latency function, as well as the waveform, are abnormal. There is a tendency to form multiple peaks, which may be a distinctive characteristic of ears involved with Meniere's disease [10]. In patients with Meniere's disease, the threshold latency is much shorter than in normal patients, varying from .09 to 4.6 msec. The threshold latency in cases of Meniere's disease is nearly the same as latency at an equivalent intensity level in normals. The amplitude in Meniere's disease at high intensity varies from 4 to 40 μv with a mean of 17 μv. These values do not vary greatly from those of normal ears. The reason suggested for these discrepancies is that at low intensities the external hair cells do not function and do not produce an eighth nerve action potential. No response is obtained until suddenly the inner hair cells become active at the patient's threshold. The neurons that go to the inner hair cells have a very short unmyelinated fiber and thus have a very short latency. At threshold the latency is short, approximately the same as it would be for a normal patient at the level at which the inner hair cells would be first excited.

The amplitude curve changes in a similar fashion for the same reason. From threshold to high intensity, the amplitude builds up very rapidly to that of a normal patient, presumably because at high intensity in the normal and in the Meniere's patient the neurons stimulated by the internal hair cells are primarily responsible for the action potential.

Brain stem audiometry accomplished in patients with Meniere's disease has objectively demonstrated that recruitment originates within the inner ear. Patients without distortion or recruitment as measured by conventional means are found to have a linear response to sound. In cases with active disease and clear-cut recruitment, no response is found until threshold is reached. As the sound level is increased, the brain stem response increases at a disproportionate and rapid rate to the normal expected level or beyond [10].

VESTIBULAR FINDINGS
AND CHANGES
The dynamic nature of Meniere's disease makes change in vestibular function and test results commonplace. Stahle [13] has documented and reported these changes. Any type of vestibular finding can occur. Nystagmus is found during the vertiginous attack and remains for several days after the attack. Directional preponderance is frequently present. Using the simultaneous bilateral bithermal test, changes on the involved ear are more frequently seen [10]. The test has increased sensitivity in finding more caloric vestibular abnormalities than the regular bithermal stimulation alone. The simultaneous bilateral bithermal test does not reliably localize the affected end-organ in two instances. The first occurs when the central vestibular mechanism is producing maximum suppression to reduce the patient's symptoms, even during the attack-free interval. In this instance, the test has no advantage over the regular bithermal test in that both stimuli fail to demonstrate responses of value in the investigation of the vestibular system. The second

occurs when the vestibular end-organ demonstrates the apparent recruitment phenomenon.

During the time of active disease, caloric responses may be reduced bilaterally as a result of vestibular suppression, or in the early stages of the disease the involved side may show a hyperactive response to caloric stimulation, possibly because caloric stimulation of the endolymph is more effective when the dilated saccule is in contact with the footplate of the stapes. Permanent reduction of the caloric response often accompanies disease of longer duration.

RADIOLOGY IN MENIERE'S DISEASE

Radiographic contribution to the diagnosis of Meniere's disease has two purposes [10]: (1) to exclude disease simulating Meniere's, such as acoustic neuroma, meningioma, or congenital cholesteatoma of the petrous apex; and (2) to identify cases of Mondini deformities of the inner ear. The Mondini deformity involves a radiologically demonstrable dilated vestibule and absence of the apical portion of the cochlea. Demonstration of this defect makes it possible to consider an endolymphatic subarachnoid shunt operation to arrest the progressive sensorineural hearing loss associated with the condition.

Special views using polydirectional tomography are necessary to assess the size of the cochlear and vestibular aqueducts. Both the endolymphatic and perilymphatic ducts are seen radiographically to be narrowed or absent in 52% of temporal bones of ears with Meniere's disease against 9% of ears in a control group. Patients with unilateral Meniere's disease usually have a similarly narrowed or absent endolymphatic duct if present on each side. This suggests that stenosis of the duct is not necessary for the development of Meniere's disease but probably predisposes an ear to the condition. We have found no correlation between the radiologic appearance of the endolymphatic or perilymphatic duct and the success of the endolymphatic subarachnoid shunt procedure. For this reason, radiographic examination of these ducts is not routinely made for clinical purposes.

MEDICAL TREATMENT

In those patients for whom no specific etiology can be determined, such as allergy, hypometabolic state, myxedema, syphilis, or a small internal auditory canal, treatment involves the initial use of vasodilators in an attempt to control symptoms. This vasodilator regimen is frequently successful in stopping a severe series of attacks and restoring hearing to useful level [12].

Histamine

Histamine is given intravenously on three consecutive days. This solution contains 2.75 mg of histamine phosphate in 250 ml of normal saline. The solution is administered at an initial rate of 20 to 30 drops per minute, and if well tolerated this dosage may be increased to 50 to 60 drops per minute after five minutes. The time of administration is 90 minutes in the average case. The patient is made aware that mild flushing, headache, and increased head noise may develop. Following completion of this intravenous series, 0.1 ml of a 1 : 100,000 dilution of histamine phosphate is administered subcutaneously twice weekly. The patient is instructed to take 2 drops of 1 : 10,000 histamine phosphate sublingually twice daily.

Nicotinic Acid

Nicotine acid tablets, 50 mg, are prescribed 30 to 45 minutes before breakfast and before dinner. The dose is adjusted by the patient up to 200 mg until a definite flush is obtained. Frequently a flush is obtained by a dose before breakfast smaller than that required before dinner. It is important that this drug be administered before meals, when the stomach is empty, to ensure rapid absorption and maximum effect. Roniacol may be substituted in patients who have difficulty taking nicotinic acid. One significant action of nicotinic acid may be to reduce atherosclerosis.

In addition, the patient is asked to take Pro-Banthine four times daily; Benadryl, 50 mg at bedtime; Lipoflavonoid, two capsules three times daily; and occasionally other medications. There seems to be little question that this form of treatment provides relief of the symptoms of Meniere's disease, although different patients may or may not respond well to each specific medication. No clear pattern is evident by which the clinician may select or predict which medication will be successful in each given situation.

A significant number of patients whose symptoms suggest a diagnosis of Meniere's disease to the otologist are found to have hyperglycemia or hypoglycemia detected only by the five-hour glucose tolerance test done after the patient is properly prepared by eating a high-carbohydrate diet of at least 3000 calories on three successive days preceding the tests. These diagnoses usually cannot be made by history alone or by relying on an internists's examination. The otologist must order and interpret the five-hour glucose tolerance test findings. The hypoglycemia is readily treated by placing the patient on a low-carbohydrate, high-protein diet with frequent meals. Strict attention to diet or control of diabetes with oral medication or insulin frequently resolves the otologic symptoms. Lipoprotein phenotyping should be accomplished, and patients with abnormalities should be given appropriate diets. Often symptoms will subside and hearing will improve a few weeks after the onset of dietary control.

SURGICAL TREATMENT

Patients who have progressive hearing loss or disabling symptoms despite medical treatment after a minimum of 2 months are candidates for surgical treatment. The operation of choice is the endolymphatic subarachnoid shunt [10]. We have preferred this procedure because it is not destructive and acts to relieve the endolymphatic hydrops and return the ear to normal. The risk of hearing loss as a result of the operation is less than 2%. Analysis of long-term results with the shunt operation reveals a successful outcome in 62% of patients, with stabilization or improvement of hearing in approximately half.

Total ablation of cochlear and vestibular function is recommended for patients who have useless cochlear and vestibular function and who are unresponsive to medical treatment or the endolymphatic subarachnoid shunt operation. Labyrinthectomy can be accomplished under local anesthesia through the external auditory canal by elevating a tympanomeatal flap and removing the incus, stapes, and bone between the round and oval windows. This allows the placement of a long, 3-mm hook into the vestibule so that the hook can be inserted into each ampulla for removal of the neurosensory epithelium of each ampulla, as well as the utricle and saccule. Aspiration of the contents of the vestibule through the oval window is unsuccessful in 15% of the cases, resulting in persistent vestibular dysfunction because the uninjured endolymphatic space seals over while healing. Careful removal with a long hook adds little time to the operative procedure and increases the success rate to 95%.

Patients who retain vestibular function following a local transcanal labyrinthectomy may be relived by a postauricular labyrinthectomy. This procedure is carried out under general anesthesia through a postauricular incision. The semicircular canals and posterior half of the vestibule are completely excised with the drill. In this way the area heals with fibrous tissue so that when the efferent vestibular nerves grow into this fibrous tissue during the postoperative period, there is no movement and usually the patient remains free of vertigo.

The most effective technique for total ablation of cochlear and vestibular function is translabyrinthine eighth nerve section. This technique is required when other types of labyrinthectomy have failed and is the surgical treatment of choice in most of the more severe cases. The procedure allows investigation of the internal auditory canal to confirm the absence of tumor. It also allows section of the cochlear nerve as well as excision of the vestibular nerves medial to Scarpa's ganglion so that there is degeneration to the brain stem and no chance for the survival of residual vestibular or cochlear function. Pressure in the ear resulting from cochlear hydrops in an otherwise destroyed ear does not occur following this procedure unless the cochlear nerve is left intact. Section of the cochlear nerve by this technique offers the best chance for relief of tinnitus. Success is in the 96% range [9]. Total eighth nerve section is also indicated for patients who have severe distortion in an otherwise asymptomatic ear, which makes it difficult for a patient to hear adequately with the normal side. Occasionally cochlear suppression in the opposite uninvolved ear associated with Meniere's disease is difficult to distinguish from bilateral Meniere's disease. The apparent sensorineural hearing loss can be as great as 25 dB. The true nature of the problem can be suspected when the ear is free of pressure and there are no audiometric findings of recruitment. Translabyrinthine eighth nerve section on the involved side will often result in a return to normal of both hearing and vestibular function in the innocent ear.

Rarely a middle fossa vestibular nerve operation is undertaken in the patient who has disabling vertigo despite all other forms of conservative treatment and who also has useful hearing. Disconnection of the vestibular labyrinth by this technique prevents the occurrence of vertigo in the symptomatic ear. It has no effect, however, on the other symptoms of Meniere's disease, including tinnitus, pressure, and fluctuating hearing. Because these symptoms persist and often are very disturbing for the patient, middle fossa vestibular nerve section is not routinely recommended for patients with Meniere's disease.

Long-term follow-up of cases has shown that those of idiopathic etiology will almost always eventually continue to have symptoms requiring surgery [10]. Approximately 15% are ultimately adequately controlled by medical treatment or spontaneous prolonged remission.

REFERENCES

1. Alfaro, V. R. Diagnostic significance of fullness in the ear. *J.A.M.A.* 166:239, 1958.

2. Collart, P. Persistence of *Treponema pallidum* in late syphilis in rabbits and humans, notwithstanding treatment. *Proceedings of the Forum on Syphilis and Other Treponematosis.* Public Health Service Publication No. 997. Washington, D.C.: U.S. Government Printing Office, 1964. Pp. 285–294.

3. Hallpike, C. S., and Cairns, H. Observations on the pathology of Ménière's syndrome. *J. Laryngol.* 53:625, 1938.

4. Karmody, C. S., and Schuknecht, H. F. Deafness in congenital syphilis. *Arch. Otolaryngol.* 83:18, 1966.

5. Ménière, P. Mémoire sur des lésions de l'oreille interne donnant lieu à des symptômes de congestion cérébrale apoplectiforme. *Gaz. Med.* [Paris] s.3, 16:597, 1861.

6. Pulec, J. L. Ménière's disease: Results of a 2½-year study of the etiology, natural history, and results of treatment. *Laryngoscope* 82:1703, 1972.

7. Pulec, J. L. Ménière's disease. Etiology, natural history, and results of treatment. *Otolaryngol. Clin. North Am.* 6:25, 1973.

8. Pulec, J. L., and House, W. F. Ménière's disease study: Three-year progress report. *Equilibrium Res.* 3:1, 1973.

9. Pulec, J. L. Labyrinthectomy: Indications, technique and results. *Laryngoscope* 84:1552, 1974.

10. Pulec, J. L. (Ed.) *Ménière's Disease: Research and Clinical Advances.* Los Angeles: Palisades Press, 1980.

11. Report of subcommittee on equilibrium and its measurements. *Trans. Am. Acad. Ophthalmol. Otolaryngol.* 76:1462, 1972.

12. Sheehy, J. L. Vasodilator therapy in sensoryneural hearing loss. *Laryngoscope* 70:885, 1960.

13. Stahle, J. Electronystagmographic results in Ménière's disease. *Otolaryngol. Clin. North Am.* 1:509, 1968.

12

Noise-Induced Hearing Loss

W. Dixon Ward

With the Industrial Revolution came louder machines and a significant increase in the number of persons suffering hearing loss from exposure to noise. Thus, some 100 years ago, the stage was set for noise-induced hearing loss (NIHL) to become a problem of social welfare. Today the impact of industrial hearing loss is a matter of tremendous concern—to the federal government, to the armed forces, to industrial giants, and even to small business owners.

It is now regarded as the obligation of the employer to prevent NIHL, either by keeping noise exposures down to acceptable harmless values or by providing ear protection for each employee. If an employee develops a hearing loss attributable to noise in his working environment, the employer is bound to pay an amount of money commensurate with the degree of hearing loss, within limits determined by state compensation laws. In view of the recent growth of claims by workers against their employers, at least some of which may be contestable, the otolaryngologist and the audiologist need to know as much as possible about the diagnosis of NIHL. For more complete discussions of noise-induced hearing loss and the technical aspects of noise, readers are referred to the proceedings of a recent symposium on noise as a public health problem [13].

Despite the fact that we know quite a bit about the characteristics and causes of NIHL, there is still no convincing evidence that any sort of medication or treatment can "cure" it or even slow its development. The clinician's task is to identify the symptoms of NIHL, rule out all other possible causes of the hearing loss except noise exposure, and indicate to the patient the alternatives available to him to avoid additional hearing loss caused by noise. The diagnosis of NIHL is not as simple as it may first appear—it is often quite difficult to answer the ultimate question that is asked in a court of law, "Is the patient's

This chapter is adapted from W. D. Ward, The identification and treatment of noise-induced hearing loss, *Otolaryngol. Clin. North Am.* 90:89, 1969; and W. D. Ward, Effects of Noise Exposure on Auditory Sensitivity, in D. K. Lee (Section Ed.), *Handbook of Physiology, Section 9: Reactions to Environmental Agents.* Baltimore, Md.: Williams & Wilkins, 1977.

hearing loss caused by the noise in question?"

CLASSIFICATION OF NOISE-INDUCED HEARING LOSS

There are two main types of noise-induced hearing loss: hearing loss that occurs gradually over a period of years and hearing loss that can be attributed to a single brief but intense exposure to noise. The latter is generally termed *acoustic trauma*. Noise exposure produces both temporary and permanent effects consisting of changes in the morphologic, biochemical, and electrophysiologic characteristics of one or more elements of the auditory pathway from the eardrum to the cortex. However, in spite of hundreds of research studies and publications, the precise relations between the parameters of the acoustic exposure and the resultant loss of auditory capability is still a matter of uncertainty and dispute.

EFFECTS OF NOISE

It is important to distinguish clearly between the concepts of noise *level* and noise *exposure*. A noise level is a measure of the acoustic intensity at some time and is measured with a sound level meter. For certain purposes we do not express the level of the noise in terms of its actual physical sound pressure level; instead, we use weighted filter networks built into the sound level meter. Present standards require three such networks to be provided: scales A, B, and C. When sound measurements are made using one of these filter scales, this fact is indicated by expressing the result as so many dBA, dBB, or dBC, respectively. These numbers are actually overall sound pressure levels in which low- and high-frequency components have been deemphasized relative to the presence of middle-frequency (1000–4000 Hz) components. Originally this was done to simulate the loudness of sounds as judged by human listeners; however, the A-weighting filter network is commonly used for measuring industrial noises because this scale happens to deemphasize low-frequency components of noise to an extent that research indicates to be commensurate with their potential hazard to hearing. Routine environ-

mental average noise levels, expressed in dBA, are shown in Table 12-1.

The noise *exposure* of an ear, on the other hand, is some joint function of the acoustic intensity of the sound entering the ear and its duration. Just what this function should be is a matter of some dispute. Ideally, exposures should be expressed in terms such that all exposures of the same magnitude produce an equal effect. If, for example, the damage to hearing depended on the simple product of intensity and time, which is the acoustic energy entering the ear, then doubling the exposure time could be balanced by reducing the intensity by half (i.e., by 3 dB). Indeed, this trading relation, the so-called equal energy principle, has been adopted by the International Standards Organization (ISO 1999) because it is so simple and easy to use. Unfortunately, it is valid only under very special circumstances, namely, for single uninterrupted exposures. If the noise level fluctuates, then during the quiet periods some of the adverse effects of the previous noise will recover, so that the final damage is less than if the same amount of total energy had been delivered to the ear by a steady noise over the same time period. So if a single scheme *must* be used to cover both steady and variable or intermittent exposures, a trading relation higher than 3 dB per halving must be employed. In the United States, the trading relation adopted by the Occupational Safety and Health Administration to account for the fact that most industrial noise exposures are not steady, is 5 dB per halving: thus exposures of 90 dBA for eight hours per day, 95 dBA for a total of four hours, 100 dBA for two hours, and so on, are decreed to be equal. A "compromise" between the 3 dB and 5 dB rules, 4 dB per halving, has been adopted by the United States Air Force, and in East Germany a 6 dB trading relation is advocated (this could be termed the equal pressure principle). None of these can be universally correct, because the amount of reduction of effect caused by interrupting the noise exposure depends on the *specific* temporal pattern of the interruptions. In short, no method has yet been devised for condensing the parameters of noise exposure—level, duration, temporal pattern, and spectrum—to a single

Table 12-1. Sample Noise Levels, Expressed in dBA

Overall level, dBA*	Industrial, military	Community (outdoor)	Home (indoor)
130	Armored personnel carrier (123)		
Uncomfortably loud			
120	Scraper-loader (117) Compactor (116)		Rock band (108–114)
110	Riveting machine (110) Textile loom (106)	Chain saw (110) Snowmobile (105) Jet flyover, 1000 ft (103)	Symphony orchestra (110)
100 Very loud	Electric furnace area (100) Farm tractor (98) Newspaper press (97)	Power mower (96) Compressor, 20 ft (94) Rock drill, 100 ft (92)	Subway car, inside 35 mph (95)
90		Motorcycle, 25 ft (90)	Cockpit—light aircraft (90)
	Cockpit—prop aircraft (88) Milling machine (85) Cotton spinning (83) Lathe (81)	Propeller aircraft flyover, 1000 ft (88) Diesel truck, 40 mph, 50 ft (84)	Food blender (88)
80			Garbage disposal (80)
Moderately loud		Passenger car, 65 mph 25 ft (77)	Clothes washer (78) Living room music (76) Dishwasher (75)
70			TV-audio (70)
		Auto traffic, freeway (64)	Conversation (65)
60		Air conditioning unit, 20 ft (60) Transformer, large 200 ft (53)	
50 Quiet		Traffic, light, 100 ft (50)	
40			
30 Very quiet			
20			
10 Just audible Threshold of hearing			
0 (1000–4000 Hz)			

* Unless otherwise specified, listed sound levels are measured at typical operator-listener distances from source.

Source: Adapted from A. Cohen, J. R. Anticaglia, and J. H. Jones, Noise-induced hearing loss. *Arch. Environ. Health* 20:614, 1970 (a publication of the Helen Dwight Reid Foundation).

valid index. Exposures are therefore generally specified by stating all four of these characteristics, except that, as just mentioned, the effect of different spectra is assumed to be accounted for by specifying levels in dBA.

The most common way to describe the effect of noise exposures on a person is by noting its effect on his auditory threshold. Ideally, the auditory threshold is established prior to and following the exposure; the difference between these two measurements is the *threshold shift* (TS), which may be either temporary (TTS) or permanent (PTS). The term *noise-induced* should be applied only if it can be firmly established that no other reason for the threshold shift exists.

Actually, the change in auditory threshold from one time to another, especially over a period of a year or more, is a complex function of many agents, because noise is not the only cause of PTS. The aging process may play a role; changes attributed to aging as such are termed presbycusis (see Chap. 14). In addition, diseases such as mumps, blows to the head, and exposure to industrial toxins may affect the sensory mechanism; a technical term to describe threshold changes other than those ascribable to either noise or aging might be *nosoacusis* (Greek *nosos:* disease). Furthermore, that portion of the observed change in threshold that can be attributed to noise is produced not only by industrial noise but also (at least partly) by the noises of everyday life, such as from chain saws, power mowers, gunfire, or amplified music. The PTS produced by noises of everyday living has been labeled *sociacusis*. Thus any given PTS is some complicated interaction of presbycusis, sociacusis, nosoacusis, and industrial noise exposure. Extracting PTS caused by industrial noise exposure alone is obviously a precarious process; for example, estimation of sociacusis over a period of years is nearly impossible. Most people are not able to recall the loud noises they heard during the past week, much less the previous 5 years.

With the vast number of uncertainties that surround most research data for noise-induced permanent threshold shift (NIPTS), we have not been able to develop a succinct formula for determining the hazard implied by a particular episode of noise exposure. So in the absence of data on known *permanent* threshold shift, we attempt to derive empirical conclusions from data on *temporary* threshold shift.

TEMPORARY THRESHOLD SHIFT

Temporary threshold shift is generally classified in terms of how the ear recovers with time. One type of TTS develops almost immediately and disappears within a second. This rapid TTS depends mainly on the level of the noise and is independent of the duration. A second type of TTS persists for about one minute following cessation of the fatiguing stimulus, and is to some extent independent of the level of the fatiguer. If TTS persists for more than two minutes, however, its value will depend on the level, duration, and temporal pattern of the noise exposure, and is thus regarded as *auditory fatigue*. The amount of TTS that persists two minutes after cessation of the exposure is referred to as TTS_2. A recent discussion of the present state of knowledge regarding TTS has been presented elsewhere [12].

Unlike the short-duration TTS, the frequency distribution of long-lasting TTS does not show a maximum at the exposure frequency. When pure tones are used as fatiguers, the maximum TTS_2 is found at a progressively higher frequency as the intensity is raised, sometimes as much as two octaves above the stimulation frequency [12]. For frequencies below 1000 Hz, the TTS_2 produced by a pure tone is somewhat larger than that produced by a noise of the same level, probably because noise is better able to cause a sustained contraction of the middle ear muscles than is a pure tone [9].

Both the growth of TTS_2 and its recovery are exponential processes [1, 3]; in the presence of a constant noise level the growth of TTS_2 reaches its asymptote in 8 to 12 hours [5]. The magnitude of TTS_2 grows in an approximately linear fashion as a function of the average sound pressure level (SPL), once the level has exceeded a certain base value below which only short-duration effects are produced. This "basic"

SPL appears to be about 70 to 75 dB [16]. Thus, a 75 dB SPL octave-band noise will not produce much TTS_2 no matter how long it is on; a 105 dB SPL noise will create about twice as much TTS_2 as one of 90 dB SPL for the same duration of exposure; a 100 dB SPL noise will produce a value of TTS_2 midway between that generated by 90 dB and 110 dB SPL, and so on. The actual rate of growth with level depends on the duration and the frequency composition of the fatiguing noise; high frequencies induce a more rapid rate of growth than low frequencies, even though the basic intensity is independent of frequency. Because the recovery of TTS is exponential with time, it is difficult to determine when recovery is effectively complete. The problem is further compounded by the fact that the variability of audiometric measurement does not ordinarily permit confidence in an individual TTS smaller than 5 dB.

The TTS_2 produced by a given exposure will be greater for normal ears than for those with elevated thresholds. There are two explanations for this empirical fact, depending on the type of hearing loss involved [14]. If the problem is one of conductive hearing loss, then the effective intensity of the sound will be reduced by the magnitude of the loss. Thus, if a TTS of 10 dB is produced in a normal ear by a given exposure at 100 dB SPL, then a person with a 25 dB conductive loss will show the same 10 dB TTS only after the same exposure to 125 dB SPL. A patient with a sensory hearing loss (an already damaged inner ear) will also show less TTS than normal hearing persons, but in this case because the ear has less left to lose. The energy entering the cochlea of such a person is no different from that entering the normal ear. But if the patient in question already has a considerable loss of hearing sensitivity, then the threshold shift produced by a given noise will be less than in normal persons, even though the shifted threshold—that is, the threshold hearing level after exposure—is always higher. In other words, after exposure to a given noise, the ear with sensory loss will still require more signal energy for hearing than will the normal ear. So the fact that he shows less TTS does not mean that he

is less affected by the noise. Accordingly, the acquisition of a permanent loss from noise cannot be considered as protection against further loss.

These examples illustrate why the following question is probably unanswerable: Is a noise-damaged ear more susceptible to further injury than an undamaged one? It would be naive indeed to postulate that a 10 dB additional PTS in an ear that already has a hearing loss of 40 dB is the same as a 10 dB change in a previously normal ear.

PERMANENT THRESHOLD SHIFT

As discussed earlier, to convert PTS to noise-induced permanent threshold shift (NIPTS), or even to determine a given PTS, is a perilous process. In addition to the practical difficulties of determining the exact conditions of the noise exposure, and of measuring accurately the hearing of persons who will receive an amount of compensation that is a direct function of the degree of their hearing loss, other problems exist. In cross-sectional studies of persons working for many years in a given noise environment, valid preexposure audiograms are seldom available. Furthermore, even if preexposure audiograms are available, one cannot overlook the effect on threshold, over the time period concerned, of such things as gradual hearing loss from the onset of increasing age, the influence of industrial chemicals, ototoxic drugs, chronic middle ear disease, infections, hereditary hearing loss of a progressive nature, head trauma, and, of course, the influence of noises outside the work environment. Sorting out these various influences has proved to be nearly impossible and has been the major stumbling block in longitudinal studies of permanent noise-induced hearing loss.

It should come as no surprise that despite the millions of audiograms that have been taken on workers since the invention of the audiometer, we still have only a rather imprecise grasp of the relations between noise exposure and NIPTS. We are able to make, however, a few general statements about NIPTS that seem reasonably well established.

In most broad-spectrum noises of industry and the military, NIPTS at 4000 and 6000 Hz will tend to appear more quickly and be larger than those at lower or higher frequencies [14]. The changes in threshold at 4000 and 6000 Hz associated with a noise that has octave-band SPLs of more than 90 dB and is substantially invariant from day to day will increase rapidly in the first few years, reaching an asymptote by 10 years or so, after which further increases occur only about as fast as in a control group of workers of the same age [1, 12]. If the noise is intense enough to develop PTS at 2000 Hz and less, however, such an asymptote does not seem to be reached [6]. It is assumed that if a worker whose NIPTS at 4000 Hz has reached an asymptote is shifted to a noisier environment, a further increase will occur; however, no evidence to either support or refute such an assumption is actually at hand.

There is some evidence that women are more resistant to NIPTS than men [11], but this evidence is usually based on cross-section studies in which initial hearing levels were not really known. Only the fact that the women's postexposure hearing levels were better than a control group of men has been substantiated. There is little doubt that both nosoacusic and sociacusic influences are greater in men than in women, and furthermore it may be easier economically for a woman who is sensitive to noise to seek quieter employment, so the question is really still open.

Whether a very young or an aged person is more susceptible to noise on the average is also unknown. Actually, for the older person the question is probably untestable. It seems unlikely that we can find an industrial population in which some workers began working at a much older age than others, and in which there were enough older workers who began the work with normal hearing, so that equal PTSs in the two groups would necessarily indicate equal susceptibility. Also, even if such a normal population could be obtained, one could argue that the older patients represented a sample biased in the direction of low susceptibility, since they had obviously been able to withstand sociacusic influences until time of employment.

The answers to many problems are still far in the future. We still have no index of noise exposure that will succinctly characterize the relative noxiousness of different noise exposures. Although, on the average, we can say that the threshold limiting value for a measurable damage from steady industrial noise is about 85 dBA for an ordinary eight-hour exposure, we do not yet have any idea of the relative hazard associated with briefer or interrupted exposures. Indeed, even the eight-hour 90 dBA value now used as the daily exposure limit by the United States is in question because of the impossibility of eliminating sociacusic and nosoacusic influences from the data on hearing loss in industry. The prospects are dim, at this time, for selecting individuals in advance of employment in noisy industries who are unusually susceptible to NIPTS by means of any index based on NITTS. Although extensive information on the temporary effects of noise exists, the relation between temporary and permanent effects is still unknown. Finally, since no satisfactory method of characterizing noise exposures has been devised, we are in the uncomfortable position of having an undefined independent variable, an undependable dependent variable, and many potent irrelevant variables! A conservative approach seems therefore in order. On the other hand, we must be aware of the antipollution activists who wish to set too-strict limits on noise levels. These people fail to realize that noise pollution differs from air and water pollution. Although our stomachs were not designed to digest mercury compounds, nor were our lungs designed to absorb sulfur dioxide, the normal function of our ears is to process sounds.

AUDIOLOGIC CONSIDERATIONS

The classic audiometric manifestation of noise-induced hearing loss and acoustic trauma is a moderate loss of sensitivity in the 4000 Hz region (Fig. 12-1). With greater exposure the 4000 Hz tonal gap grows deeper and broader, the high frequencies being affected more rapidly than the low frequencies, until finally high-frequency perception is lost entirely. After this the low frequencies are affected more and more, but typically there is always greater loss at higher than at lower frequencies.

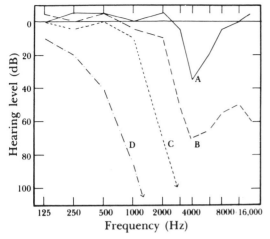

Figure 12-1. Typical audiograms illustrating the gradual progression of noise-induced hearing loss with time, from A, a narrow loss centered at 4000 Hz to D, a severe high-frequency hearing loss. (From W. D. Ward, The identification and treatment of noise-induced hearing loss. Otolaryngol. Clin. North Am. 90:89, 1969.)

The maximum loss tends to occur in the neighborhood of 4000 Hz even when the energy in the noise is more concentrated in low frequencies. An early explanation for this fact was that possibly the hair cells in the 4000 Hz region were simply more susceptible to noise damage than other hair cells. Lehnhardt [4] refuted this notion by showing that auditory fatigue and recovery at 4000 Hz were no different from fatigue and recovery at other test frequencies. The main reason therefore seems to be that the average outer ear canal resonates at approximately 3000 Hz, so that in ordinary broad-spectrum noises, the most energy will be transmitted to the inner ear in the 3000 Hz region; indeed, there is actually a 10 dB or greater amplification of sounds at that frequency. That fact, coupled with the observation that the frequency most affected by a narrow-band noise will be half an octave to an octave above the frequency of the noise itself, would predict that 4000 and 6000 Hz would be first and most strongly affected by noise.

The fact that a beginning NIHL is called the *4000 Hz notch* should not be taken to mean that the maximum is *always* at 4000 Hz. Individuals differ in sensitivity and in the characteristics of their outer and middle ears, resulting in different amounts of energy reaching the cochleas of different ears for a given frequency. So the maximum loss may often be found at 3000 or 6000 Hz and occasionally at 2000 or 8000 Hz in an individual ear.

Noise-induced hearing loss always shows loudness recruitment. Although the threshold may be as high as 70 or 80 dB HL, once the threshold is exceeded the loudness grows more rapidly than loudness grows in a normal ear. The basis of recruitment in the ear with NIPTS is open to question. The most likely explanation is the following: Permanent NIHL corresponds to a "dead" area on the basilar membrane. The hair cells are therefore unresponsive and a deficit will exist in the total neural firing at higher centers when the cochlea is stimulated. As the stimulus intensity is increased, more and more of the unaffected sensory units adjacent to the dead area are stimulated. Thus the relative contribution to the normal total firing by the dead area becomes *proportionately* less and less, so that at higher levels the total firing in the dead area is not *perceptibly* different from the firing of a normal ear.

Diplacusis is also often found in patients who exhibit NIHL. Diplacusis exists when a single frequency, presented alternately to the two ears, appears to have a different pitch in the respective ears. If the threshold of one ear is clearly normal and the other abnormal, the difference in frequency required to produce equal pitch is assumed to reflect the shift in pitch in the abnormal ear at that test frequency. The physiologic basis of diplacusis in cochlear deafness is conjectural, although it seems reasonable that if an area of the basilar membrane is dead, as previously suggested, then the first fibers to be fired as the intensity is raised will be those that correspond normally to a higher (or possibly lower) frequency.

DIFFERENTIAL DIAGNOSIS OF NOISE-INDUCED HEARING LOSS

Suppose that an elderly man seen in a clinic complains that he is not able to understand conversation as well as he used to. Threshold testing reveals a sloping bilateral sensorineural hearing loss beginning at 1000 Hz and increasing to 80 dB at 4000

Hz. There is no earlier audiogram against which to compare the present results. He indicates that it is quite noisy where he has worked for the past 10 years and now wonders if the noise might be the cause of his hearing problems.

The diagnostic audiometric work-up (see Chap. 3) will identify the cochlea as the site of lesion if it is involved in the hearing loss. One would certainly expect to see signs of loudness recruitment in NIHL. In fact, if no recruitment is noted, the loss is probably not noise-induced. On the other hand, NIHL is not the only type of sensory hearing loss. For completeness in the differential diagnosis, other possible causes of sensory damage must be considered.

History of exposure to some single explosion, such as gunfire or a firecracker, can produce a sensory hearing loss that is audiometrically indistinguishable from hearing loss developed only after years of exposure to steady industrial noise. Several years ago we studied hearing loss in a group of professional policemen who had never been exposed to high-level industrial noise and a group of men who had worked in steady noise for many years but who had little exposure to gunfire [15]. We could not distinguish between these two groups of men on the basis of any audiologic tests. The clinician can never be absolutely sure, without a series of audiograms, whether a given bilateral loss was produced by industrial noise or by a single explosion. Figure 12-2 shows three audiograms with nearly identical characteristics, of hearing losses caused by a single firecracker, steady noise, and gunfire, respectively. Only when the hearing loss is unilateral can steady industrial noise be reasonably excluded as the cause.

Questions that have been found to be of value in identifying possible causes of high-frequency hearing loss include those dealing with the onset of tinnitus, difficulty in understanding ordinary conversation, and the direct query as to whether the patient can remember a particular incident that may have damaged his hearing. Temporary difficulty in understanding speech is of course not conclusive—a loss may already have been present at the time of a particular incident that merely produced an over-

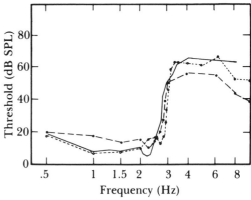

Figure 12-2. Audiograms in SPL showing threshold sensitivity in three patients with hearing losses of different causes. The solid line shows loss caused by a single firecracker explosion; the long broken line shows loss caused by several years of work in a factory with noise that exceeded 100 dB SPL; the short broken line shows hearing loss caused by regular gunfire exposure in a pistol range of a police academy. (From W. D. Ward and A. Glorig, A case of firecracker-induced hearing loss. Laryngoscope 71:1590, 1961.)

lay of auditory fatigue which drew attention to the hearing loss.

Head trauma is an important consideration. As far as the ear is concerned, a severe blow to the head is the same as an explosion and can produce the same type of hearing loss. In both cases, the stapes moves suddenly inward, sending an intense traveling wave down the cochlear partition. When the head is struck, the skull moves, but the ossicles do not because they are not connected directly to the skull. Hence the cochlea on the opposite side of the head is, as it were, driven into the stapes, and a high-frequency hearing loss is produced in that ear.

Another type of hearing loss that may masquerade as NIHL is the bilateral, progressive, hereditary high-frequency loss. In its intermediate stages the hereditary hearing loss may be quite indistinguishable from an NIHL that has progressed to the point where the loss is no longer just a notch but is as great at all frequencies above 4000 Hz as it is at 4000 Hz. Huizing and associates [2] have discussed bilateral, progressive, hereditary high-frequency loss and noted that, in the stages of the disease in which normal low-frequency hearing is present and the hearing loss is confined to frequencies above 2000 Hz, loudness recruitment is always present. Thus, a careful family history for hearing loss is an important part of the differential diagnosis of NIHL.

Other possible causes of high-frequency hearing loss that may mimic noise-induced hearing loss include exposure to industrial chemicals, ototoxic drugs, and some types of illness. Lehnhardt [4] concludes that the most convincing evidence for industrial chemicals points to benzene and carbon disulfide as producing high-frequency hearing losses. Although carbon monoxide produces high-frequency loss also, Lehnhardt concludes that its origin is probably retrocochlear. While aniline dyes may also produce a hearing loss, Lehnhardt questions whether the action is direct or a by-product of a general anemia induced by the toxin.

In regard to illness and drugs, one must again be careful in attributing a cause-effect relation to a joint occurrence. Although it was once thought that tuberculosis produced sensory hearing loss, the actual cause turned out to be a drug used in treatment—one of the various ototoxic aminoglycosides (see Chap. 10). A similar situation existed for malaria and quinine. Lehnhardt's summary [4] of the evidence of high-frequency sensory cell lesions possibly induced by diseases gives credibility only to dysentery, although some other diseases such as typhus and spotted fever may lead to high-frequency losses without recruitment.

A common result of high-intensity noise exposure is tinnitus. It may be a type of rushing noise or a high-pitched tinnitus that lasts for some time [12]. Although it has been speculated that exposures producing tinnitus are more likely to cause permanent loss than those that do not, no convincing evidence to support this notion can be found.

An occasional patient will have a recruiting high-frequency loss but no suggestive history except that he works in a steady moderate-level noise. The temptation is great, under such circumstances, to conclude that the moderate noise was responsible and that this patient may be unusu-ally susceptible to noise injury. But if the average noise level was less than 80 dBA, there is little justification for this conclusion. Individual difference in susceptibility—if such a thing really exists—apparently enters the picture only when the noise level exceeds 80 dBA. On the other hand, certain data show that a noise level of approximately 104 dBA gives everyone who works with unprotected ears in the noise a high-frequency hearing loss after a few years of exposure [11]. Thus, if this patient worked in a steady noise of 100 dBA or more, you can state just as confidently that the industrial noise was responsible as you can say that if the noise was 80 dBA or less, it was not responsible.

ADVICE FOR THE NOISE-INDUCED HEARING LOSS PATIENT

When it has been determined that the patient indeed has a permanent NIHL, there are a few statements that should be made to the patient for his best interests. The basis for the following is discussed in more detail elsewhere [10]:

1. He should wear some type of ear protection at work, or consider changing his work to quieter duties.

2. If he does so, his hearing will not get any worse until nosoacusic, presbycusic, or sociacusic factors intervene. No evidence exists that there is any sort of degenerative process that, once set in motion, will eventually wipe out the whole cochlea. If noise exposure stops, progression of NIHL stops.

3. On the other hand, no medications will make the hearing better, although at various times vitamin A, Hydergine, dextran, and other substances have been touted as ameliorative agents on the basis of poorly controlled studies.

4. The fact that he already has a hearing loss does not prove that he is any more "susceptible" to damage than the average worker, since he may have merely been more unlucky in his exposure on a couple of days. On the other hand, it is unlikely that he has unusually resistant ears. Hence, the desirability of reasonable precautions,

in his particular case, should be strenuously reiterated.

REFERENCES

1. Botsford, J. H. Theory of TTS. *J. Acoust. Soc. Am.* 44:352, 1968.
2. Huizing, E. H., van Bolhuis, A. H., and Odenthal, D. W. Studies on progressive hereditary perceptive deafness in a family audiological results. *Acta Otolaryngol.* 61:35, 1966.
3. Keeler, J. S. Compatible exposure and recovery functions for temporary threshold shift—Mechanical and electrical models. *J. Sound Vib.* 7:220, 1968.
4. Lehnhardt, E. Die Berufsschäden des Ohres. *Arch. Ohr. Nas. Kehlkopfheilk.* 185:11, 1965.
5. Melnick, W., and Maves, M. Asymptotic threshold shift (ATS) in man from 24-hour exposure to continuous noise. *Ann. Otol. Rhinol. Laryngol.* 83:820, 1974.
6. Reger, S. N., and Lierle, D. M. Changes in auditory acuity produced by low and medium intensity level exposures. *Trans. Am. Acad. Ophthalmol.* 58:433, 1954.
7. Taylor, W., Pearson, J., Mair, A., and Burns, W. Study of noise and hearing in jute weaving. *J. Acoust. Soc. Am.* 38:113, 1965.
8. Tobias, J. V., Jansen, G., and Ward, W. D. (Eds.). *Proceedings of the Third International Congress on Noise as a Public Health Problem. ASHA Reports 10.* Rockville, Md.: American Speech-Language-Hearing Association, 1980.
9. Van Dishoeck, H. A. E. The continuous threshold or detailed audiogram for recording stimulation deafness. *Acta Otolaryngol.* [Suppl.] 78:183, 1948.
10. Ward, W. D. Adaptation and Fatigue. In A. B. Graham (Ed.), *Sensorineural Hearing Processes and Disorders.* Boston: Little, Brown, 1967.
11. Ward, W. D. The identification and treatment of noise-induced hearing loss. *Otolaryngol. Clin. North Am.* 90:89, 1969.
12. Ward, W. D. Adaptation and Fatigue. In J. Jerger (Ed.), *Modern Developments in Audiology* (2d ed.). New York: Academic Press, 1973.
13. Ward, W. D. (Ed.). *Proceedings of the International Congress on Noise as a Public Health Problem.* Washington, D.C.: U.S. EPA Document 550/9-73-006, 1974.
14. Ward, W. D. Effects of Noise Exposure on Auditory Sensitivity. In D. K. Lee (Section Ed.), *Handbook of Physiology, Section 9: Reactions to Environmental Agents.* Baltimore, Md.: Williams & Wilkins, 1977.
15. Ward, W. D., Fleer, R. E., and Glorig, A. Characteristics of hearing losses produced by gunfire and by steady noise. *J. Aud. Res.* 1:325, 1961.
16. Ward, W. D., Glorig, A., and Sklar, D. Temporary threshold shift from octave-band noise: Applications to damage-risk criteria. *J. Acoust. Soc. Am.* 31:522, 1959.

SUGGESTED READING

Cantrell, R. W. (Ed.). Noise—Its effects and control. *Otolaryngol. Clin. North Am.* 12:3, 1979.

Hamernik, R. P., Henderson, D., and Salvi, R. (Eds.). *New Perspectives on Noise-Induced Hearing Loss.* New York: Raven, 1982.

Olishifski, J. B., and Harford, E. R. (Eds.). *Industrial Noise and Hearing Conservation.* Chicago: National Safety Council, 1975.

Sulkowski, W. J. *Industrial Noise Pollution and Hearing Impairment.* Springfield, Va.: U.S. Department of Commerce National Technical Information Service, 1980.

13

Congenital Hearing Loss

LaVonne Bergstrom

The term *congenital deafness* must be modified and made somewhat inaccurate to put it in a practical clinical framework. Strictly speaking, *congenital* denotes "present at birth." However, from a functional standpoint there is no substantive difference between the child whose deafness was indeed present at birth and the one who suffered a significant loss of hearing in the prespeech period. In fact, in many children it is not possible to determine whether the hearing loss was present at birth or was of somewhat later onset. In either instance, the child will fail to develop normal speech and language to a degree roughly proportional to the severity of his hearing loss. I will, therefore, arbitrarily define congenital hearing loss to include losses occurring in the prespeech period. The word *deafness* usually is inaccurate; *hearing loss* is better and will be used throughout the remainder of this chapter. True deafness or total loss of hearing is present in less than 1% of children having profound congenital hearing loss (CHL). The term *deaf-mute* is archaic.

GENERAL PRINCIPLES

CHL varies in degree and type from mild to profound and includes bilateral and unilateral sensorineural, conductive, and mixed deficits. CHL may become progressively worse. The overall incidence of CHL is unknown, probably since individuals with milder losses tend to blend with the normal population educationally and socially. Only the prevalence of profound sensorineural CHL is well established and averages from 1 : 1000 to 1 : 2000 live births.

There is considerable urgency to detect the more severe congenital hearing losses early in the prespeech period. Ideally all major losses should be detected and habilitation begun by 3 months of age. The most compelling reason for early detection is so that the young deaf child may, with amplification, have optimum opportunity to hear the sounds of his environment, particularly his native language. The unfortunate experience of our referral clinic has been that the hearing loss of the severely to profoundly deaf child is first suspected, on the average, at age 10 months, detected at age 21 months, and training and amplification first begun at 27 months of age. This is disgraceful and subjects such a handicapped child to severe language deprivation from which he is unlikely to fully recover. The effects of this early deprivation follow the child throughout his life, arresting his reading skills at the fourth-grade level, limiting his educational opportunities, and thwarting his vocational and personal achievement.

Other reasons for early detection include the relative ease of putting a hearing aid on an unopinionated infant rather than on a "terrible 2-year-old" who must demonstrate his autonomy by "rejecting" his hearing aid. Also the parents early become accustomed, although not resigned, to the realization that their child has a hearing loss. The hearing aid becomes the symbol of active intervention to combat their infant's handicap and to keep a hearing loss from developing into a concomitant language loss.

What are the reasons for delay in detecting congenital hearing loss? The first delay is due to the deceptive "normality" of the deaf baby's responses up to about 9 months of age, although the mother may suspect hearing loss very early, long before she verbalizes her worst fears. She notices that the infant does not startle to loud sounds, that the 6-month-old playing quietly does not hear his mother call his name when she is out of the range of his peripheral vision. The second delay usually occurs in the doctor's office where the ears are examined, some inadequate estimate of hearing made on the basis of stimuli which the infant *sees*, and reassurance given that the child, his ears, and his responses look normal. It is still not realized by most physicians, despite the numerous writings during the past 30 years, that it is possible to test hearing in infants, which is a reflection of the totally inadequate teaching time allotted to otolaryngology and related disciplines in most medical schools. The final delay in the severely or profoundly deaf child's life is a reflection of parental delay, and various delays in agencies to which the parents apply for help.

ETIOLOGY

There are a number of practical reasons for determining the etiology or cause of a given patient's CHL. To understand these reasons it is necessary to classify CHL by cause. In general, causes may be broadly divided into *hereditary* (genetic) and *nonhereditary* (nongenetic). Other terms used are *endogenous* and *exogenous* or *acquired*, which are approximately synonymous to genetic and nongenetic. Endogenous encompasses genetic and certain other inborn defects of a nonhereditary nature, which may, however, still be genetic, for example, mutations and chromosomal defects.

Heredity

Recessive inheritance occurs when each apparently normal parent carries one abnormal gene for the condition. Statistically, one of every four of their children may have an abnormal gene from each parent, thus allowing the trait to be expressed. The affected child is homozygous or has two abnormal genes for the trait while his parents are heterozygous or have only one abnormal gene. The homozygous child, who has two abnormal genes, is capable of passing on the trait to his children, but only if his mate either has the same trait or is a carrier for it. The likelihood of this combination of circumstances occurring is about 15% greater than in the normal population. Theoretically two of his normal siblings would be heterozygous, or carriers, and one would be entirely free of the gene, having been fortunate to inherit a normal gene from each parent. Thus a recessive trait may appear among siblings, but it is highly unlikely that the same trait would appear in other relatives or other generations unless there is intermarriage.

On the other hand, dominantly inherited traits tend to appear in each generation of an affected family. A dominant gene usually produces the trait even when the individual also carries a normal gene, because in this instance the dominant gene is "stronger." However, a genetic trait may show variable *penetrance*, that is, even though the individual has a dominant gene for a trait, for some reason the trait fails to be manifest. Genes may also show variable *expressivity*, that is, only some of the characteristics of a syndrome may appear, and they may vary in severity.

X-linked inheritance is quite rare, and is

characterized by mother-to-son transmission of the trait. An affected male then may produce daughters who are carriers but who are themselves essentially unaffected.

Environmental

Exogenous or acquired causes are those resulting from environmental influences. Evidence suggests some interplay of endogenous and exogenous factors, but these relationships, where they exist, need further clarification. *Environment* encompasses all milieux an individual encounters, from that within the uterus to those circumstances during and after birth that could deafen him. The relative distribution of these etiologies is shown in Table 13-1. In a fairly substantial percentage of cases the etiology is unknown. For those persons for whom the cause of CHL is known the prognosis for eventual outlook may be predicted. The patient or his parents will want to know the likelihood of the condition being inherited and therefore of its recurrence in the family. They would also need to know whether the loss is progressive or whether other defects or disorders might occur later in life. Hence the importance assigned to determining the cause of a given child's CHL.

Certain other terms perhaps require definition before continuing with our topic. The infant's life is divided arbitrarily into four periods: prenatal (from conception until onset of labor); perinatal (encompassing labor and delivery); neonatal (the first four weeks of extrauterine life); and postnatal. Certain environmental abnormalities during any of these periods may cause CHL as we have broadly defined it.

EMBRYOLOGY AND CONGENITAL DEAFNESS

The human embryo has three primitive tissue layers from which all organs of the body are formed: ectoderm, entoderm, and mesoderm.

1. *Ectoderm* is the surface layer that, logically, becomes the skin and various skin appendages: hair, teeth, nails, sweat glands. This surface layer also thickens and then sinks in or invaginates in cer-

Table 13-1. Etiology of Prelinguistic Hearing Loss (795 patients)

Cause	Number
GENETIC (29.3%)	233
Dominant	
CHL alone	60
With syndrome	54
Recessive	
CHL alone	70
With syndrome	32
X-linked	3
Polygenic	1
Chromosomal defect	13
NONGENETIC (21.6%)	172
Prenatal	
Rubella	85
Cytomegalovirus	5
Other viruses	1
Ototoxicity	2
Miscellaneous	6
Perinatal	
Hypoxia and prematurity	24
Erythroblastosis fetalis	10
Ototoxicity	1
Multiple factors	8
Miscellaneous	18
Postnatal	20
Neonatal meningitis	12
UNKNOWN (27.8%)	221
CHL alone	166
CHL with miscellaneous associated defects	55
SPECIFIC OTIC DEFECTS, ETIOGENESIS UNKNOWN (21.3%)	169
Conductive lesions	97
Microtia/atresia	54
Sensorineural lesions	
Michel	1
Mondini	18*
Others	16
Mixed lesions	37

* Exclusive of familial Mondini defects.

tain areas to form (a) the neural groove, which is the precursor of the entire central nervous system; (b) the optic cup, which forms the eye; and (c) the otic pit, which forms the endolymphatic part of the ear.

2. *Entoderm* may be considered the internal surface area of the embryo and forms structures that interface with the outside world. These include pharynx and its pouches, which form the eusta-

chian tube, middle ear and mastoid cavities, the thyroid gland, the larynx, trachea, and bronchi, and the intestinal tract and its various outpouchings.

3. *Mesoderm* comprises the "meat in the sandwich" between ectoderm and entoderm and ultimately forms bone, muscle, cartilage, vasculature, and such specific organs as heart, kidney, and the organs of reproduction.

It is a simplification but nevertheless helpful to remember, for example, that a congenital abnormality of the eye involves a structure whose origin is ectoderm, an origin shared by the endolymphatic portions of the inner ear—organ of Corti, stria vascularis, semicircular canals, utricle, saccule, and endolymphatic duct and sac. Therefore, the presence of a congenital eye anomaly suggests that the infant might also have a congenital inner ear abnormality. Similar analogies can be made for other tissue layer derivatives, and, in fact, many clinical disorders illustrate this principle. In general, multiple or diffuse abnormalities of the organs of a particular tissue layer imply a genetic disorder. However, it should be pointed out that sensorineural CHL occurring alone may be a genetic disorder appearing in a given family, sometimes over many generations.

The branchial arch system deserves special attention. The first branchial groove of embryologic life forms the external auditory canal; the external ear or pinna is formed from hillocks derived from branchial arches one and two. The middle ear ossicles derive from branchial arches one and two. The facial (seventh cranial) nerve's destiny is linked with that of the second branchial arch, because it is the nerve of that arch. This close relationship is shown by its passage through the temporal bone, and, of practical interest to this discussion, by the association between anomalies of middle ear and facial nerve. Most branchial anomalies occur sporadically (nongenetically) but a few are clearly genetic. However, the presence of one branchial anomaly, for example, a mandibular anomaly or microtia, increases the likelihood of a middle ear defect.

Another embryologic principle that is helpful to recall is that of timing. During the first 6 to 12 weeks of embryologic life organs are being formed. Any *teratogen,* or factor capable of causing deformity, may cause malformations of organs and systems developing during that period. A disorder that exemplifies this principle is rubella. Maternal rubella contracted during the first 3 months (first trimester) of pregnancy is capable of causing cardiac defects, cataracts, microcephaly, mental retardation, retardation both of overall growth and of organ growth, CHL, and sometimes other defects. Rubella occurring in the second and last trimesters of pregnancy may cause only CHL. Examples of teratogens are x-rays, viruses, and drugs.

These embryologic principles may alert the clinician to the need for high-risk follow-up evaluations for certain infants until the presence of CHL is established or until normal speech and language has developed.

PATHOLOGY
Embryonic Clinical Correlations
It is not within the scope of this paper to describe in detail the many CHL syndromes and the varying genetic and audiometric patterns that CHL may assume. Instead, each category will be discussed and an exemplary syndrome or two described. Others presently known will be merely listed.

Ectodermal Disorders. Ectodermal disorders, which include pigmentary disorders, are frequently genetic, the hearing loss usually sensorineural, and the mode of transmission often recessive. A representative recessive disorder is Usher's syndrome, which is characterized by profound sensorineural CHL, retinitis pigmentosa, later onset of night blindness, progressive visual loss, and ataxia. This syndrome is classic in its involvement of inner ear, eye, and central nervous system. Other recessively inherited CHL syndromes affecting ectodermal derivatives are Eldridge's syndrome of congenital severe myopia and retardation; Cockayne's syndrome; Hallgren's syndrome; Laurence-Moon-Bardet-Biedl syndrome, the congenital hearing loss associated with myoclonic epilepsy; progressive opticocochleodentate degeneration; piebaldness;

partial albinism; Richards-Rundle syndrome; Refsum's disease, Norrie's disease; Möbius syndrome; albinism-deafness; onychodystrophy; pili torti; congenital atopic dermatitis; cerebral palsy; Friedreich's ataxia; and severe infantile muscular dystrophy.

Probably the most common of the dominantly inherited syndromes of ectodermal origin is Waardenburg's. A patient with all the manifestations has outward or lateral displacement (dystopia) of the medial canthi of the eyes; heterochromia irides (one iris may be pale blue, the other brown, or a blue iris may have a brown quadrant); median white forelock of the hair; areas of depigmentation of the skin; confluence of the eyebrows over the bridge of the nose; premature graying; obstruction of the nasolacrimal duct; a rather pinched-together appearance of the nostril area of the nose; a small, downturned mouth; and sensorineural CHL. The only constant feature of the syndrome is the dystopia of the medial canthi of the eyes. The only handicapping characteristic is hearing loss, which shows diminished penetrance (present in only 20% of patients) and variable expressivity (ranging from mild or unilateral loss to profound CHL). Up to 50% of persons having inner ear involvement show vestibular manifestations. This syndrome shows predominantly ocular, auditory, and pigmentary abnormalities.

Other dominant CHL or later-onset syndromes of ectodermal derivatives include hidrotic ectodermal dysplasia, the syndrome of keratopachydermia and digital constrictions; albinism with blue irides, lentigines, or leopard syndrome; Flynn-Aird; Herrmann's; sensory radicular neuropathy; familial acoustic neuromas; knuckle pads—leukonychia; and Stickler's arthro-ophthalmopathy.

Entodermal. Not many associations of CHL with anomalies of entodermal origin have been described. Occasionally aplasia of the middle ear occurs, but most middle ear defects are of branchial origin. One recessive syndrome, that of sporadic goiter and sensorineural CHL, or Pendred's syndrome, is a common cause of recessive CHL. The thyroid gland is an outpouching of the primitive pharynx. The goiter usually occurs in adolescence, is more common in females than in males, and is due to an enzymatic defect of thyroid hormone synthesis. However, the association of these two maladies may be chance segregation of two separate genes. An alternate explanation, that the thyroid hormone defect may exert its influence early in fetal life to alter the structure and function of the inner ear, has not been proved. Only one temporal bone report is available, and the defect was a Mondini aplasia.

Other entodermal syndromes associated with CHL include Groll's congenital deafness with intestinal diverticulosis (dominant), and DiGeorge's thymic agenesis (recessive).

Mesodermal. Mesodermal derivatives comprise the bulk of bodily tissue. Associated hearing losses may be conductive or sensorineural. Many mesodermal defects are recessively inherited. An uncommon recessive syndrome, but one that manifests severe abnormalities of mesodermal derivatives, is Fanconi's syndrome. The affected patient may show absent or deformed finger-like thumbs, short stature, cardiac and kidney malformations, and pancytopenia. Mental retardation and abnormal skin pigmentation may also be present. The hearing loss is conductive owing to congenital fixation of the stapes footplate.

Other recessively inherited mesodermal syndromes and symptoms in which CHL or late-onset genetic deafness may occur are Klippel-Feil syndrome (may also be dominant); absent tibia, split-hand and foot, stippled epiphyses–deaf-mutism (De Wind et al., cited in Hemenway and Bergstrom); otopalatodigital syndrome, orofaciodigital syndrome II of Mohr; Goldenhar's syndrome; renal-genital syndrome; Taylor's syndrome; van Buchem's syndrome; osteogenesis imperfecta; osteopetrosis (Albers-Schönberg disease); and Hurler's syndrome.

Acrocephalosyndactyly (Apert's syndrome) is a dominantly inherited mesodermal complex of findings characterized by craniosynostosis, or premature closure of sutures of the skull, conductive hearing loss owing to stapes footplate fixation, and bony syndactyly or fusion of fingers and toes. The obvious defects in this syndrome involve skeletal structures.

Other dominantly inherited mesodermal defects that may be associated with CHL include cleidocranial dysostosis; hand-hearing syndrome; Treacher Collins syndrome; otofaciocervical syndrome; proximal symphalangism; Madelung's deformity; Pierre Robin syndrome; Marfan's syndrome; Crouzon's syndrome (craniofacial dysostosis); achondroplasia; Pyle's craniometaphyseal dysplasia; Alport's syndrome; the syndromes of amyloidosis, nephritis, and urticaria; diaphyseal dysplasia (Engelmann's disease); and the cardioauditory syndrome of Jervell and Lange-Nielsen.

Branchial Arch Deformities. Branchial derivative anomalies that may be associated with CHL, usually conductive in type, range from mild anomalies of the pinna, including preauricular fistulas and appendages, to severe, deforming defects, which may include severe microtia and atresia, congenital facial nerve paralysis, hypoplasia of the mandible, zygoma, branchial cysts, and fistulas and macrostomia. Other abnormalities of dubious relationship to the branchial system, such as cleft palate, epibulbar dermoids, colobomata of the lower eyelid, and absence of the parotid gland may accompany them.

Inner Ear Congenital Malformations
The pathology of CHL has been classified in a very general sense, but the student of this subject will soon become aware that in this area, as in all inner ear diseases, there is a paucity of information.

Michel anomaly of the inner ear is exceedingly rare, comprising about 1% of profoundly deaf persons. There is total absence of the inner ear, and the acoustic nerve may be absent. The facial nerve is present.

Mondini anomaly has variable manifestations, but in general there is dysplasia and hypoplasia of the cochlear duct and its contents, so that the cochlea may be considerably shortened. The modiolus is deficient. Other labyrinthine spaces and their associated nervous structures may be maldeveloped.

Scheibe malformation is believed to comprise the pathology of about 70% of profound CHL. It may be either genetic, acquired in prenatal life as a result of rubella or in postnatal life from mumps, measles, or other viruses. All the bony labyrinthine spaces and the membranous structures of the labyrinth, with the exception of the saccule, are normal. The saccule is collapsed and its sensory epithelium degenerated. The cochlea shows the following changes, most severe at the basal end of the cochlea: atrophy of the stria vascularis and organ of Corti, rolling up and epithelial encasement of the tectorial membrane in the limbus so that contact with the organ of Corti is lost, and either collapse or distention of Reissner's membrane.

Alexander anomaly is poorly defined as partial membranous cochlea aplasia.

Bing-Siebenmann anomaly is said to have abnormalities of the membranous vestibular labyrinth with or without cochlea involvement, degeneration of vestibular nerves and vessels, and dark-staining concretions in the stria vascularis of the cochlea.

DIAGNOSIS AND DETECTION
Detection is merely discovering the presence of CHL and getting some idea of type and degree of loss. Diagnosis implies establishing cause, finding associated defects, and establishing prognosis for the patient.

Detection may be effected by hearing screening or by using a high-risk register. These techniques may be applied in the newborn nursery, well-baby clinic, or doctor's office; it is hoped that only a few patients will be discovered in school or on draft board physical examinations.

Diagnosis is a more involved procedure. Central to its success is meticulous history-taking, including detailed histories of known hearing loss, speech or language delay, "retardation," and congenital defects that may be part of known congenital deafness syndromes for *every known maternal and paternal family member.* It includes prenatal history to look for the possible effects of viral infections, drugs, irradiation, and hypoxia; perinatal history with special reference to hypoxia, extreme

Table 13-2. Laboratory Evaluation of the Congenitally Hearing-impaired Child

ROUTINE STUDIES

Family audiometrics (routine, high-frequency, Bekesy, and impedance studies)
Complete blood count
Urinalysis
Serum and urine amino acids
Ophthalmologic examination

STUDIES DONE AS INDICATED

Antibody titers for rubella, cytomegalovirus, toxoplasmosis, and herpes simplex (routine if less than age 1), measles and mumps, serum immunoglobulins
Viral cultures of urine, throat, and nasopharynx for rubella and cytomegalovirus
Electrocardiography
Electroretinography
PBI, T_4, perchlorate discharge test
Petrous pyramid polytomograms
CT scan with edge enhancement
Mucopolysaccharide screening of the urine
Karyotype, buccal smear
Dermatoglyphics
VDRL and other tests for syphilis
Roentgenograms (skull, chest, long bones, cervical spine, intravenous pyelogram)
Developmental or psychologic testing
Serum pyrophosphate
Serum uric acid

Source: Adapted from J. M. Stewart, The pediatric management of the congenitally deaf child, *Otolaryngol. Clin. North Am.* (G. Hemenway and L. Bergstrom, Eds.), 4:2, 337, 1971.

blood loss, and prolonged rupture of fetal membranes; and neonatal history of hypoxia, severe erythroblastosis fetalis, and sepsis (see Table 13-1). Physical examination of the affected child includes a thorough pediatric and neurologic evaluation. The head and neck examination, which is best done by the otolaryngologist, includes inspection of the ears under the microscope, looking carefully for associated head and neck anomalies, and assessment of the vestibular system. Only then is the child referred to the laboratory and radiology for carefully selected tests as shown in Table 13-2.

After the initial workup is completed, referral is made for fitting of a hearing aid and for a training program. The audiologist and otologist should advise the family that periodic hearing tests are important because some losses may progress, perhaps making necessary a change in training. Repeat tests should be scheduled at about 3-month intervals during the period of speech and language acquisition; later, annual tests should be sufficient. The otologist must schedule the child for periodic ear, nose, and throat examinations because the child with hearing loss also may suffer from bouts of serous otitis media and from impacted cerumen. The family should be counseled in hearing conservation: (1) avoidance by the child of excessive noise or sudden loud sounds that may further damage his hearing; (2) avoidance of ototoxic medications if at all possible; (3) prompt attention to any ear complaint; and (4) no self-cleaning or self-medication of the ear. At some time before vocational training is begun a thorough evaluation of the vestibular system should be done.

It must be emphasized that follow-up by the same clinician who did the initial evaluation has considerable value to the patient. New physical findings or progression of hearing loss may provide a specific diagnosis that could not be ascertained at the first visit. Transfer of records from one institution or group of clinicians to another has value, but continuity of care, when possible, is crucial in the early years of the young child with CHL. Interdisciplinary cooperation and communication among the various specialists who are looking after the child is essential to his progress and well-being.

SUGGESTED READING

Bergstrom, L. Anomalies of the Ear. In G. English (Ed.), *Otolaryngology*, Vol. 1. Hagerstown, Md.: Harper & Row, 1979.

Black, F. O., Bergstrom, L., Downs, M. P., and Hemenway, W. *Congenital Deafness: A New Approach to Early Detection of Deafness Through a High Risk Register.* Boulder, Col.: Colorado Associated University Press, 1971.

Feingold, M., and Pashayan, H. *Genetics and Birth Defects in Clinical Practice.* Boston: Little, Brown, 1983.

Hemenway, W. G., and Bergstrom, L. (Eds.) Symposium on congenital deafness. *Otolaryngol. Clin. North Am.* Vol. 4, 1971.

Konigsmark, B., and Gorlin, R. *Genetic and Metabolic Deafness*. Philadelphia: Saunders, 1976.

Northern, J. L., and Downs, M. P. *Hearing in Children* (2d ed.). Baltimore: Williams & Wilkins, 1978.

Simmons, F. B. Identification of hearing loss in infants and young children. *Otolaryngol. Clin. North Am.* 11:19, 1978.

Ward, P. H., and McConnell, F. (Eds.) *Deafness in Childhood*. Nashville: Vanderbilt University Press, 1967.

14

Presbycusis

Charles A. Mangham
C. Thomas Yarington, Jr.

The peculiar attitude toward deafness in the United States, and indeed throughout the world, is of primary importance in considering the dilemma of persons with auditory disabilities. Hearing aids are designed to be hidden, hearing conservation programs are difficult to establish and frequently do not have widespread support, and few organized programs exist beyond childhood for detecting early hearing loss. By contrast, considerable effort is directed toward sophisticated rehabilitative measures for those without vision. In general, the person with slowly deteriorating hearing is faced with the prospect of gradual estrangement from associates and family.

Perhaps no group faces this problem to such an extent as the elderly. At least 13% [3], and perhaps as many as 60% [22], of America's 24 million elderly [67] have impaired hearing. The form of hearing loss that classically appears in the elderly is termed *presbycusis,* literally meaning "old age hearing" (Fig. 14-1).

We are all familiar with hearing aid advertisements that ask, "Can you hear, but not understand?" We are also quite familiar with the senior citizen who has difficulty hearing but when the statement is repeated in a loud voice, answers, "Don't shout, I'm not deaf." Discrimination loss and recruitment are characteristic signs of hearing loss attributed to aging [13].

PATHOPHYSIOLOGY

Diagnosis comes from correlating pathologic changes in human temporal bones with the results of hearing tests [54]. Temporal bone studies are particularly difficult in the aging ear because many pathologic processes related to aging are not accompanied by changes in hearing function [62].

For discussion purposes we grouped our analysis of pathophysiology into anatomic units beginning at the auditory periphery.

Middle Ear

The eardrum and ossicles with their joints and muscular attachments serve to transmit sound vibrations from low-impedance air to high-impedance cochlear fluids [5, 32, 65, 66]. Age-related arthritic changes occur at the joint between ossicles, but

161

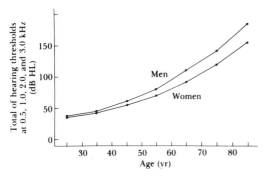

Figure 14-1. Total of pure-tone thresholds at four speech frequencies for men and women as a function of age [34]. Average threshold at each frequency is obtained by dividing the total threshold by four.

these changes are not associated with detectable conductive hearing loss [9].

Inner Ear

Two sites of inner ear dysfunction causing presbycusis have been identified: the stria vascularis and the organ of Corti.

Stria Vascularis. The stria vascularis is a separate compartment sealed off from the endolymphatic space and spiral ligament [23, 60]. This separation allows the stria to function as the power plant that generates the endolymphatic potential [7].

Strial atrophy begins in the first to second decades [29]. Atrophy may be focal or diffuse [63] and typically involves the middle and apical turns of the cochlea [30]. (Strial atrophy may be an important cause of degeneration of the organ of Corti.) Isolated strial atrophy is uncommon (Fig. 14-2). More typical is strial atrophy and degeneration of the organ of Corti at the same site along the basilar membrane (Fig. 14-3). Although there is clinical evidence of familial occurrence [54], this has not been documented histologically.

Human beings with the histopathologic finding of strial atrophy at postmortem examination typically have hearing loss during life that is equal across frequency (often termed a flat hearing loss), mild recruitment, and good speech discrimination (see Fig. 14-1). Strial atrophy may also cause dysfunction of frequency analysis. Data from animals suggest that strial atrophy may decrease the ability to differentiate between the pitch of tones of different

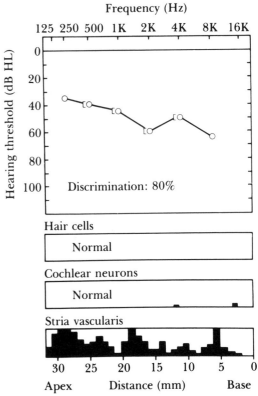

Figure 14-2. Strial presbycusis. This woman had a bilaterally symmetric hearing loss. The audiogram at age 68 years and histologic studies after her death at 72 years show results from the right ear. She had severe patchy atrophy of the stria vascularis throughout the cochlea, most severe at the apex. (Adapted from H. F. Schuknect, Pathology of the Ear. Cambridge, Mass.: Harvard University Press, 1974.)

frequencies because of impaired place-pitch specificity (frequency selectivity). Although we are not aware of an animal model for strial atrophy, there is evidence of an association between increased threshold and decreased frequency selectivity. For example, single cochlear nerve fiber recordings from hypoxic animals show loss of the low threshold, sharply tuned portion of the frequency threshold (tuning) curve at the characteristic frequency leaving a high threshold and broad tuning curve [10, 11]. High threshold and sharp tuning curves were not detected. Critical bandwidth data from subjects with strial atrophy would be of interest to test the hypothesis of impaired frequency selectivity.

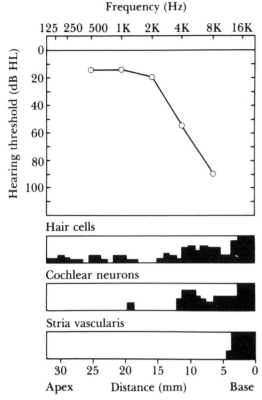

Figure 14-3. Sensory presbycusis. This 70-year-old man had a bilaterally symmetric high-frequency hearing loss. The audiogram and temporal bone histology show results from the right ear. The loss of hair cells is greatest at the basal end of the cochlea. The loss of cochlear neurons probably is secondary to degeneration of supporting cells of the organ of Corti. (Adapted from H. F. Schuknect, Pathology of the Ear. *Cambridge, Mass.: Harvard University Press, 1974.)*

Organ of Corti. The organ of Corti is on the scala medial side of the basilar membrane adjacent to the bony spiral lamina. Its sensory cells, the inner and outer hair cells, convert the mechanical energy of sound vibration into electrical impulses that ascend the central auditory pathway.

Degeneration of the organ of Corti begins in childhood, progresses slowly, and even in advanced age is typically limited to the basal end of the cochlea [16, 29]. Degeneration begins with distortion and flattening, followed by a loss of hair cells and supporting cells necessary for viability of spiral ganglion nerve fibers [4]. The loss of supporting cells causes a secondary neural degeneration.

Subjects with atrophy of the basal end of the organ of Corti at postmortem examination usually had in life an increased threshold for high-frequency pure tones and reduced speech discrimination (see Fig. 14-2). The discrimination loss may be due to decreased sensitivity for the high-frequency content in speech or to impaired frequency selectivity [38]. The anatomic lesion responsible for impaired frequency selectivity may be in the cochlea [31] or cochlear nucleus [45].

Assuming applicability of data from animals, single cochlear nerve fiber recordings from animals with kanamycin-associated hair cell loss in the basal end of the cochlea show elevated thresholds at the characteristic frequency and either broad tuning curves or sharp tuning curves [6] from fibers innervating the area adjacent to the injury. Areas in the cochlea innervated by fibers with broad tuning curves should have poorer frequency selectivity than areas with sharp tuning curves. Variability in the width of the tuning curves may account for variability in frequency selectivity in patients with presbycusis who were otherwise matched by age and audiometric configuration [38].

Another possible explanation for discrimination loss may be that fibers coded for high frequencies above the speech range may contribute speech information in the presence of noise. In cochlear nerve fiber recordings from animals, broad-band noise causes an increase in threshold that is greater at the characteristic frequency than in the low-frequency tail of the tuning curve [10]. These data may apply, for example, to the task of synthetic sentence identification with competing spoken babble. Stimulus intensity may be suprathreshold for the low-frequency tail of fibers coded for high frequencies. In normal ears, these fibers may contribute to speech understanding by carrying information to more central auditory centers. Presbycusic ears with hair cell loss at the cochlear base cannot activate these fibers coded for high frequencies. These presbycusics would have a smaller population of auditory nerve fibers carrying speech information, even though their fiber counts may be normal.

Central Auditory Pathways

The central auditory pathways begin in the spiral ganglion efferent fibers in the cochlea and proceed to the brain stem, midbrain, and auditory cortex. Generally, anatomic material is limited to temporal bones because access to material that includes the whole auditory system, including central nervous system tissue, is uncommon [18].

How central relay stations function in the coding of speech information is only partly known. The cochlear nucleus may accentuate amplitude and frequency modulation, decode low-frequency pitch information, and provide temporal integration [41–46]. The role of higher relays (inferior colliculus, medial geniculate, and auditory cortex) for speech processing is not known.

The degree of hearing impairment is greater in central than in peripheral (inner ear) presbycusis. In peripheral presbycusis, cochlear nerve fibers innervating the basal end of the cochlea may degenerate secondary to the loss of supporting and sensory cells in the organ of Corti. This loss differs from central auditory presbycusis, in which the cochlear nerve fiber loss is greater than can be explained by organ of Corti degeneration (Fig. 14-4).

The losses in the mid-frequency region of the cochlear apex associated with central auditory presbycusis cause greater decrement in speech discrimination than losses confined to the high-frequency region of the base [50]. Gaeth [12] used the words *phonemic regression* to describe the poor speech understanding associated with central presbycusis.

DIFFERENTIAL DIAGNOSIS

Presbycusis is a diagnosis of exclusion. Other forms of treatable or recognizable pathology must first be excluded (e.g., head trauma, ototoxicity drugs, ear disease, noise exposure, ear surgery, and family history of hearing loss). Criteria suggesting the diagnosis include symmetric hearing loss, conductive loss less than 10 dB, and age more than 65 years [35].

The configuration of the audiogram may be helpful in differentiating between fa-

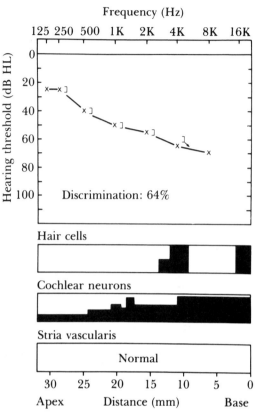

Figure 14-4. *Central auditory presbycusis. This man had a bilaterally symmetric hearing loss. The audiogram at age 80 years and temporal bone histology after his death at 81 years show results from the left ear. He had diffuse loss of cochlear neurons that was greater than could be accounted for by degeneration of supporting cells of the organ of Corti. (Adapted from H. F. Schuknect,* Pathology of the Ear. *Cambridge, Mass.: Harvard University Press, 1974.)*

milial hearing loss and presbycusis. In a retrospective review of 99 persons more than 65 years old, 38 of the 85 patients without a family history of hearing loss had a loss that increased in frequency at greater than 10 dB per octave. Of the 14 subjects with a family history of hearing loss, 13 had a slope less than 10 dB per octave. Subjects with a familial hearing loss had better speech discrimination for a given pure-tone average threshold [35].

The hearing loss is flat or gradually sloping in both familial hearing loss in the elderly and in central auditory presbycusis. However, patients with central presbycusis tend to be older (average, 74 years) and have difficulty understanding speech in the presence of background noise [21].

Presbycusis is generally associated with increasing hearing loss at high frequencies. By contrast, noise-induced hearing loss is generally a pure-tone hearing loss occurring between 3.0 to 6.0 kHz with return to near normal hearing at higher levels. Differentiation of age-related hearing loss from noise-induced hearing loss is best done by comparing prenoise and postnoise exposure audiograms, but if this is not possible, a correction for age-related hearing loss can be made from normative data [14, 15, 46]. Guidelines for calculating age-adjusted hearing impairment have been published [2, 34].

Ideally, normative data on the effects of aging on auditory sensitivity should be obtained from a defined population to eliminate potential bias associated with self-selection. For example, the hearing thresholds of volunteers at the Wisconsin State Fair were elevated compared to those of Mabaans, a primitive African tribe in the Sudan (Fig. 14-5), whereas American men selected on the basis of lack of noise exposure had thresholds similar to those of Mabaan men (see Fig. 14-5). Well-defined population studies are limited. Pooled data

Figure 14-5. Hearing thresholds for men in their sixth decade. Closed circles indicate mean hearing threshold for the better and poorer hearing ear for American men without noise exposure [46]. Open squares indicate mean hearing thresholds for men of the Mabaan tribe, Sudan, Africa [51].

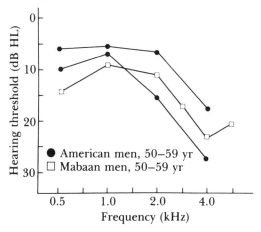

from the better surveys [61] indicate that age-related hearing impairment more than 25 dB HL begins at 62 years in men and 68 years in women (see Fig. 14-1).

AUDIOLOGIC TESTS

Audiometric evaluation of thresholds for pure tones provides only an estimate of the degree of hearing loss as threshold apparently reflects the activity of only a few auditory nerve fibers. Up to 75% of auditory nerve fibers can be lost without an increase in the threshold for pure tones [56].

Tests of discrimination of phonetically balanced monosyllable words (PB speech discrimination) add further information about the function of the auditory system under ideal signal-to-noise conditions. These tests identify gross functional impairment but cannot reliably differentiate between peripheral and central presbycusis [20, 33].

Several tests can be used to evaluate patients with clinical evidence of central auditory dysfunction: acoustic reflexes, brief tone audiometry, frequency selectivity, speech with competing noise or reverberation, and time-compressed speech.

Parameters of the acoustic reflex response are threshold, latency, rate of rise, amplitude, amplitude decay, and relaxation. Thresholds for pure-tone stimuli are similar among elderly patients with peripheral and central auditory dysfunction [20] and in normal hearing young and elderly patients [58, 64]; therefore reflex thresholds for pure-tone stimuli appear to be insensitive to central auditory dysfunction. On the other hand, thresholds for broad-band noise stimuli are elevated in normal-hearing elderly persons compared to young adults [58]; therefore reflex thresholds for broad-band noise stimuli may be sensitive to identification of central auditory dysfunction.

The amplitude (magnitude) of the reflex response is reduced in normal hearing elderly persons when compared to young adults [17, 58, 59, 64], possibly from age-related fiber atrophy and splitting of the stapedius muscle [19]. However, reduction in magnitude also occurs in animals with auditory nerve compression [37] and in human beings with acoustic tumors suggesting that age-related decreases in the numbers of functioning auditory nerve fibers can also account for reduction in magnitude with age. Reflex magnitude may be difficult to apply clinically in presbycusis because it exhibits considerable variability.

The latency of the reflex response is less variable than reflex magnitude and therefore may be useful clinically. Our preliminary studies indicate that reflex latency is prolonged in some elderly patients. Reflex rate of rise, amplitude decay, and relaxation have not been studied in persons with presbycusis.

Brief tone audiometry measures the ability of the auditory system to integrate sound energy over time. This is done typically by (1) determining the threshold-duration function for pure tones and (2) determining the shortest duration at which tones still have some pitch character [1]. Further shortening of the signal results in the patient's hearing only a click.

Brief tone audiometry is abnormal in patients with a clinical diagnosis of peripheral auditory dysfunction [1, 52] but normal in patients with an acoustic tumor [53]. To our knowledge, brief tone audiometry has not yet been used to evaluate presbycusis but has been used to screen elderly persons for cerebral circulatory impairment in the selection of patients for arteriography [4]. Abnormal temporal integration in patients with vertebral artery insufficiency suggests that brief tone audiometry potentially can be used to screen persons for central auditory evaluation. Temporal integration at least in part is a function of the cochlear nucleus [45] so that persons with central presbycusis should have impaired integration.

Determination of critical bandwidth may be of benefit in determining disorders of frequency selectivity [38]. The test can be done with tonal or complex maskers. Tonal masking involves measuring threshold for one tone in the presence of a second tone as a function of the frequency interval between tones. The results are similar in configuration to threshold tuning curves recorded from single auditory nerve fibers [68].

The most important part of the audio-metric evaluation of presbycusis is to determine how the auditory system functions in the real world environment of poor acoustics and unfavorable signal-to-noise ratios. This determination can be done by using speech with competing noise [27, 49], time-compressed speech [33], or speech with reverberation [8].

One method for testing speech discrimination in noise is by determining scores for performance versus intensity functions (PI) for synthetic sentence identification (SSI). The test is composed of ten third-order sentences recorded in nine permutations. The sentences are presented in the presence of competing discourse at the same intensity, a signal-to-noise ratio of 0 dB [28]. There is a decrement in the PI-SSI function compared to the PI-phonetically balanced monosyllable word (PB) function that begins in the seventh decade and is greater for the right ear than the left. This decrement in the PI-SSI function tentatively has been attributed to central auditory dysfunction [57].

Another test is time-compressed speech, which may be considered the speech equivalent of brief tone audiometry. Lists of words are presented at a normal rate and then the duration is compressed, typically by 20, 40, and 60% [33].

REHABILITATION

In general, rehabilitation in presbycusis is centered around amplification with a hearing aid [21, 24, 26, 48]. Hearing aids use filtering and input and output compression to even intensity across frequency at threshold and suprathreshold levels. Therefore, hearing aids only compensate for loss of sensitivity. There have been no developments for treating loss of frequency selectivity. A trial period of hearing aid use is essential prior to purchase because only 44% (N = 604) of elderly persons use aids more than eight hours per day [25]. Frequent counseling of the patient and the family is necessary to determine whether the instrument fits the individual's capabilities and requirements. Eyesight should be evaluated because it affects adjunctive skills such as lipreading, which can reduce the overall communication handicap [47].

Coordination and other health problems that may affect the ability to adjust to a hearing aid should be considered.

Although presbycusis does not cause middle ear hearing loss, elderly persons may have middle ear dysfunction from other causes. For middle ear hearing loss, the hearing aid need only increase intensity to compensate for impairment in the middle ear transformer mechanism. Hearing aid failures usually occur in elderly patients whose hearing loss is too mild to warrant the inconvenience of wearing an aid [40].

Patients with inner ear presbycusis have intermediate success with hearing aids. Some hearing aid users complain of excessive loudness recruitment and difficulty in hearing in the presence of competing noise. Patients with hearing loss from strial atrophy may have better success than patients with sensory degeneration [55].

Hearing aid requirements are greatest in central auditory presbycusis because of the need for performing complex functions such as decoding of place pitch, periodicity pitch, and temporal integration [45]. This group has the largest percentage of hearing aid nonusers (89%; N = 18), usually because the hearing aid actually decreases speech discrimination [40], perhaps because of increased distortion with increased loudness. Persons with impaired binaural interaction may be expected to have difficulty using binaural aids. Since central dysfunction frequently is asymmetric, the best ear for central auditory function should be selected for fitting of a monaural aid. Family members should be counseled to reduce speech rate if there is a disorder in temporal integration or to provide optimum listening conditions if there is impaired discrimination with competing noise. Adjunctive measures such as facing the subject to facilitate lipreading may be helpful.

Certain communication problems involving the use of telephone, radio, and television cannot be solved by the use of a hearing aid or by lipreading. Special instruments have been developed to help solve these problems [39]. Not all of these instruments are appropriate for every hearing-impaired person. The instruments are available either through the telephone company business office, hearing aid dispenser, or radio and television repair service.

Telephone conversation may offer the hearing-impaired person considerable difficulty. Devices have been incorporated into the hearing aid or telephone handset to increase the desired signal without increasing noise, which is an advantage over the standard hearing aid. Most hearing aids have a telephone switch that turns off the aid's microphone and activates an induction coil. When the telephone receiver is placed in contact with the hearing aid, the magnetic field of the receiver induces an electrical current in the hearing aid coil. However, new telephone receivers have eliminated electromagnetic leakage that prevents the signal from activating the hearing aid induction coil. The telephone company has provided an adapter for the newer telephone receivers that permits the hearing aid telephone switch to work.

Another approach is to increase the intensity of the signal in the telephone handset. Some handsets are equipped with a thumb-operated wheel that permits adjustment of the loudness of the incoming signal. A portable pocket-sized battery-operated amplifier is available that simply clips to the telephone receiver.

Some hearing-impaired persons have difficulty hearing the telephone bell. The typical presbycusic patient with a hearing loss for high frequencies should substitute a low-frequency bell for the standard bell. The telephone company offers the following alerting devices: bells enclosed in the telephone set ranging from 805 to 4060 Hz, bells not enclosed in the telephone set ranging from 580 to 1500 Hz, a low-frequency tone ringer (580–1500 Hz), a plastic gong that makes a buzzer-like sound, and a unit called "signalman" that activates a flashing lamp when the telephone rings.

Families watching television may have conflicts over sound intensity when the group includes normal-hearing and hearing-impaired members. A frequently successful solution is to fit the hearing-impaired listener with a hearing aid. However, an aid is not satisfactory when other household sounds are distracting. If the aid is equipped with a telephone switch, an induction coil can be connected to the loudspeaker of the television and the signal routed to a second coil placed close to the aid similar to using the aid's telephone switch with a telephone receiver. A variation of this approach is to produce a magnetic field in the room by a wire loop running from the television set around the baseboard of the viewing room. An alternative to hearing aids is placement of a remote amplifier and speaker near the hearing-impaired listener allowing the listener to control loudness from his seat.

The true measure of success or failure of rehabilitation is the long-term satisfaction manifested by the patient, his family, and associates, which may or may not correspond with objective test results. An illustration of one problem infrequently recognized may be pertinent. A past president of the United States was suffering from advanced hearing loss, possibly due to otosclerosis. The patient would not use a hearing instrument. When it was suggested that stapes surgery might offer some increase in hearing, the president replied, "All my life I have worked to attain peace in the world, and now while I have it, you want to alter the situation." The anecdote demonstrates that some elderly patients do not really desire to enter the hearing world. Obviously, rehabilitation efforts on their behalf will generally meet with failure.

REFERENCES

1. Abramovich, S. J. Hearing investigation in relation to the duration of acoustic signals. *Laryngoscope* 88:334, 1978.
2. American Academy of Otolaryngology Committee on Hearing and Equilibrium. Guide for the evaluation of hearing handicap. *J.A.M.A.* 241:2055, 1979.
3. Corso, J. F. Presbycusis, hearing aids and aging. *Audiology* 16:146, 1977.
4. Creel, W., Powers, S. R., and Boomsliter, P. C. Tonal sensation as a criterion of vertebral artery insufficiency. *Arch. Surg.* 98:309, 1969.
5. Dallos, P. *The Auditory Periphery.* New York: Academic Press, 1973.
6. Dallos, P., Ryan, A., Harris, D., McGee, T., and Ozdamar, O. Cochlear Frequency Selectivity in the Presence of Hair Cell Damage. In E. F. Evans and J. P. Wilson (Eds.), *Psychophysics and Physiology of Hearing.* London: Academic Press, 1977.
7. Davis, H. A model for transducer action in the cochlea. *Cold Spring Harbor Symp. Quant. Biol.* 30:181, 1965.
8. Duquesnoy, A. J., and Plomp, R. Effect of reverberation and noise on the intelligibility of sentences in cases of presbycusis. *J. Acoust. Soc. Am.* 68:537, 1980.
9. Etholm, B., and Belal, A. Senile changes in the middle ear joints. *Ann. Otol. Rhinol. Laryngol.* 83:49, 1974.
10. Evans, E. F. Auditory Frequency Selectivity and the Cochlear Nerve. In E. Zwicker and E. Terhardt (Eds.), *Facts and Models in Hearing.* New York: Springer Verlag, 1974.
11. Evans, E. F., and Klinke, R. Reversible effects of cyanide and furosemide on the tuning of single cochlear fibers. *J. Physiol.* [*London*] 242:129, 1974.
12. Gaeth, J. H. A study of phonemic regression in relation to hearing loss. Northwestern University. Ph.D. Dissertation. Chicago, 1948.
13. Gilad, O., and Glorig, A. Presbycusis: The aging ear. *J. Am. Audiol. Soc.* 4:195, 1979.
14. Glorig, A., and Davis, H. Age, noise and hearing loss. *Ann. Otol. Rhinol. Laryngol.* 70:556, 1961.
15. Glorig, A., and Nixon, B. A. Distribution of hearing loss in various populations. *Ann. Otol. Rhinol. Laryngol.* 69:497, 1960.
16. Guild, S. The progression of impaired hearing for high tones during childhood. *Laryngoscope* 60:885, 1950.
17. Habener, S. A., and Snyder, J. M. Stapedius reflex amplitude and decay in normal hearing ears. *Arch. Otolaryngol.* 100:294, 1974.
18. Hansen, C. C. The aetiology of perceptive deafness. *Acta Otolaryngol. Suppl.* 309, 1973.
19. Harty, M. Elastic tissue in the middle ear cavity. *J. Laryngol. Otol.* 67:723, 1953.
20. Hayes, D., and Jerger, J. Low frequency hearing loss in presbycusis. *Arch. Otolaryngol.* 105:9 (a), 1979.
21. Hayes, D., and Jerger, J. Aging and the use of hearing aids. *Scand. Audiol.* 8:33(b), 1979.
22. Herbst, K. G., and Humphrey, C. Hearing impairment and mental state in the elderly living at home. *Br. Med. J.* 281:903, 1980.
23. Jahnke, K. The fine structure of freeze-fractured intercellular junctions in the guinea pig inner ear. *Acta Otolaryngol.* [*Suppl.*] 336:1, 1975.
24. Jeffers, J. The social adequacy of two selected samples of geriatric-presbycusis with

significant hearing loss. *Int. Audiol.* 8:317, 1969.

25. Jensen, P. A., and Funch, E. The Result of Hearing Aid Treatment of Geriatric Patients. In G. Liden (Ed.), *Geriatric Audiology.* Stockholm: Alqvist and Wiksell, 1968. Pp. 110–114.

26. Jerger, J. Audiological findings in aging. *Adv. Otorhinolaryngol.* 20:115, 1973.

27. Jerger, J., and Hayes, D. Diagnostic speech audiometry. *Arch Otolaryngol.* 103:216, 1977.

28. Jerger, J., Speaks, C., and Trammel, J. A new approach to speech audiometry. *J. Speech Hear. Disord.* 33:318, 1968.

29. Johnsson, L., and Hawkins, J. Sensory and neural degeneration with aging as seen in microdissections of the human inner ear. *Ann. Otol. Rhinol. Laryngol.* 81:179(a), 1972.

30. Johnsson, L., and Hawkins, J. Symposium on basic ear research. II. Strial atrophy in clinical and experimental deafness. *Laryngoscope* 82:1105, 1972.

31. Kiang, N. Y-S., Moxon, E. C., and Levine, R. A. Auditory Nerve Activity in Cats with Normal and Abnormal Cochleas. In G. E. W. Westenholme and J. Knight (Eds.), *Sensorineural Hearing Loss.* London: Churchill, 1970.

32. Killion, M. C., and Dallos, P. Impedance matching by the combined effects of the outer and middle ear. *J. Acoust. Soc. Am.* 66:599, 1979.

33. Konkle, D. F., Beasley, D. S., and Bess, F. H. Intelligibility of time-altered speech in relation to chronological aging. *J. Speech Hear. Res.* 20:108, 1977.

34. Lebo, C. P., and Reddell, R. C. The presbycusic component in occupational hearing loss. *Laryngoscope* 82:1399, 1972. Corrected, 83:2050, 1973.

35. Lowell, S. H., and Paparella, M. M. Presbycusis: What is it? *Laryngoscope* 87:1711, 1977.

36. Mangham, C. A., Lindeman, R. C., and Dawson, W. D. Stapedius reflex quantification in acoustic tumor patients. *Laryngoscope* 90:242, 1980.

37. Mangham, C. A., and Miller, J. M. A case for further quantification of the stapedius reflex. *Arch. Otolaryngol.* 105:593, 1979.

38. Margolis, R. H., and Goldberg, S. M. Auditory frequency selectivity in normal and presbycusic patients. *J. Speech Hear. Res.* 23:603, 1980.

39. Maurer, J. F., and Rupp, R. R. *Hearing and Aging.* New York: Grune & Stratton, 1979.

40. McCandless, G. A., and Parkin, J. L. Hearing aid performance relative to site of lesion. *Otolaryngol. Head Neck Surg.* 87:871, 1979.

41. Møller, A. R. Unit responses in the rat cochlear nucleus to repetitive, transient sounds. *Acta Physiol. Scand.* 75:542, 1969.

42. Møller, A. R. Coding of sounds in lower levels of the auditory system. *Q. Rev. Biophys.* 5:59(a), 1972.

43. Møller, A. R. Coding of amplitude and frequency modulated sounds in the cochlear nucleus of the rat. *Acta Physiol. Scand.* 86:223(b), 1972.

44. Møller, A. R. Coding of time-varying sounds in the cochlear nucleus. *Audiology* 17:446, 1977.

45. Møller, A. R. Neurophysiological basis of discrimination of speech sounds. *Audiology* 17:1, 1978.

46. Nixon, J., Glorig, A., and High, W. Changes in air and bone conduction thresholds as a function of age. *J. Laryngol. Otol.* 76:288, 1962.

47. Noble, W. G. Critical factors in the assessment of deafness due to noise. Maico Audiological Library Series II, No. 8. Minneapolis: Maico Hearing Instruments, 1974.

48. Northern, J. L. Visual and Auditory Rehabilitation for Adults. In J. Katz (Ed.), *Handbook of Clinical Audiology.* Baltimore: Williams & Wilkins, 1972.

49. Orchik, D. J., and Roddy, N. The SSI and NU6 in clinical hearing and evaluation. *J. Speech Hear. Disord.* 45:401, 1980.

50. Otte, J. Estudio del ganglio espiral y su relacion con la discrimination. *Rev. Otorinolaring.* 28:89, 1968.

51. Rosen, S., Bergman, M., Plester, D., El-Mofty, A., and Satti, M. H. Presbycusis study of a relatively noise-free population in the Sudan. *Ann. Otol. Rhinol. Laryngol.* 71:727, 1962.

52. Sanders, J. W., and Honig, E. A. Brief tone audiometry. *Arch Otolaryngol.* 85:640, 1967.

53. Sanders, J. W., Josey, A. F., and Kemker, F. J. Brief tone audiometry in patients with VIIIth nerve tumor. *J. Speech Hear. Res.* 14:172, 1971.

54. Schuknecht, H. F. *Pathology of the Ear.* Cambridge, Mass.: Harvard University Press, 1974.

55. Schuknecht, H. F., and Ishii, T. Hearing loss caused by atrophy of the stria vascularis. *Jpn. J. Otol.* 69:1825, 1966.

56. Schuknecht, H. F., and Woellner, R. C. Hearing losses following partial section of the cochlear nerve. *Laryngoscope* 63:441, 1953.

57. Shirinian, M. J., and Arnst, D. J. Patterns

in the performance-intensity functions for phonetically balanced word lists and synthetic sentences in aged listeners. *Arch. Otolaryngol.* 108:15, 1982.

58. Silman, S., and Gelfand, S. A. Effect of sensorineural hearing loss on the stapedius reflex growth function in the elderly. *J. Acoust. Soc. Am.* 69:1099, 1981.

59. Silman, S., Popelka, G., and Gelfand, S. Effect of sensorineural hearing loss on acoustic stapedius reflex growth functions. *J. Acoust. Soc. Am.* 65:1406, 1981.

60. Smith, C. Structure of the stria vascularis and the spiral prominence. *Ann. Otol. Rhinol. Laryngol.* 66:521, 1957.

61. Spoor, A. Presbycusis values in relation to noise-induced hearing loss. *Int. Audiol.* 6:48, 1967.

62. Suga, F., and Lindsay, J. R. Histopathological observations of presbycusis. *Ann. Otol. Rhinol. Laryngol.* 85:169, 1976.

63. Takahashi, T. The ultrastructure of the pathologic stria vascularis and spiral prominence in man. *Ann. Otol. Rhinol. Laryngol.* 80:721, 1971.

64. Thompson, D. J., Sills, J. A., Recke, K. S., and Bui, D. C. Acoustic reflex growth in the aging adult. *J. Speech Hear. Res.* 23:405, 1980.

65. Tonndorf, J. The mechanism of hearing loss in early cases of endolymphatic hydrops. *Ann. Otol. Rhinol. Laryngol.* 66:766, 1957.

66. Tonndorf, J. Bone Conduction. In W. D. Keidel and W. D. Neff (Eds.), *Auditory System (Handbook of Sensory Physiology,* Vol. 5/3). New York: Springer-Verlag, 1976. Pp. 37–84.

67. U.S. Department of Health, Education and Welfare. Information Service Bull. No. 63-11. Washington, D.C.: Vocational Rehabilitation Administration, 1963.

68. Zwicker, E. On a Psychophysical Equivalent of Tuning Curves. In E. Zwicker and E. Terhardt (Eds.), *Facts and Models of Hearing.* New York: Springer-Verlag, 1974.

15

The Acoustic Nerve Tumor

Marlin Weaver
Steven J. Staller

The accurate identification of an acoustic nerve tumor is among the most formidable diagnostic problems facing the otolaryngologist and audiologist. Although the classic symptoms of the acoustic tumor (also known as an eighth nerve or auditory nerve tumor) have been well documented [16, 17, 32], clinicians must beware of diagnostic misadventures [11]. The purpose of this chapter is to review the basic pathology of the acoustic nerve tumor and to discuss the clinical workup necessary for its identification. Additional diagnostic considerations are explained and case reports that reflect interesting foibles in acoustic nerve tumor diagnosis are presented.

NOSOLOGY OF THE ACOUSTIC TUMOR

A description of tumors and their related symptomatology evolves from considerations of the primary body unit, the cell. The mechanics of cell division are controlled by many factors. If these controls are interrupted and normal cell division rate is exceeded, an abnormal growth known as a tumor or *neoplasm* can occur. Tumors are generally classified as benign or malignant. Benign tumors are similar in organization to the parent cell structure. As benign tumors grow they tend to occupy space by displacing other soft tissue and may even erode bone. Malignant tumors are different from benign tumors in that they are not typical of the parent structure. Malignant tumors invade the surrounding normal structures, thereby destroying them. Malignant tumors have a potential to metastasize by vascular or lymphatic transport to other parts of the body.

The acoustic nerve tumor is a benign tumor that usually arises from the vestibular nerve sheath, and thus should more accurately be called a *vestibular neurilemmoma* or *schwannoma*. These tumors develop from the nerve sheath cells rather than from the nerve itself. During the embryonic period the vestibular nerve sheath grows medially from the otic capsule vestibule toward the brain stem. Coincident nerve development occurs laterally from the brain stem toward the peripheral vestibular nerve sheath. The interface location of the meeting of the nerve sheath and nerve fiber is the most common site for potential benign neoplasms [28].

It is fortunate for the diagnostician that the acoustic tumor usually originates within the internal auditory meatus. As the tumor grows, pressure is exerted on the other nerve fibers located within the internal auditory meatus—the facial nerve, two vestibular nerves, and the cochlear nerve—thereby creating patient complaints and symptoms that lead to accurate diagnosis. Growth of the tumor in the internal auditory meatus may erode the bone of the internal auditory meatus causing a bony defect, which may be observed by x-ray study. Exceptions to the routine growth pattern exist, however: Wanamaker [41] described an acoustic tumor that originated in the inner ear vestibule; Gussen [15] reported a case in which the tumor originated in the modiolus of the cochlea; Fisch [10] presented a case where the tumor arose from the cochlear nerve rather than the vestibular nerve; Nauton and Petasnick [27] discussed six cases of acoustic tumor that originated in the cerebellopontile angle position of the posterior cranial fossa.

Acoustic nerve tumors are commonly identified during the third or fourth decade of the patient's life, and continue to grow slowly through the sixth and seventh decade. However, cases of acoustic tumors in children, although rare, have been reported [3, 5, 9, 23, 42]. The total number of published cases of children with acoustic nerve tumors is approximately ten. It is vitally important that the clinician not overlook the possibility of such tumors in children.

Naturally, the size of the tumor is most important since the risk of morbidity and mortality associated with removal of large tumors is considerable. The capsule of large tumors may compress the brain stem, creating the risk of cardiac and respiratory complications on removal. Care must be exercised to avoid damage to the displaced cerebellum at the time of surgery, creating severe postoperative complications, which may include loss of motor coordination. Large tumors are often removed at the expense of the patient's facial nerve. Ian

MacKenzie [25] studied 130 postoperative acoustic tumor patients and found that less than half were able to return to their preoperative mode of life. He was especially impressed with the devastating effect of postoperative facial paralysis in female patients who withdrew from society and family life.

Because of the numerous possible complications associated with removal of large tumors, early identification of the small tumor is essential. Small tumors are growths less than 2 cm, which may be surgically removed through the patient's ear, so that he may return to normal life and work within three weeks following surgery. As the diagnostic acumen develops, the ability to identify tumors early should increase the incidence of surgical removal of small tumors.

THE CLINICAL WORKUP

Patients with acoustic tumors may have any variety of six basic clinical symptoms: (1) hearing loss, (2) vertigo, (3) tinnitus, (4) parasthesia of the face, (5) anesthesia of the face, and (6) facial weakness or paralysis. The initial three symptoms are perhaps the most important in early tumor identification. The symptoms relating to facial feeling and movement are usually found late in the course of the disease, and are especially interesting because the facial nerve seems to have a remarkable tolerance for compression without showing signs of abnormal function. Facial function may be normal for a long time even in the presence of a large tumor. Unfortunately, the major problem in diagnosing an acoustic tumor is that despite our expected "classic" symptoms, few patients actually fit into the expected picture. Numerous patients with confirmed acoustic tumor *do not* show expected patterns of symptoms.

Patient History

The typical patient appears with a complaint of unilateral hearing loss or pressure sensations in the ear. The history of the loss of hearing is usually gradual, progressive, and unilateral. Patients are also occasionally seen with sudden unilateral sensorineural hearing loss or normal hearing. Tinnitus is a prominent symptom in nearly 75% of acoustic tumor patients. Another early symptom, and a common reason for the patient to seek help, is vertigo. The symptom is usually described by the patient as "an unsteadiness." The vertigo may be related to a particular head position or change in head position. However, some 15% of acoustic tumor patients have no vestibular symptoms. When patients describe any of the previous complaints, which are accompanied by valid clinical findings, the otolaryngologist is obliged to conduct further examination, or the audiologist must ensure otologic referral to pursue the possibility of acoustic tumor.

A general neurologic examination is necessary to focus attention on the function of those cranial nerves most likely to be affected by the presence of an acoustic tumor. Sensory function of the face and of the cornea of the eye, served by the trigeminal (fifth) nerve, is tested with cotton. Motor function of the facial musculature is noted through facial movements that show emotional expression through smiling and frowning.

Audiometric Evaluation
The systematic evaluation of the auditory effects of eighth nerve lesions constitutes an important aspect of the diagnostic regimen for acoustic tumors. In 1962 Jerger [16] proposed a battery of audiometric procedures to differentiate pathology affecting the eighth nerve from cochlear or middle ear disorders. His original battery included Bekesey audiometry, the alternate binaural loudness balance (ABLB), and the short increment sensitivity index (SISI). According to Jerger [16], the classic eighth nerve battery profile included a low SISI score (0 to 20%), normal loudness appreciation with no loudness recruitment, and a type III or IV Bekesey tracing. He strongly advocated the interpretation of overall patterns for diagnosis, because the results of individual tests within the battery tend to be somewhat unreliable.

Other audiometric tests that have been used include speech discrimination, which tends to be abnormally low in light of the hearing loss present [13, 35, 40], and tests of auditory adaptation [6, 14]. The measurement of the performance-intensity function

for phonetically balanced words [16], the threshold tone decay test (TDT) [21, 26, 30], and the suprathreshold adaptation test (STAT) [19] have been cited as indices of auditory adaptation that tend to be abnormal in patients with acoustic tumors.

Although classical audiometric site-of-lesion tests may be of value, their diagnostic accuracy has been questioned. Jerger [16] and Glasscock and colleagues [12] caution clinicians that an eighth nerve pattern in diagnostic audiometry does not necessarily mean the presence of an acoustic tumor, nor does a cochlear test battery rule out the presence of a tumor. Johnson [21] reported the results of various audiometric tests in a sample of 500 patients with confirmed acoustic tumors. He concluded that only approximately half of the tests performed yielded the expected diagnostic results. Sanders [33] presents an interesting review of eight published studies conducted over a 16-year period. In a combined group of 1271 patients with acoustic tumors, he reports a progressive decline in the predictive accuracy of audiometric site-of-lesion tests from earlier studies to the most recent. Citing a battery of tests including speech discrimination, Bekesey audiometry, SISI, ABLB, and TDT, Sanders reports that only the tone decay test was accurate in more than approximately half of the patients in the more recent studies. The TDT was accurate in 78% of this population while the other diagnostic tests in this battery ranged from 50 to 57%. Both Sanders [33] and Johnson [21] conclude that these tests are considerably less accurate in patients with small tumors, and that the decline of their predictive accuracy appears to be a function of a higher index of suspicion and the earlier stage at which these tumors are being diagnosed.

Acoustic reflexes have become a powerful component of the audiometric site of lesion test battery. Anderson and associates [1, 2] described the acoustic reflex decay test and elevated acoustic reflex thresholds as important early detectors of small acoustic tumors. Jerger and colleagues [20] examined the acoustic reflex in 30 eighth nerve lesion patients, as well as other conventional audiometric procedures. They reported elevated reflex thresholds or reflex decay in 26 of the 30 patients with eighth nerve disorders. The high predictive accuracy (87%) reported by Jerger and colleagues has been supported by several other studies [21, 37].

Recently, several investigators have evaluated the dynamic characteristics of the acoustic reflex as an adjunct to the more traditional reflex threshold and decay measures. Clemis and Sarno [8] reported significant delays in the onset latency of the acoustic reflex in 100% of their patients with acoustic tumors. They also reported a lower false-positive rate in this population, with reflex latencies than with the auditory brain stem response. Jerger [18] and Keith [22] have evaluated the entire dynamic function of the acoustic reflex in patients with lesions of the eighth nerve and brain stem. Although they reported that the onset latency is highly variable, the onset slope was noted to be significantly affected by lesions of the auditory nervous system. Clearly this area holds promise as an increasingly sensitive index of small acoustic tumors.

AUDITORY BRAIN STEM RESPONSE

The auditory brain stem response (ABR) has become the most powerful noninvasive procedure for the diagnosis of acoustic tumors. Several recent studies [36, 38, 39] have demonstrated unilateral abnormalities in ABR waveforms in very high percentages of patients with acoustic tumors. The most common waveform changes noted are latency delays or elimination of components beyond wave I on the tumor side. Presumably, pressure exerted by the tumor mass on the cochlear nerve creates a reduction in the neural conduction velocity or a desynchronization of the individual neurons within the nerve bundle, which effectively eliminates the ABR peaks.

Selters and Brackmann [36] reported an interaural wave V latency difference of greater than 0.2 msec in 91% of 46 patients with temporal bone tumors. More recently, Clemis and McGee [7] cited unilaterally abnormal ABRs in 93% of their patients with acoustic tumors, while Glasscock and associates [12] reported 98% predictive accuracy with ABR.

Although these percentages are impressive, ABR is not without limitations. The incidence of false-positive results ranges from 12% [36] to 33% [7]. False-positive results increase dramatically in patients with severe hearing losses, particularly when the diagnostic criteria are restricted to examination of the wave IV to V complex. In our experience, interaural comparison of interpeak neural conduction is the most sensitive and specific index of eighth nerve pathology.

A final consideration that should not be overlooked is that ABR is not a diagnostic test for acoustic tumors. Rather, it is an indication of the functional integrity of the auditory nervous system to the level of the midbrain. Other neurologic lesions of these pathways can create ABR changes that mimic those found in the presence of acoustic tumors. These types of findings should not be considered false-negative, but should serve to emphasize the necessity of using ABR as one component of the diagnostic battery, which when taken as a whole provides the most effective means of obtaining an accurate clinical picture.

Vestibular Tests

Evaluation of the vestibular response is commonly done with cold water caloric irrigations to identify unilateral vestibular weakness through observation of nystagmus. Bithermal calorics and electronystagmography (see Chap. 18) are better test procedures for vestibular function. As the disease progresses with extracanalicular extension, tumors of the posterior fossa and cerebellopontile angle produce systematized vertigo often accompanied by spontaneous and/or positional nystagmus [4].

Linthicum and Churchill [24] reported vestibular findings from 200 patients with proved acoustic neuromas tested with minimal icewater caloric irrigations and electronystagmography. They found that 82% of the patients showed reduced caloric vestibular response on the affected ear. The incidence of positive response was found to be directly related to the size of the tumor. The diminished vestibular response was shown equally well with caloric irrigations and electronystagmography (ENG). The ENG technique has numerous advantages over icewater caloric examination (see Chap. 18). Again it must be pointed out that decreased vestibular function does not necessarily indicate the presence of an acoustic neuroma, nor does normal vestibular response preclude the presence of a tumor. ENG may hold much for the future in terms of diagnostic potential through improved techniques of stimulation or computer analysis of tracings.

A recent development in the evaluation of vestibular disorders is the application of low-frequency harmonic acceleration (HA) through the use of a "rotary chair." Olson and colleagues [29] reported the results of HA on 24 patients with surgically confirmed acoustic tumors. Sixty-seven percent of this group demonstrated abnormalities in the HA test. When combined with caloric evaluation, 91% of these patients demonstrated vestibular abnormalities.

Additional Diagnostic Considerations
When routine clinical examination of the patient does not rule out the presence of an acoustic tumor; or if a patient has a positive history of unilateral, progressive sensorineural hearing loss suggesting acoustic tumor; or if the audiologic vestibular evaluation results in positive tumor signs, additional diagnostic workup must be considered. Additional testing procedures include the computerized tomography (CT) scan, CT scan with air, petrous pyramid polytomography, posterior fossa myelogram, pneumoencephalogram, and angiography. Radiographic procedures are employed for the following two reasons: (1) to determine the presence or absence of a tumor and (2) to determine the size and extent of a tumor. Cost-benefit considerations must be addressed.

Computerized Tomography (CT) Scan. CT scan produces an image by computer analysis of x-ray beams passed through a portion of the body (e.g., the temporal bone). "Fourth generation" equipment (General Electric 8800 series) is now available giving detail not previously visible. Tumors extending less than 1.0 cm into the posterior cranial fossa can be identified. The size of the internal auditory canal (IAC) can be assessed.

CT Scan with Air. For x-ray contrast, 5.0 cc of air is injected into the subarachnoid space by lumbar puncture using a small (22 or 25 gauge) needle [31]. The head is positioned to move the air into the IAC. In the absence of tumor, the IAC is filled with air and the nerve trunks are readily visible. With a tumor present, the air will outline the margins of the mass. This procedure can be done on an outpatient basis with virtually no morbidity or complications because a small spinal needle is used and no fluid is withdrawn.

Petrous Pyramid Polytomograms. This x-ray modality focuses on a 1-mm "slice" of the temporal bone. Approximately 12 such x-ray films are produced of each ear, which are viewed in sequence. Of special interest in these films is a comparison of the diameter of the internal auditory meatus of the patient's temporal bone. Often, acoustic tumors erode bone in the affected internal auditory meatus creating a widening of the canal itself. Analysis of the films is done by viewing the shape of the questionable canal, which is classically "trumpet-shaped" in the presence of an acoustic tumor.

Posterior Fossa Myelogram. An iodine dye is used for x-ray contrast for the myelogram. The dye (Metrizamide or Pantopaque) is injected in the subarachnoid space by a lumbar puncture. Again, the patient is positioned to move the contrast material to the temporal bone. A normal IAC will be filled with dye or a small- to medium-sized tumor will be outlined.

Pneumoencephalography. Pneumoencephalography is especially helpful in outlining a large tumor and in identifying displacement of the brain stem, cerebellum, or both. A sizeable volume of air is injected into the subarachnoid space and moved into the posterior cranial fossa.

Angiography. An iodine dye is injected in the vertebral artery. Images of the intra-arterial dye assist in assessing the size of large tumors and in identifying the blood supply to the tumor.

The choice of diagnostic tests from a cost-benefit standpoint is difficult. Many clinicians believe that if noninvasive clinical testing suggests the possibility of a tumor, the most definitive x-ray study should be employed, namely, a CT scan with air contrast.

TREATMENT

Acoustic neuromas do not respond to x-ray therapy, so surgery is the only treatment. Not all patients with acoustic tumors undergo surgery; an individual decision must be made with consideration of circumstances, age, and symptoms of each patient. Since this tumor generally grows slowly, many patients outlive the tumor.

The classic neurosurgical approach to remove an acoustic neuroma requires a craniotomy. A 3- to 4-inch panel of bone is removed from the back of the skull. Part of the cerebellum must be removed or displaced to gain access to the posterior fossa and the acoustic tumor. This operation is complex and risks of mortality and of morbidity (e.g., facial nerve paralysis) are quite high.

A middle cranial fossa approach is advocated under certain circumstances. This surgical approach involves removing a small panel of bone from above the ear. The dura mater and the temporal lobe of the brain are displaced, exposing the superior surface of the temporal bone. The tumor is exposed by drilling the bone from above until the internal auditory meatus is opened. The disadvantage to this surgical technique is that the facial nerve is at greater risk because drilling into the internal auditory meatus from above may involve inadvertent trauma to the facial nerve. The advantage to this procedure is that it can be accomplished without sacrificing the cochlea and vestibular apparatus of the involved ear. The blood supply to the cochlea must be preserved during the operation or the patient's hearing will be lost. A final consideration is that few tumors are small enough to be completely removed with this surgical procedure.

The translabyrinthine approach is the surgical technique of choice for removal of small and medium-sized acoustic tumors. In this technique the surgeon operates essentially through the patient's ear. The mastoid air cells and the vestibular portion of the inner ear are drilled out to gain access to the internal auditory meatus. The advantage to this procedure is the direct access to the internal auditory meatus; the disadvantage to this procedure is that the hearing must be sacrificed. This technique was originally described by German physicians in the early 1900s. The Otologic Medical Group of Los Angeles refined the procedure and popularized its use in recent years [10].

REFERENCES

1. Anderson, H., Barr, B., and Wedenberg, E. Intra-aural Reflexes in Retrocochlear Lesions. In C. Humberger and J. Wersall (Eds.), *Disorders of the Skull Base Region.* Stockholm: Almqvist and Wiksell, 1969.
2. Anderson, H., Barr, B., and Wedenberg, E. Early diagnosis of VIIIth nerve tumors by acoustic reflex tests. *Acta Otolaryngol.* Suppl. 263, 1970.
3. Anderson, M. S., and Bentinck, B. R. Intracranial schwannoma in a child. *Cancer* 29: 231, 1972.
4. Battin, R. R. Vestibulography. Springfield, Ill.: Thomas, 1974.
5. Bjorkesten, G. Unilateral acoustic tumors in children. *Acta Psychiatr. Scand.* 32:1, 1957.
6. Carhart, R. Clinical determination of abnormal adaptation. *Arch. Otolaryngol.* 65: 32, 1957.
7. Clemis, J., and McGee, T. Brainstem electric response audiometry in the differential diagnosis of acoustic tumor. *Laryngoscope* 89:31, 1979.
8. Clemis, J., and Sarno, C. The acoustic reflex latency test: Clinical application. *Laryngoscope* 90:601, 1980.
9. Craig, W., Dodge, H., and Ross, P. Acoustic neuromas in children: Report of two cases. *J. Neurosurg.* 11:505, 1954.
10. Fisch, U. Transtemporal surgery of the internal auditory canal. Report of 92 cases, technique, indications and results. *Adv. Otorhinolaryngol.* 17:203, 1970.
11. Glasscock, M., and Hays, J. Pitfalls in the diagnosis of acoustic and other cerebellopontine angle tumors. *Laryngoscope* 83: 1038, 1973.
12. Glasscock, M., et al. Brainstem evoked response audiometry in a clinical practice. *Laryngoscope* 89:7, 1979.
13. Goetzinger, C., and Angell, S. Audiological assessment in acoustic tumors and cortical

lesions. *Eye Ear Nose Throat Mon.* 44:39, 1965.

14. Green, D. The modified tone decay test (MTDT) as a screening procedure for eighth nerve lesions. *J. Speech Hear. Disord.* 28:31, 1963.

15. Gussen, R. Intramodiolar acoustic neurinoma. *Laryngoscope* 81:1979, 1971.

16. Jerger, J. Hearing tests in otologic diagnosis. *Asha* 4:139, 1962.

17. Jerger, J. Review of diagnostic audiometry. *Ann. Otol. Rhinol. Laryngol.* 77:2, 1968.

18. Jerger, J. Site specificity of diagnostic audiometry. Presented to The Colorado Otology-Audiology Workshop, Vail, March 10, 1982.

19. Jerger, J., and Jerger, S. A simplified tone decay test. *Arch. Otolaryngol.* 101:403, 1975.

20. Jerger, J., et al. The acoustic reflex in eighth nerve disorder. *Arch. Otolaryngol.* 99:409, 1974.

21. Johnson, E. W. Auditory test results in 500 cases of acoustic neuroma. *Arch. Otolaryngol.* 103:152, 1977.

22. Keith, R. A study of acoustic reflex latency and ABR tests in multiple sclerosis patients. Presented to The Colorado Otology-Audiology Workshop, Vail, March 10, 1982.

23. Krause, C. J., and McCabe, B. F. Acoustic neuroma in a seven-year-old girl. *Arch. Otolaryngol.* 94:359, 1971.

24. Linthicum, F. H., Jr., and Churchill, D. Vestibular test results in acoustic tumor cases. *Arch. Otolaryngol.* 88:604, 1968.

25. MacKenzie, I. Consequences of removing an acoustic neuroma by conventional surgical means. *Proc. R. Soc. Med.* 58:1071, 1965.

26. Moules-Garcia, C., and Hood, J. D. Tone decay test in neurootological diagnosis. *Arch. Otolaryngol.* 96:231, 1972.

27. Naunton, R., and Petasnick, J. Acoustic neurinomas with normal auditory meatus. *Arch. Otolaryngol.* 91:437, 1970.

28. Netter, F. *The Nervous System,* Vol. 1 (The CIBA Collection of Medical Illustrations). New York: CIBA Pharmaceutical Co., 1962.

29. Olson, J., Wolfe, J., and Engelken, E. Responses to low frequency harmonic acceleration in patients with acoustic neuromas. *Laryngoscope* 91:1270, 1981.

30. Owens, E. Tone decay in eighth nerve and cochlear lesions. *J. Speech Hear. Disord.* 29:14, 1964.

31. Penley, M. W., et al. Diagnosis of cerebellopontine angle tumors with small quantities of air. *Otolaryngol. Head Neck Surg.* 89:457–462, 1981.

32. Pulec, J. When to Suspect the Possibility of an Acoustic Neuroma—Diagnostic Tests. In *Otolaryngologic Clinics of North America Symposium on Hearing Loss.* Philadelphia: Saunders, 1969.

33. Sanders, J. W. Diagnostic Audiology. In N. J. Lass et al. (Eds.), Speech, Language, and Hearing: Normal Processes and Clinical Disorders. Philadelphia: Saunders, 1982. Pp. 944–967.

34. Saunders, J., Josey, A., and Glasscock, M. Audiologic evaluation in cochlear and eighth nerve disorders. *Arch. Otolaryngol.* 100:283, 1974.

35. Schuknecht, H., and Woeliner, R. An experimental and clinical study of deafness from lesions of the cochlear nerve. *J. Laryngol. Otol.* 69:75, 1955.

36. Selters, W., and Brackmann, D. Acoustic tumor detection with brain stem electric response audiometry. *Arch. Otolaryngol.* 103:181, 1977.

37. Sheehy, J., and Inzer, B. The acoustic reflex test in neurootologic diagnosis. *Arch. Otolaryngol.* 102:11, 1976.

38. Starr, A., and Hamilton, A. Correlation between confirmed sites of neurological lesions and abnormalities of far field auditory brainstem responses. *Electroencephalogr. Clin. Neurophysiol.* 41:595, 1976.

39. Stockard, J., Stockard, J., and Sharbrough, F. Detection and localization of occult lesions with brainstem auditory responses. *Mayo Clin. Proc.* 52:761, 1977.

40. Walsh, T., and Goodman, A. Speech discrimination in central auditory lesions. *Laryngoscope* 65:1, 1955.

41. Wanamaker, H. Acoustic neuroma: Primary arising in the vestibule. *Laryngoscope* 82:1040, 1972.

42. Weaver, M. Cited in J. Northern and M. Downs, *Hearing in Children* (2nd ed.). Baltimore: Williams & Wilkins, 1978.

16

Detection and Localization of Central Auditory Disorders

George E. Lynn

John Gilroy

The traditional behavioral measures of auditory functions, such as those described in Chapters 2 and 3, provide useful information about the localization of disturbed auditory functions associated with peripheral lesions. However, these procedures are usually less useful in locating abnormalities of the central auditory system. Bocca, Calearo, and Cassinari [6] pioneered the use of specialized speech discrimination tests to evaluate auditory functions of patients with temporal lobe lesions. They found that conventional audiometry failed to detect impaired function, yet when they made their speech discrimination tests more difficult by low-pass filtering, understanding of the material was significantly reduced in the ear contralateral to the affected side of the brain. These findings were subsequently confirmed in later studies in Italy [1, 4, 7] and in the United States [21, 22].

Since that time, a number of audiologic procedures have been developed and used to detect and to localize the site of central auditory dysfunction. At first, the emphasis was on the use of speech stimuli; however, more recent applications have included pure-tone binaural interaction studies (alternate binaural loudness balance; ABLB, and simultaneous binaural median plane localization; SBMPL) [48], the pitch pattern test [42, 43, 46, 55, 56], and the binaural pure-tone masking level difference (MLD) test [18, 48, 49, 52]. The application of impedance audiometry and evoked potentials are discussed in Chapters 4 and 5.

CENTRAL AUDITORY SYSTEM

The central auditory nervous system arises at the junction of the neuroglial-neurilemmal junction of the eighth nerve within the internal auditory canal [47]. This junction is usually located 10 to 13 mm distal to the brain stem in the man and approximately 7 to 10 mm in the woman. Occasionally, it may be located more distally, nearer to the fundus of the internal auditory canal, or at times it may be located medial to the porus acusticus outside the petrous bone. The physiologic origin of the afferent central auditory nervous system is usually considered to begin at the first synapse located in the cochlear nuclei in the upper medulla. From this point, the central auditory system consists of crossed and uncrossed multisynaptic projections that connect nuclear centers at different levels and on both sides of the brain stem. These include the (1) cochlear nuclei in the upper part of the medulla, (2) decussating fiber tracts and cells of the trapezoid body, (3) the several superior olivary nuclei in the caudal pons, (4) ipsilateral and contralateral axons and cell groups of the ascending lateral lemniscus in the middle and rostral regions of the pons, and (5) the inferior colliculi and commissure at the caudal midbrain level. From this level, the brachium of the inferior colliculi project to the medial geniculate body of the thalamus and from there, auditory radiations (geniculocortical projections) follow a sublenticular course to reach Heschl's transverse gyri buried in the sylvian fissure of both cerebral hemispheres. Heschl's gyri give origin to transverse interhemispheric pathways that connect homologous as well as heterologous regions of the cerebral hemispheres through the posterior portion of the body of the corpus callosum.

Lesions caused by various diseases of the central nervous system may affect auditory functions at any level, unilaterally or bilaterally. The purpose of the neuroaudiologic evaluation is the anatomic localization of the region or regions involved in the central auditory system. The test results do not reveal information about the type or nature of the lesion, but when considered with the clinical findings and other abnormal findings of diagnostic procedures, results often confirm the site and the pathologic changes present in the affected person.

SPECIALIZED SPEECH DISCRIMINATION TESTS

Speech discrimination tests of central auditory function may be classified as monotic low-redundancy, binaural fusion, and dichotic procedures.

Monotic Low-Redundancy Tests

Monotic low-redundancy tests include tests in which distorted or degraded speech stimuli are presented to each ear one at a time. Various methods of distorting speech have been used to increase difficulty in perception for the listener and added difficulty in the presence of central auditory disturbances. Some investigators have used low-pass filtering [23, 24, 31, 33, 35, 37], while others have used temporally interrupted, accelerated, or time-compressed speech [5, 11, 12, 15, 31, 32]. Other methods include the presentation of noise or of continuous discourse as ipsilateral competing messages in the same ear with the primary (attended) signal at various signal-to-competing-message intensity ratios [25, 26, 53]. All of these methods for degrading speech have been used with various degrees of success in the detection of the site of central auditory dysfunction.

Monotic low-redundancy test results are usually abnormal in patients with temporal lobe lesions involving the auditory system who obtain poor test scores in the ear opposite the affected side of the brain. However, patients with involvement of the interhemispheric auditory pathways may demonstrate no abnormality with monaural low-pass filtered material [16, 34, 37, 44, 45, 46]. Presumably, similar findings may be expected with other forms of monaural low-redundancy speech test material. Patients with brain stem lesions have shown a number of findings including an absence of abnormality in either ear or depressed scores in either the contralateral, ipsilateral, or both ears.

Binaural Fusion Tests

Binaural fusion tests are tests in which different components or segments of the speech sample are delivered to the two ears simultaneously, one segment to each ear. This type of test assesses the patient's ability to fuse or synthesize the different portions of the same signal (which are unintelligible under monaural conditions) into easily understood messages. Low- and high-frequency narrow bands of speech have been used [39, 50, 54, 59]. Patients with brain stem lesions may demonstrate poor performance under binaural conditions, indicating disturbed binaural integration processes. A similar disturbance in binaural integration has been shown with swinging or rapidly alternating speech in patients with brain stem pathology [5, 11, 37].

Another procedure that may be included

in this category of central tests is the binaural MLD test for speech [51, 52]. In this procedure, binaural speech thresholds or discrimination scores are obtained with a 180-degree interaural phase difference in the presence of in-phase binaural masking noise (antiphasic condition). These scores are compared to scores obtained with the same amount of noise when the speech is in-phase at the two ears (homophasic condition). The difference between the scores obtained under the two conditions is the MLD. Binaural MLDs are not affected by hemispheric lesions [14, 38, 49]; however, abnormally small MLDs have been reported in patients with pontile lesions, particularly those located at the medullopontile level of the brain stem [18, 38, 48, 57].

Dichotic Tests
Dichotic tests are tests in which different speech samples, such as syllables, words, or sentences, are presented binaurally and simultaneously with a different message in each ear. This type of test evaluates the patient's ability to separate the two completely different speech messages arriving simultaneously. Some tests require the listener to repeat only the primary message in one ear while attempting to ignore the competing message in the other ear. For example, phonetically balanced (PB) words and synthetic sentences have been used as the primary message in the test ear and continuous discourse from one or more speakers in the other ear [24–26]. Also, familiar sentences have been used as the test material in one ear while meaningful and related sentences were competing for attention in the opposite ear [66].

It is possible to increase the difficulty of the listening task by requiring the listener to attend to different stimuli in both ears and to repeat each message heard. Kimura [30] used a technique in which a series of different digits were presented in pairs to both ears. The staggered spondaic word (SSW) test [8, 29] consists of two-syllable words staggered in time so that a portion of each word in the pair arrives at the two ears at about the same time. Berlin and associates [2, 3] among others have used nonsense consonant-vowel (CV) syllables presented in pairs; a different CV syllable to

each ear simultaneously and under various lead and lag times.

The results of dichotic tests generally have shown them to be sensitive to the effects of lesions involving auditory areas of the temporal lobe and the interhemispheric auditory pathways [16, 19, 30, 34–37, 40, 43, 44, 46, 60, 61]. In patients with temporal lobe lesions, abnormal performance with dichotic tests usually occurs in the ear contralateral to the involved hemisphere. In patients with lesions involving the interhemispheric auditory pathways, abnormal dichotic test scores occur in the ear ipsilateral to the dominant hemisphere for speech and language (left ear in most people) regardless of the hemisphere involved. Findings in patients with brain stem lesions have not been well documented, although cases have been reported that show little or no deficit with the dichotic synthetic sentence identification–contralateral competing message (SSI–CCM) test [26].

AUDITORY EVOKED
BRAIN STEM POTENTIALS
Auditory evoked brain stem potentials (AEP) are far-field, volume-conducted reflections of evoked electrical activity generated in the central auditory nervous system. The response, when recorded with a midline scalp electrode referred to either a mastoid or earlobe electrode located on the same side as the stimulated ear, consists of seven waves that occur within 10 to 12 msec following click stimulation [13]. Wave I represents electrical activity of the auditory nerve. Subsequent waves II, III, IV, and V reflect activity at different regions or levels of the auditory pathways of the brain stem [9, 20, 28]. The generator regions for waves VI and VII are less well recognized; however, the region of the medial geniculate body and the auditory cortex may be the primary contributors to these potentials [10]. These waves have been shown to have abnormally prolonged latencies, reduced amplitudes, and distorted waveforms on one or both sides in patients with a variety of diseases affecting the brain stem [17, 58, 63, 64, 65], but not in patients with hemispheric lesions [38]. Latency and amplitude differences between

the two ears also may be abnormal in the presence of brain stem abnormalities.

A neuroaudiologic battery of tests including behavioral and evoked potential measurements may be used effectively to identify and to localize abnormalities of the central auditory nervous system. The main criterion for determining if monaural low-redundancy and dichotic test scores are abnormal is whether the test scores of the two ears are significantly different. Binaural fusion test scores are considered abnormal if binaural performance is not significantly improved over the scores obtained under monotic conditions. The MLD test score is abnormal when there is no significant difference in test scores obtained under the antiphasic condition compared to the homophasic. Auditory evoked brain stem potentials are considered abnormal when there are prolonged absolute and interpeak latencies, reduced amplitudes, and significant distortion in wave morphology. It is important to keep in mind that test findings may vary owing to factors that may have little to do with the effects of central lesions. These factors include hearing loss, reduced phonemic discrimination associated with peripheral auditory disorders, and stimulus and procedural differences. Thus, the possible effects of other variables related to the patient or to the test procedures used should be considered carefully when interpreting test findings [41, 62].

Neuroaudiologic findings are presented from seven well-documented cases with neurologic disorders. The findings are illustrative and should not be viewed as all inclusive of the varieties of central auditory disorders or test findings that may be seen in a clinical population.

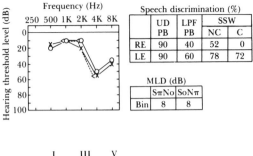

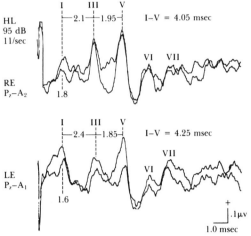

Figure 16-1. Audiogram, speech discrimination scores, masking level difference (MLD) scores, and auditory evoked potential (AEP) results in a patient with an astrocytoma of the left temporal lobe. Low-pass filtered (LPF) PB and staggered spondaic word (SSW) scores are poorer in the right (contralateral) ear than in the left. MLDs and AEPs are normal. PB = phonetically balanced; UD = undistorted; NC = noncompeting; C = competing; SπNo = noise in-phase/signal out-of-phase; SoNπ = signal in-phase/noise out-of-phase; Bin = binaural.

CASE REPORT: A 45-year-old man complained of pressure in his head and neck extending down into his shoulders, arms, and hands. The pressure was of 3 weeks' duration. The neurologic examination revealed impaired mentation with forgetfulness, impaired insight, and poor judgment. He was agitated and vociferous. Examination of the cranial nerves and motor and sensory systems was negative.

Audiometric findings and AEPs are shown in Figure 16-1. There was a moderate high-frequency sensorineural hearing loss of 50 to 55

dB centered at 4000 Hz, which may have been related to past noise exposure. Phonemic discrimination for undistorted PB material was normal and bilaterally symmetric (90% correct for each ear at 40 dB SL). Monaural low-pass filtered speech discrimination scores obtained at 50 dB sensation levels showed significantly reduced performance in the right ear (40%) compared to the left (60%). Similarly, performance of the right ear under the noncompeting and competing conditions of the SSW test (52 and 0%, respectively) was significantly poorer

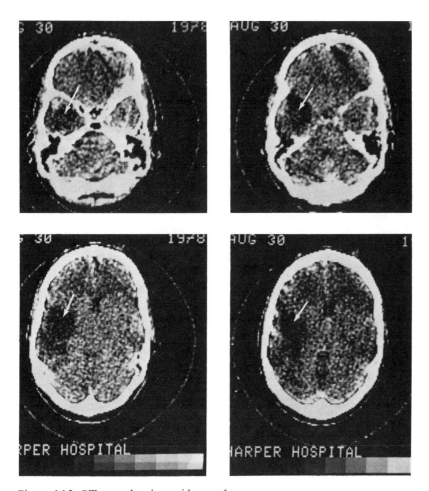

Figure 16-2. CT scan showing evidence of a large left temporal lobe tumor (arrow).

than in the left ear. The left ear score was also impaired, but not to the extent noted in the right. Binaural speech MLD scores of 8 dB were normal.

Monaural AEP recordings demonstrated seven Jewett waves, bilaterally. Wave I latency for each ear was slightly delayed for the stimulus intensity used (95 dB HL), which was consistent with the bilateral sensorineural hearing loss recorded on the audiogram. Interpeak latencies between waves I, III, and V were within normal limits, bilaterally. There were no significant changes in amplitudes or waveform for the various components.

The normal evoked potential recordings and MLD scores failed to demonstrate involvement of auditory pathways of the brain stem. Therefore, the abnormal test performance in the right ear (with some reduction in the left ear scores as well) with monaural low-redundancy and dichotic speech material suggested the presence of a left temporal lobe abnormality.

The electroencephalogram (EEG) was abnormal with a focus of continuous irregular very slow activity in the left temporal area. Computed tomography (CT) of the brain demonstrated a large, left temporal lobe lucency that did not enhance with iodine (Fig. 16-2). The lateral ventricles were not dilated, but there was a slight ventricular shift from left to right side. The posterior fossa was normal in appearance. At surgery, an astrocytoma was found to occupy the middle and posterior regions of the left temporal lobe.

CASE REPORT: A 27-year-old woman was admitted to the hospital for evaluation of headaches and progressive personality changes of about 3 months' duration. On neurologic examination, she demonstrated a mild disturbance in mentation with some loss of past and recent memory. There was constructional apraxia but no agnosia. The cranial nerve examination was normal. Examination of the motor system showed some increased tone and weakness on the left side. Coordination was markedly impaired in the left lower extremity. The gait was hemiparetic on the left side and the Romberg test was positive with a tendency to fall to the right. Sensory examination revealed an area of decreased sensation over the left side of the forehead.

Audiometric findings and AEP recordings are shown in Figure 16-3. Hearing sensitivity for pure tones and discrimination for undistorted PB material were bilaterally normal. However, discrimination for low-pass filtered PB material at 40 dB SL was abnormal for the left ear (36%) and normal in the right ear (52%). Performance scores on the SSW for both the noncompeting and competing conditions (85 and 65%, respectively) were abnormal in the left ear and unimpaired in the right. Binaural speech MLD scores of 10 and 8 dB were normal.

AEPs recorded during monaural click stimulation revealed seven well-defined waves on each side. Absolute and interpeak latencies for all waves were well within normal limits, bilaterally, with normal amplitudes and waveform. Recordings were bilaterally symmetric and repeatable among trials.

Test results in this case showed no evidence of brain stem disturbance; binaural speech MLDs and AEPs were normal bilaterally. The consistent deficit in the left ear with monaural low-pass filtered PB and dichotic SSW material with a normal audiogram and normal undistorted PB speech discrimination therefore suggested involvement of the right temporal lobe. A CT scan (Fig. 16-4) showed the presence of foreign body material, scar tissue, and atrophy of the right side of the brain believed to be related to a gunshot wound to the right temporoparietal area 5 years earlier.

CASE REPORT: This patient was a 38-year-old woman who had a history of epileptic seizures for approximately 5 years. She developed left hemiparesis and was admitted to the hospital for further evaluation. The neurologic examination revealed a left-sided facial weakness. Examination of the motor system showed a spastic left hemiparesis and a loss of pin-prick sensation over the whole of the left side of the body. Audiometric findings are shown in Figure

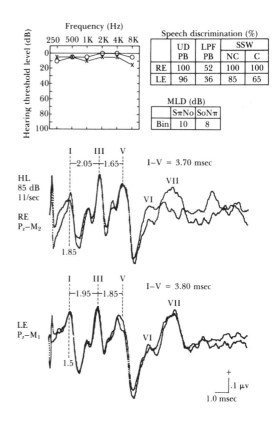

Figure 16-3. Audiogram, speech discrimination scores, masking level difference (MLD) scores, and auditory evoked potential (AEP) results in a patient with atrophy of the right temporoparietal lobe. Low-pass filtered (LPF) PB and staggered spondiac word (SSW) scores are poorer in the left (contralateral) ear than in the right. MLDs and AEPs are normal. PB = phonetically balanced; UD = undistorted; NC = noncompeting; C = competing; SπNo = noise in-phase/signal out-of-phase; SoNπ = signal in-phase/noise out-of-phase; Bin = binaural.

16-5. Results revealed normal hearing for pure tones bilaterally. Discrimination for undistorted and low-pass filtered material was normal and bilaterally symmetric. Binaural speech MLDs were normal. However, SSW was abnormal in the left ear for both the noncompeting and competing conditions (86 and 78%, respectively) and normal in the right ear. AEPs were not recorded.

This study showed no evidence of pontile involvement; MLDs were normal. The normal monaural low-pass filtered PB scores and abnor-

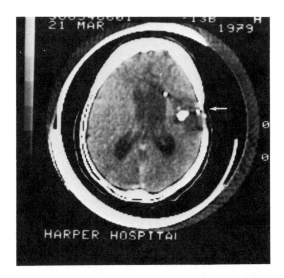

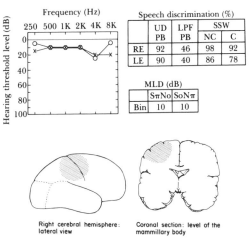

	Frequency (Hz)						Speech discrimination (%)			
							UD PB	LPF PB	SSW NC	SSW C
RE							92	46	98	92
LE							90	40	86	78

	MLD (dB)	
	SπNo	SoNπ
Bin	10	10

Right cerebral hemisphere: lateral view

Coronal section: level of the mammillary body

Figure 16-5. Audiogram, speech discrimination scores, and masking level difference (MLD) scores in a patient with an astrocytoma of the right frontoparietal lobe. Low-pass filtered (LPF) PB and MLD scores are normal. Staggered spondaic word (SSW) scores are abnormal in the left ear. Localization of the tumor is illustrated by the stippled area in the drawings of the right lateral and coronal views of the brain. PB = phonetically balanced; UD = undistorted; NC = noncompeting; C = competing; SπNo = noise in-phase/signal out-of-phase; SoNπ = signal in-phase/noise out-of-phase; Bin = binaural.

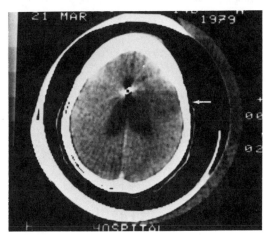

Figure 16-4. CT scan showing evidence of foreign body, scar tissue, and atrophy (arrow) of the right hemisphere from a previous gunshot wound to the right temporoparietal region of the brain.

mal dichotic SSW test findings in the left ear indicated disturbed auditory function of the interhemispheric auditory pathways. However, the tests did not indicate the side of the brain in which the lesion was located.

Radiographic studies including a pneumoencephalogram and an arteriogram revealed the presence of a mass occupying the frontoparietal region of the right hemisphere. The branches of the middle cerebral artery were depressed with a slight forward displacement. The cortical veins were abnormal in the right parietal region, and the right internal cerebral vein was shifted 8 mm to the left. The roof of the right lateral ventricle was depressed compared to the

left, which indicated pressure on the right side of the corpus callosum. The interhemispheric auditory pathways on the right side of the corpus callosum would have been involved. At surgery, an astrocytoma was found in the right frontoparietal region of the brain.

CASE REPORT: This 49-year-old woman was admitted to the hospital because of right focal seizures involving the right upper and lower extremities. Mentation was impaired with memory loss, confusion, and olfactory hallucinations. The neurologic examination revealed a right homonymous hemianopia. The left pupil was larger than the right but both were reactive. There was bilateral nystagmus. There were no weaknesses and plantar responses were flexor, bilaterally.

Audiometric findings are shown in Figure 16-6. The audiogram shows normal hearing sensitivity bilaterally. Speech discrimination scores for undistorted and low-pass filtered PB material obtained at 40 dB sensation level were bilaterally normal and symmetric. The dichotic SSW test showed a definite abnormality in discrimination scores for the left ear under both the noncompeting and competing conditions;

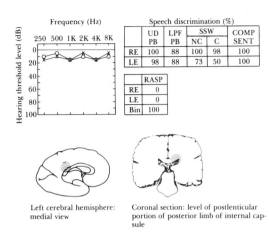

Frequency (Hz)		Speech discrimination (%)				
		UD PB	LPF PB	SSW NC	SSW C	COMP SENT
	RE	100	88	100	98	100
	LE	98	88	73	50	100

	RASP
RE	0
LE	0
Bin	100

Left cerebral hemisphere: medial view   Coronal section: level of postlenticular portion of posterior limb of internal capsule

Figure 16-6. Audiogram, speech discrimination, and rapid alternating speech (RASP) scores in a patient with an astrocytoma involving the left side of the corpus callosum. Low-pass filtered (LPF) PB, competing sentence (COMP SENT), and RASP scores are normal. Staggered spondaic word (SSW) scores are abnormal in the left ear. Localization of the tumor is illustrated by the stippled area in the drawings of the medial view of the left hemisphere and the coronal section of the brain. PB = phonetically balanced; UD = undistorted; NC = noncompeting; C = competing; MLD = masking level difference; SπNo = noise in-phase/signal out-of-phase; SoNπ = signal in-phase/noise out-of-phase; Bin = binaural.

73 and 50% correct, respectively. Right ear scores were normal. The dichotic competing sentence test was bilaterally normal. The ability to understand speech alternating rapidly between the two ears was normal as indicated by the binaural score of 100% correct. The MLD test was not given and AEPs were not recorded.

This patient demonstrated no difficulty in understanding monaural low-pass filtered speech in either ear; however, a definite disturbance was present in the left ear with the dichotic SSW test. Assuming there was no involvement of auditory pathways in the brain stem, the pattern of responses on monaural low-pass filtered PB and dichotic SSW indicated abnormal function of the interhemispheric auditory pathways.

The EEG showed abnormal slow activity in the left parietal region. Radioisotope brain scan was abnormal showing increased radioactive uptake in the left posterior parietal region. A left carotid angiogram was normal. A pneumoencephalogram was not conclusive; however, a ventriculogram revealed a mass depressing the left lateral ventricle in its posterior region. The patient had a left temporoparietal craniotomy, and an astrocytoma was found deep in the pa-

rietal lobe involving the left side of the corpus callosum, posterior region.

CASE REPORT: This 52-year-old man was admitted to the hospital because of difficulties with speech described as an inability to name simple objects, such as a fork, spoon, or knife, and difficulty completing simple sentences with the appropriate words. Two days before admission, he had transient blurring of vision followed by the development of an episode of expressive dysphasia associated with transient dyscalculia, dysgraphia, right-left confusion, and finger agnosia (Gerstmann's syndrome). Cranial nerve examination showed bilateral papilledema, but the other cranial nerves were normal. There was no motor weakness, and coordination was intact. There was loss of sensation to pin-prick over the right upper extremity. Deep tendon reflexes were hyperactive in the right upper limb.

Audiometric findings and AEP recordings are shown in Figure 16-7. There was a mild high-frequency, sensorineural hearing loss above 1000 Hz, which occurred bilaterally and symmetrically. Speech discrimination was normal bilaterally for undistorted PB material. Discrimination for low-pass filtered PB material was slightly poorer in the right ear than the left, but only by 8% (which was not considered significant). The dichotic SSW test, competing condition, showed a definite abnormality in the left ear (55% correct) but was normal in the right ear. There was no abnormality noted under the noncompeting condition of this test. Binaural speech MLDs were 10 dB with both antiphasic conditions, which were normal.

AEP recordings showed normal wave I latency and normal interpeak latencies, bilaterally. Amplitudes and waveform for all components were normal on both sides.

The neuroaudiologic studies in this case showed normal evoked electrical activity from the brain stem with normal MLDs. Undistorted and monaural low-pass filtered PB speech discrimination was normal and bilaterally symmetric. The only abnormality shown in this study was on dichotic stimulation, in which the left ear score was significantly reduced (55%) compared to the right. These findings were interpreted as evidence of disturbed auditory function of the interhemispheric auditory pathways. The hemisphere in which the lesion was located could not be determined from these tests.

The EEG was abnormal showing a focus of continuous high voltage irregular very slow activity in the left frontal region. This indicated that a significant lesion involved the anterior portion of the left hemisphere. A CT scan with

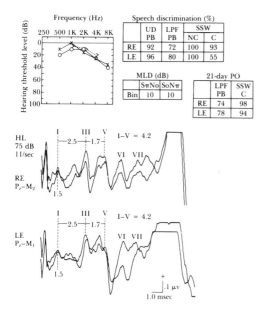

Figure 16-7. Audiogram, preoperative and 21-day postoperative speech discrimination scores, masking level difference (MLD) scores, and auditory evoked potential (AEP) results in a patient with a meningioma of the left frontal lobe. Low-pass filtered (LPF) PB scores show no significant difference between the two ears. Preoperative staggered spondaic word (SSW) score (competing condition) for the left ear is abnormal and normal 21 days postoperatively. MLDs and AEPs are normal. PB = phonetically balanced; UD = undistorted; NC = noncompeting; C = competing; SπNo = noise in-phase/signal out-of-phase; SoNπ = signal in-phase/noise out-of-phase; Bin = binaural.

iodine enhancement (Fig. 16-8) revealed the presence of a large left frontal lobe lesion with pressure effects. An arteriogram also revealed a large mass lesion in the left frontal lobe of the brain. At surgery, a large benign meningioma was removed from the surface of the left frontal lobe of the brain.

Postoperative audiometric studies 21 days after surgery (see Fig. 16-7) showed a normal SSW score for the left ear (94%) under the competing condition. All other test findings were unchanged.

This case demonstrates that auditory function of the interhemispheric auditory pathways located in the posterior region of the brain may be affected by the secondary effects of pressure from a tumor located at some distance from the auditory pathway. In this case, there was a tumor in the left frontal lobe of the brain. In-

stances of abnormal auditory functions associated with secondary effects of frontal lobe mass lesions have been reported by others [16, 34, 36, 37, 43].

CASE REPORT: A 36-year-old woman was admitted to the hospital for treatment of a neurogenic bladder and multiple sclerosis. She gave a history of ataxia and weakness involving the lower extremities for 2 years prior to admission. Neurologic examination revealed normal mentation and a mild right facial weakness of the central type with other cranial nerves within normal limits. Examination of the motor system was abnormal showing severe weakness of the proximal muscles of the lower extremities, which was greater on the right side. Deep tendon reflexes were hyperactive but bilaterally symmetric, and there were bilateral extensor plantar responses. Examination of the sensory system revealed diminished vibration in the lower extremities and diminished pin-prick sensation at level T-9 bilaterally.

Audiometric test findings and AEP recordings are shown in Figure 16-9. Sensitivity for pure tones was bilaterally elevated to the upper limit of normal. Discrimination for undistorted PB material, 60% time-compressed monosyllabic word lists, and the SSW, both noncompeting and competing conditions, was normal bilaterally. Binaural speech detection MLD scores of 3 and 1 dB for both antiphasic conditions were abnormal.

AEP recordings revealed a bilaterally normal wave I latency. The I to III interpeak latency was 2.5 msec on both sides. This latency was prolonged and exceeded three standard deviations when related to the normal latency values for women and is definitely abnormal. The I to V interpeak latency on the right side and I to IV on the left was prolonged. Wave V was absent on the left side. The III to IV (V) interpeak latencies were normal bilaterally. Amplitudes were normal.

Results of the audiometric tests and AEP recordings indicated the presence of disturbed functions involving the auditory pathways in the brain stem, bilaterally at the level of the medullopontile region. The test findings are compatible with involvement in the region of the cochlear nuclei, trapezoid body, and superior olivary nuclei.

CASE REPORT: A 30-year-old woman was admitted to the hospital for evaluation of multiple sclerosis of 2 years' duration. At this time her chief complaint was progressive weakness, difficulty with fine movements of the hands, especially when writing, and difficulty walking. She also had experienced occasional numbness of both legs, left more than right. Neurologic examina-

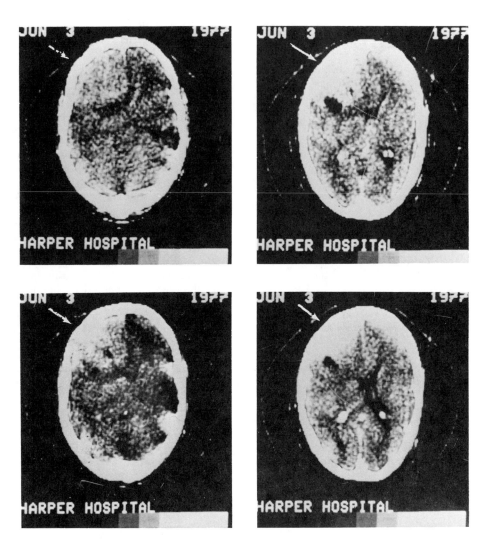

Figure 16-8. CT scan showing evidence of a large frontal lobe mass with pressure effects, left hemisphere.

tion revealed normal mentation and normal cranial nerve findings. Examination of the motor system showed decreased tone in the lower extremities with bilateral weakness. Rapid alternating movements were poorly performed with the left hand. The gait was spastic and ataxic. The deep tendon reflexes were hyperactive with bilateral ankle clonus. There were bilateral extensor plantar responses. Sensory examination revealed decreased sensation to pinprick in the lower extremities and decreased sensation to vibrations in the right upper and both lower extremities.

Audiometric findings and AEP recordings are shown in Figure 16-10. Threshold sensitivity for pure tones and discrimination for undistorted PB material was normal bilaterally. Discrimination scores for low-pass filtered PB material were 52% correct in the right ear and 44%

correct in the left. Although the interaural difference was only 8% and probably not significant, the left ear score was somewhat reduced, suggesting possible abnormal performance. SSW test findings showed a significant impairment of discrimination in the left ear under the competing condition (20% less than the right ear), but no significant difference between the two ears under the noncompeting condition. Competing sentence discrimination was bilaterally normal. The ability to understand rapidly alternating speech was normal; binaural masking level differences were abnormal (2 and 1 dB).

AEPs revealed normal wave I latency bi-

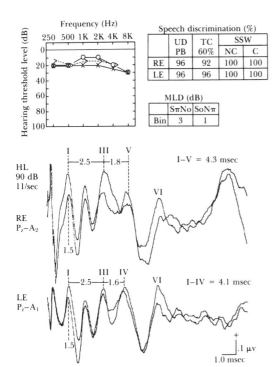

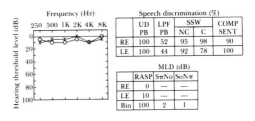

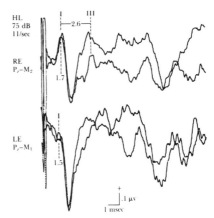

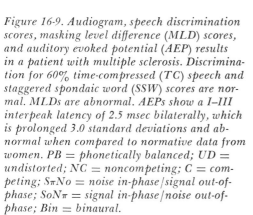

Figure 16-9. Audiogram, speech discrimination scores, masking level difference (MLD) scores, and auditory evoked potential (AEP) results in a patient with multiple sclerosis. Discrimination for 60% time-compressed (TC) speech and staggered spondaic word (SSW) scores are normal. MLDs are abnormal. AEPs show a I–III interpeak latency of 2.5 msec bilaterally, which is prolonged 3.0 standard deviations and abnormal when compared to normative data from women. PB = phonetically balanced; UD = undistorted; NC = noncompeting; C = competing; SπNo = noise in-phase/signal out-of-phase; SoNπ = signal in-phase/noise out-of-phase; Bin = binaural.

laterally. Waves II through V were severely distorted in waveform and bilaterally reduced in amplitude, making them hard to positively identify. On the right side, a probable wave III had an abnormally prolonged latency of 2.6 msec. IV and V could not be identified on either side.

Auditory test findings and AEP recordings indicated disturbed function involving the auditory pathways in the brain stem bilaterally at the medullopontile level. The possible abnormal low-pass filtered PB score and definitely abnormal SSW score in the left ear could be either an effect of the bilateral brain stem disorder, which for some obscure reason affected performance only in the left ear, or an indication of a hemispheric abnormality localized to

Figure 16-10. Audiogram; speech discrimination, rapid alternating speech (RASP), and masking level difference (MLD) scores; and auditory evoked potential (AEP) results in a patient with multiple sclerosis. Low-pass filtered (LPF) PB scores show no significant difference between the two ears. Staggered spondaic word (SSW) score (competing condition) for the left ear is abnormal. Competing sentence (COMP SENT) discrimination and RASP are normal. MLDs are abnormal. AEPs are abnormal for all components above wave I bilaterally. PB = phonetically balanced; UD = undistorted; NC = noncompeting; C = competing; SπNo = noise in-phase/signal out-of-phase; SoNπ = signal in-phase/noise out-of-phase; Bin = binaural.

either the right temporal lobe or the interhemispheric auditory pathways depending on how the low-pass filtered PB scores are interpreted. However, because of the brain stem abnormality, it is not possible to tell the extent to which hemispheric auditory functions are involved.

The EEG was compatible with the presence of demyelination involving the deep portions of the left temporal or frontal lobes of the brain. The visual evoked potentials (VEP) were abnormal. Neuropsychologic studies revealed patchy bilateral cerebral disturbances associated with dementia suggesting predominant left hemisphere dysfunctions.

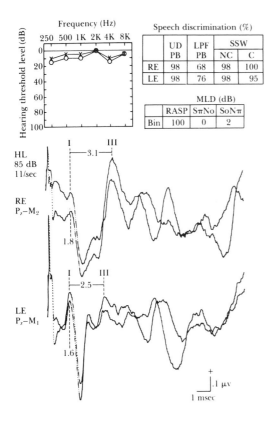

Speech discrimination (%)

	UD PB	LPF PB	SSW NC	SSW C
RE	98	68	98	100
LE	98	76	98	95

MLD (dB)

	RASP	SπNo	SoNπ
Bin	100	0	2

Figure 16-11. Repeat studies (3 months later) from patient shown in Fig. 16-10. Low-pass filtered (LPF) PB and staggered spondaic word (SSW) scores (competing condition) are significantly improved. MLDs and AEPs remain abnormal. AEP tracings from left ear stimulation are improved compared to the previous recordings. PB = phonetically balanced; UD = undistorted; NC = noncompeting; C = competing; SπNo = noise in-phase/signal out-of-phase; SoNπ = signal in-phase/noise out-of-phase; Bin = binaural.

The patient was seen for further testing 3 months later. The EEG was normal. There was some overall improvement in her clinical picture and VEP. Audiometric and AEP studies are shown in Figure 16-11. Monaural low-pass filtered PB discrimination scores were improved for both ears, especially in the left (32% improved). However, the interaural difference was still only 8%.

The dichotic test scores with the SSW also showed improvement in the left ear under the competing condition (17%). RASP and binaural MLD scores were unchanged. AEP recordings were still abnormal bilaterally; however, the left ear recordings showed improvement in

waveform configuration. Waves II and III could be identified; however, the I-III interpeak latency of 2.5 msec was still definitely abnormal with reduced voltage. Waves IV and V still could not be identified on either side.

The improved low-pass filtered PB and SSW test scores in the left ear (and the right ear to some extent) could be either the result of improved hemispheric functions, as the EEG also suggested, or a reflection of changes in the brain stem as indicated by the AEP recordings on the left side. However, as on the first study, since there is such extensive involvement of the brain stem, it is not possible to tell whether the low-pass filtered PB and SSW test scores reflect hemispheric or brain stem abnormality.

Some tests (e.g., MLDs, evoked potentials) reveal abnormalities specific to certain regions of the brain, whereas other tests (monaural low redundancy, dichotic) may be less specific, making localization more difficult. Abnormal test results may be caused by secondary pressure effects of a lesion far from auditory areas, which could lead to false localization of the primary abnormality. Test findings may also suggest more than one localization. Accuracy of identification and localization is enhanced by tests specific to functions mediated at different levels or regions of the brain. Effects of lesions of the peripheral auditory system on test results must be recognized and applied in appropriate cases. The importance of well-defined normative data and abnormal criteria cannot be over emphasized.

REFERENCES

1. Antonelli, A., and Calearo, C. Further investigations on cortical deafness. *Acta Otolaryngol.* 66:97, 1968.
2. Berlin, C. I., et al. The construction and perception of simultaneous messages. *Asha* 10:397, 1968.
3. Berlin, C. I., et al. Central auditory deficits after temporal lobectomy. *Arch. Otolaryngol.* 96:4, 1972.
4. Bocca, E. Clinical aspects of cortical deafness. *Laryngoscope* 68:301, 1958.
5. Bocca, E., and Calearo, C. Central Hearing Processes. In J. Jerger (Ed.), *Modern Developments in Audiology.* New York: Academic, 1963. Pp. 337–370.
6. Bocca, E., Calearo, C., and Cassinari, V. A

new method for testing hearing in temporal lobe tumors. *Acta Otolaryngol.* 44:219, 1954.

7. Bocca, E., et al. Testing "cortical" hearing in temporal lobe tumors. *Acta Otolaryngol.* 45:289, 1955.

8. Brunt, M. The Staggered Spondaic Word Test. In J. Katz (Ed.), *Handbook of Clinical Audiology* (2d ed.). Baltimore: Williams & Wilkins, 1978. Pp. 262–275.

9. Buchwald, J. S., and Huang, C.-M. Far-field acoustic response: origins in the cat. *Science* 189:382, 1975.

10. Buchwald, J. S., et al. Middle- and long-latency auditory evoked responses recorded from the vertex of normal and chronically lesioned cats. *Brain Res.* 205:91, 1981.

11. Calearo, C., and Antonelli, A. R. Audiometric findings in brainstem lesions. *Acta Otolaryngol.* 66:305, 1968.

12. Calearo, C., and Lazzaroni, A. Speech intelligibility in relation to the speed of the message. *Laryngoscope* 67:410, 1957.

13. Chiappa, K. H., Gladstone, K. J., and Young, R. R. Brainstem auditory evoked responses: Studies of wave form variations in 50 normal hearing subjects. *Arch. Neurol.* 36:81, 1979.

14. Cullen, J. K., and Thompson, C. L. Masking release for speech in subjects with temporal lobe resections. *Arch. Otolaryngol.* 100:113, 1974.

15. de Quiros, J. Accelerated speech audiometry, an examination of test results (transl. by J. Tonndorf). *Hear. Res.* Chicago: Beltone Institute, 1964.

16. Gilroy, J., and Lynn, G. E. Reversibility of abnormal auditory findings in cerebral hemisphere lesions. *J. Neurol. Sci.* 21:117, 1974.

17. Gilroy, J., et al. Auditory evoked brainstem potentials in a case of "locked-in" syndrome. *Arch. Neurol.* 34:492, 1977.

18. Hannley, M., Jerger, J. F., and Rivera, V. M. Relationships among auditory brainstem responses, masking level differences and the acoustic reflex in multiple sclerosis. *Audiology* 22:20, 1983.

19. Heilman, K. M., Hammer, L. C., and Wilder, B. J. An audiometric defect in temporal lobe dysfunction. *Neurology* 23:384, 1973.

20. Henry, K. Auditory brainstem volume-conducted responses: Origins in the laboratory mouse. *J. Am. Audiol. Soc.* 4:173, 1979.

21. Hodgson, W. R. Audiological report of a patient with left hemispherectomy. *J. Speech Hear. Disord.* 32:39, 1967.

22. Jerger, J. Audiological manifestations of lesions in the auditory nervous system. *Laryngoscope* 70:417, 1960.

23. Jerger, J. Observations on auditory behavior in lesions of the central auditory pathways. *Arch. Otolaryngol.* 71:797, 1960.

24. Jerger, J. Auditory Tests for Disorders of the Central Auditory Mechanism. In B. R. Alford and W. S. Fields (Eds.), *Neurological Aspects of Auditory and Vestibular Disorders.* Springfield: Thomas, 1964. Pp. 77–86.

25. Jerger, J., and Jerger, S. Auditory findings in brainstem disorders. *Arch. Otolaryngol.* 99:324, 1974.

26. Jerger, J., and Jerger, S. Clinical validity of central auditory tests. *Scand. Audiol.* 4:147, 1975.

27. Jerger, S., and Jerger, J. Extra- and intra-axial brainstem auditory disorders. *Audiology* 14:93, 1975.

28. Jewett, D. Volume-conducted potentials in response to auditory stimuli as detected by averaging in the cat. *Electroencephalogr. Clin. Neurophysiol.* 28:609, 1970.

29. Katz, J. The Staggered Spondee Word Test. In R. W. Keith (Ed.), *Central Auditory Dysfunction.* New York: Grune & Stratton, 1977. Pp. 103–128.

30. Kimura, D. Some effects of temporal-lobe damage on auditory perception. *Can. J. Psychol.* 15:156, 1961.

31. Korsan-Bengtsen, M. Distorted speech audiometry: A methodological and clinical study. *Acta Otolaryngol.* [Suppl.] 310:7, 1973.

32. Kurdziel, S., Noffsinger, D., and Olsen, W. Performance by cortical lesion patients on 40% and 60% time-compressed materials. *J. Am. Audiol. Soc.* 2:3, 1976.

33. Lundborg, T., et al. Information abundance of speech and distorted speech testing in topical diagnosis within the C.N.S. *Scand. Audiol.* 4:9, 1975.

34. Lynn, G. E., and Gilroy, J. Auditory manifestations of lesions of the corpus callosum. *Asha* 13:566, 1971.

35. Lynn, G. E., and Gilroy, J. Neuro-audiological abnormalities in patients with temporal lobe tumors. *J. Neurol. Sci.* 17:167, 1972.

36. Lynn, G. E., and Gilroy, J. Effects of Brain Lesions on the Perception of Monotic and Dichotic Speech Stimuli. In M. D. Sullivan (Ed.), *Central Auditory Processing Disorders.* Omaha: University of Nebraska, 1975. Pp. 47–83.

37. Lynn, G. E., and Gilroy, J. Evaluation of Central Auditory Dysfunction in Patients with Neurological Disorders. In R. W. Keith (Ed.), *Central Auditory Dysfunction.* New York: Grune & Stratton, 1977. Pp. 177–221.

38. Lynn, G. E., et al. Binaural masking-level differences in neurological disorders. *Arch. Otolaryngol.* 107:357, 1981.

39. Matzker, J. Two new methods for the assessment of central auditory functions in cases of brain disease. *Ann. Otol. Rhinol. Laryngol.* 68:1185, 1959.

40. Milner, B., Taylor, L., and Sperry, R. Lateralized suppression of dichotically presented digits after commissural section in man. *Science* 161:184, 1968.

41. Miltenberger, G. E., Dawson, G. J., and Raica, A. N. Central auditory testing with peripheral hearing loss. *Arch. Otolaryngol.* 104:11, 1978.

42. Musiek, F. E., Pinheiro, M. L., and Wilson, D. H. Auditory pattern perception in "split brain" patients. *Arch. Otolaryngol.* 106:610, 1980.

43. Musiek, F. E., and Sachs, E., Jr. Reversible neuroaudiologic findings in a case of right frontal lobe abscess with recovery. *Arch. Otolaryngol.* 106:280, 1980.

44. Musiek, F. A., and Wilson, D. H. SSW and dichotic digit results pre- and post-commissurotomy: A case report. *J. Speech Hear. Disord.* 44:528, 1979.

45. Musiek, F. E., Wilson, D. H., and Pinheiro, M. L. Audiological manifestations in "split-brain" patients. *J. Am. Audiol. Soc.* 5:25, 1979.

46. Musiek, F. E., Wilson, D. H., and Reeves, A. G. Staged commissurotomy and central auditory function. *Arch. Otolaryngol.* 107:233, 1981.

47. Nager, G. T. Acoustic neurinomas: Pathology and differential diagnosis. *Arch. Otolaryngol.* 89:252, 1969.

48. Noffsinger, D., Kurdziel, S., and Applebaum, E. L. Value of special auditory tests in the latero-medial inferior pontine syndrome. *Ann. Otol. Rhinol. Laryngol.* 84:384, 1975.

49. Noffsinger, D., et al. Auditory and vestibular aberrations in multiple sclerosis. *Acta Otolaryngol.* [Suppl.] 303:1, 1972.

50. Ohta, F., Hayashi, R., and Morimoto, M. Differential diagnosis of retrocochlear deafness: Binaural fusion test and binaural separation test. *Int. Audiol.* 6:58, 1967.

51. Olsen, W. O., and Noffsinger, D. Masking level differences for cochlear and brainstem lesions. *Ann. Otol. Rhinol. Laryngol.* 85:820, 1976.

52. Olsen, W. O., Noffsinger, D., and Carhart, R. Masking level differences encountered in clinical populations. *Audiology* 15:287, 1976.

53. Olsen, W. O., Noffsinger, D., and Kurdziel, S. Speech discrimination in quiet and in white noise by patients with peripheral and central lesions. *Acta Otolaryngol.* 80:375, 1975.

54. Palva, A., and Jokinen, K. The role of the binaural test in filtered speech audiometry. *Acta Otolaryngol.* 79:310, 1975.

55. Pinheiro, M. Auditory pattern perception in patients with right and left hemisphere lesions. *Ohio J. Speech Hear.* 12:9, 1976.

56. Pinheiro, M. L. Tests of Central Auditory Function in Children with Learning Disabilities. In R. W. Keith (Ed.), *Central Auditory Dysfunction.* New York: Grune & Stratton, 1977. Pp. 223–256.

57. Quaranta, A., and Cervellera, G. Masking level differences in central nervous system diseases. *Arch. Otolaryngol.* 103:482, 1977.

58. Rowe, M. J. The brainstem auditory evoked response in neurological disease: A review. *Ear Hear.* 2:41, 1981.

59. Smith, B., and Resnick, D. An auditory test for assessing brainstem integrity: Preliminary report. *Laryngoscope* 82:414, 1972.

60. Sparks, R., and Geschwind, N. Dichotic listening in man after section of neocortical commissures. *Cortex* 4:3, 1968.

61. Sparks, R., Goodglass, H., and Nickel, B. Ipsilateral versus contralateral extinction in dichotic listening resulting from hemisphere lesions. *Cortex* 6:249, 1970.

62. Speaks, C. Evaluation of Disorders of the Central Auditory System. In M. M. Paparella and D. A. Shumrick (Eds.), *Otolaryngology,* Vol. II, *The Ear.* Philadelphia: Saunders, 1980. Pp. 1846–1860.

63. Starr, A., and Achor, L. J. Auditory brain stem responses in neurological disease. *Arch. Neurol.* 32:761, 1975.

64. Starr, A., and Hamilton, A. E. Correlation between confirmed sites of neurological lesions and abnormalities of far-field auditory brain stem responses. *Electroencephogr. Clin. Neurophysiol.* 41:595, 1976.

65. Stockard, J. J., and Rossiter, V. S. Clinical and pathologic correlates of brain stem auditory response abnormalities. *Neurology* 27:316, 1977.

66. Willeford, J. Central auditory function in children with learning disabilities. *Audiol. Hear. Educ.* 2:12, 1976.

III

Vestibular Evaluation, Disorders, and Treatment

17

Vestibular Anatomy and Physiology

David L. Asher

The inner ear contains one peripheral sensory organ for hearing and five sensory organs for balance. The nonauditory structures make up the vestibular system and respond to movements and positional changes in space. Such responses to static tilt and angular and linear acceleration in three-dimensional planes require rather elaborate anatomic and physiologic consideration. The functional significance of the vestibular system is seemingly so important to animals' survival that the system's neural responsibilities are intimately shared with the organisms' visual system and postural motor feedback mechanisms.

ANATOMY OF THE VESTIBULAR SYSTEM

Bony Labyrinth

The peripheral vestibular system is located in the petrous portion of the temporal bone (Figs. 17-1 and 17-2). The continuous series of interrelated cavities and channels formed within this extremely hard bone are called the bony (osseous) labyrinth. Three component regions can be identified in the bony labyrinth: the vestibule, the semicircular canals, and the cochlea [1]. The vestibule is a relatively large chamber in the bony labyrinth. The anteroinferior portion of this chamber extends into the cochlea, and the posterosuperior side accepts the end of the three semicircular canals. After forming approximately two thirds of a circle, the three osseous semicircular canals connect with the vestibule at five openings, with the superior and posterior canals sharing a short segment of a single canal, the common osseus crus, which has a single orifice in the vestibule. The bony cochlea resembles a snail shell, the base of which is continuous with the medial and anteroinferior wall of the vestibule.

The inner surface of the bony labyrinth is meagerly lined with epithelium and filled with perilymph, a fluid comparable in chemistry and consistency with cerebrospinal and extracellular fluid. The origin of perilymph remains speculative, although evidence of communication between cerebrospinal fluid and perilymph in the vestibular system has been found in mammals [2, 11]. Two recognized communication routes are through the cochlear aqueduct,

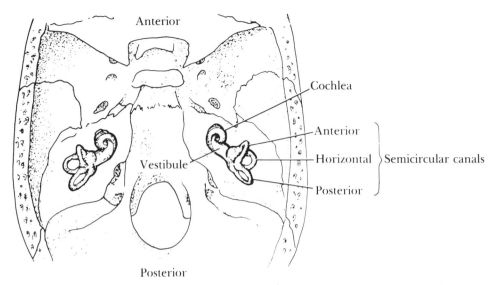

Figure 17-1. Drawing of the bony labyrinths located in the temporal bones of the skull, superior view. The horizontal semicircular canals of each temporal bone are seen in opposition to each other and the anterior and posterior semicircular canals of opposite sides parallel each other. (After J. Sobatta, Blood Vessels-Nervous System-Sense Organs-Integument and Lymphatics. In E. Uhlenhath (Ed.), Atlas of Descriptive Human Anatomy. New York: Hafner, 1957. P. 309.)

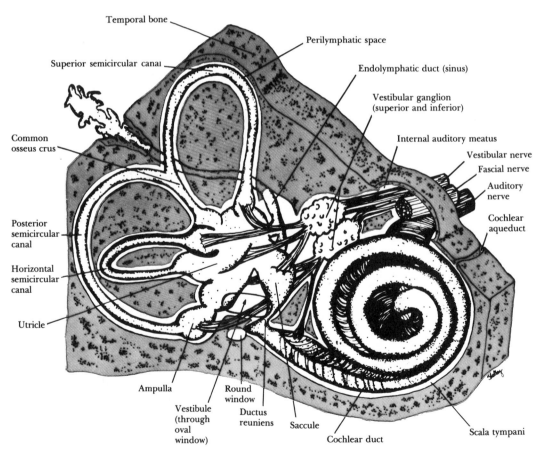

Figure 17-2. Membranous labyrinth within the bony labyrinth of the right temporal bone. The cochlear aqueduct establishes communication with perilymphatic space of the scala tympani near the round window but is depicted as drawn for reasons of simplicity.

a small canal that extends from the subarachnoid space to the scala tympani of the cochlea, and through the internal auditory meatus along eighth cranial nerve fibers that innervate the auditory and vestibular end organs. The primary perilymphatic communication route to the latter appears to be by way of the internal auditory meatus and vestibular portion of the eighth cranial nerve.

MEMBRANOUS LABYRINTH

Vestibular end organs innervated by the eighth nerve are located in the membranous labyrinth. The membranous labyrinth is scantily attached to the bony labyrinth by a thin layer of connective tissue in the perilymph; otherwise it may be considered a fluid-filled tube that generally conforms to the configuration of the bony labyrinth but remains completely sealed from surrounding perilymphatic space. The fluid inside the membranous labyrinth is endolymph and is in chemical contrast to perilymph: perilymph is high in sodium concentration and low in potassium whereas endolymph is low in sodium concentration and high in potassium. Theoretically, the different ionic compositions of these fluids creates a potential gradient across mechanoreceptor membranes of the vestibular end organs, and this difference may be important for energy transduction processes. Precisely how this occurs has not been defined.

The membranous labyrinth consists of five main parts: the cochlear duct, the saccule, the utricle, the semicircular ducts and their ampullae, and the endolymphatic duct and sac. All contain endolymph and are connected through small channels. As depicted in Figure 17-2, the cochlear duct of the membranous labyrinth is joined and continuous with the membranous vestibular labyrinth at the ductus reuniens. The narrow ductus reuniens widens from its attachment to the cochlear duct and opens into the saccule of the membranous labyrinth located in the perilymphatic space of the vestibule. The oval-shaped saccule is located in the spherical recess on the anteroinferior medial wall of the vestibule. At this area of attachment, saccular nerve fibers from the inferior division of the vestibular branch of the eighth nerve permeate the bony labyrinth and enter the sac-

cule directly below a hook-shaped region of saccular sensorineural epithelium, the macula sacculi. Because the macula sacculi is located on the medial wall of the saccule, an approximate vertical macular orientation exists when a human being is in an upright position.

A second duct from the saccule, the saccular duct, permits endolymphatic communication with the endolymphatic duct and indirectly with the utricular duct and utricle. (The saccular duct and utricular duct form two arms of a Y-shaped tube that connect with the endolymphatic duct.) In other words, one tube leaving the saccule and one tube from the utricle meet at the endolymphatic duct permitting continuous endolymphatic communication throughout the membranous labyrinth. Once joined, the endolymphatic duct forms a sinus, narrows through an isthmus according to Anson [1], and again widens into the endolymphatic sac. The sac is divided into two anatomic regions—rugose and smooth. The rugose portion is irregularly shaped and extends beyond the bony labyrinth before becoming smooth and terminating in a pouch within layers of dura mater of the brain (see Fig. 17-2).

The utricular duct extends from the endolymphatic duct superiorly to open into the utricle. The utricle is usually described as an irregular oval-shaped sac and located superior and posterior to the saccule in the perilymph-filled vestibule. Like the saccule, the utricle is also attached to the medial wall of the vestibule, and the utricular branch of the vestibular division of the eighth nerve enters the utricle and extends beneath the macula utriculi. Unlike the macula sacculi, the macula utriculi is located at the bottom of the utricle or in a horizontal plane relevant to one's normal upright posture. The oval window is located approximately 1.5 to 1.9 mm across the vestibule in opposition to the lateral membranous boundaries of the utricle and saccule [1].

Five openings in the utricle permit endolymphatic communication with the three membranous semicircular canals. These canals follow the confines of the bony semicircular canals and occupy one third of their space. The superior and posterior membranous canals also share a common membranous crus within the common os-

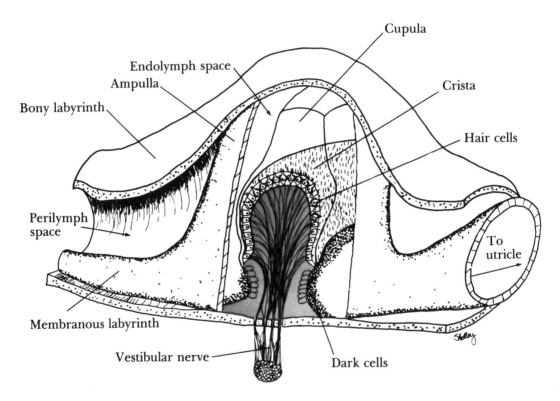

Figure 17-3. Drawing of the ampullated end of a semicircular canal and related internal structures. (Adapted from E. Mira and F. dal Negro, Die histochemischen und histoenzymologischen Eigenschapten des Epithels der Ubergangszone der Crista Ampullans. Arch. Ohr. Nas.-Kehlk-Heilk, 193:222, 1969.)

seus crus. A dilated area, called an ampulla, is located at one end of each canal near its opening into the utricle (Fig. 17-3). At the base of these dilations is a region of membranous attachments to the bony labyrinth and an extension of a crista into the membranous ampulla. Cristae are arched prominences across the base of the ampullae in the direct path of endolymphatic current moving through the semicircular canals and ampullae (Fig. 17-4).

Vestibular nerve fibers permeate the bony labyrinth at the ampullae below the cristae in a manner similar to that of the maculae. The nerve fibers then lose their myelin sheath as they pass through a basement membrane to terminate on hair cells (ciliated mechanoreceptors). The surface

epithelium of the cristae and maculae is made up of supporting cells and two kinds of hair cells, type I and type II (Fig. 17-5). Type I hair cells are shaped like a rounded flask, the neck and lower portion of which are surrounded by an afferent nerve ending of calyx shape. Type II hair cells are cylindrical, and both efferent and afferent nerve terminals are located at the base of these cells. Efferent nerve endings have also been identified contacting the nerve chalice of type I hair cells [16]. The intri-

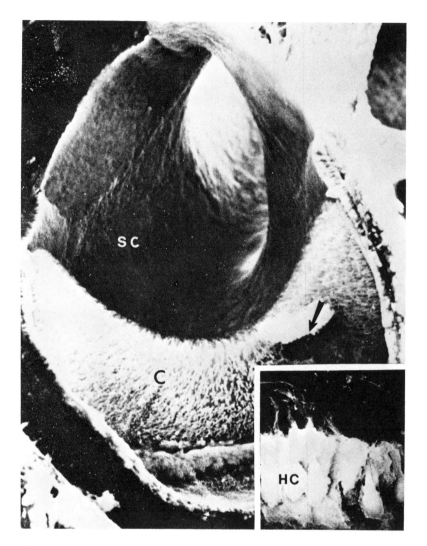

Figure 17-4. Scanning electron micrograph of a crista (C) located in the partially dissected ampulla of a semicircular canal (SC). Tufts of stereocilia and kinocilia are observed covering the surface of the crista. The gelatinous cupula is missing. The inset is a higher magnification of hair cells (HC) seen along the edges of a hole (arrow) made in the crista with a fine pick. Note the flask shape of certain hair cells.

cacies of a feedback system for suppression of hair cell response remains speculative. Both types I and II hair cells are evident on cristae. However, the crest of the crista is predominantly composed of type I hair cells. The upper surface of each hair cell is covered with an orderly array of stereocilia and a single kinocilium. Kinocilia are located on the perimeter of each hair cell surface and approximately 50 to 100 stereo-

cilia protrude adjacent to it. Kinocilia on the hair cell surface are oriented toward the utricle in the horizontal semicircular canals and away from the utricle on the superior and posterior canal cristae. The length of the stereocilia decreases as the distance from the kinocilia increases. Movement of stereocilia toward the kinocilia results in depolarization of the hair cell, and movement away from the kinocilia results in hyperpolarization. This morphologically directional response has been uniquely demonstrated by Hudspeth and Corey [10], who mechanically stimulated the hair bundles and measured intracellular changes in response to stereocilia movement. Furthermore, greater extracellular current flow occurs near the top of the stereocilia during

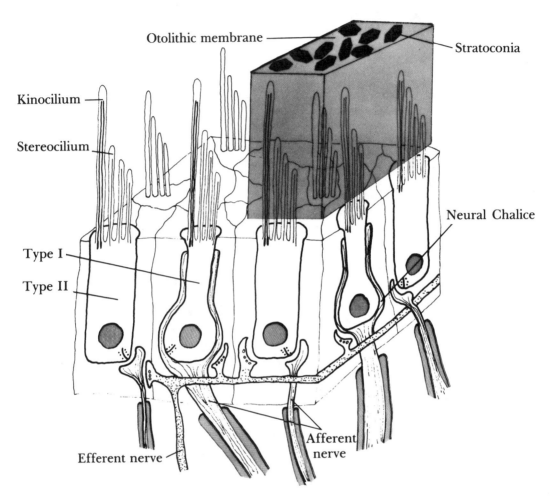

Figure 17-5. Drawing of neural distribution to types I and II hair cells in vestibular maculae. Afferent nerves innervate both type I and type II hair cells. Efferent nerve fibers terminate at type II hair cells and on afferent nerve endings. (After C. Smith and G. Rasmussen, Nerve endings in the maculae and cristae of the chinchilla vestibule, with special reference to the efferents. Third Symposium on the Role of Vestibular Organs in Space Exploration. NASA SP-152, 1967.)

mechanical stimulation, and Hudspeth [9] attributes cablelike electrical properties from the stereocilia to the hair cell as principals for the transduction process.

The kinocilia and stereocilia are not free to move in endolymph but are embedded in a cap of fixed gelatinous substance called the cupula of the ampullary crest and the otolithic membrane of the maculae (see Fig. 17-5). The otolithic membrane contains very small crystals of calcium carbonate called statoconia. These tiny rocks increase the density of the otolithic membrane that covers the maculae. Morphologically, another region can be identified in the maculae that seems to have a functional relationship with the otolithic membrane and the hair cells. This thickened region is called the striola and stretches through the

long axis of the sensory epithelium near the centers of the maculae. Type I hair cells are more numerous in the striola than type II hair cells, a condition similar to that noted for the crown of the cristae. Kinocilia on the tops of the macular hair cells are aligned and subsequently polarized toward the striola of the macula of the utricle and away from the striola of the macula of the saccule [12]. The thickness of the otolithic membrane also varies above each macula. In the region of the striola, a thin otolithic membrane is observed above the macula of the utricle while a thick membrane is observed above the striola of the saccular macula.

PHYSIOLOGY OF THE VESTIBULAR SYSTEM

The physiology of the semicircular canals and maculae is not completely understood. However, initial consideration is given to the orientation of the vestibular sense organs in the skull (see Fig. 17-1). The horizontal canals are inclined toward the utricle at an angle of approximately 30 degrees. When the skull is in an anatomically erect position, the anterior and posterior vertical canals are at right angles to it and approximate 45-degree angles to the sagittal plane of the skull. The result of this configuration is that the anterior canal on one side of the head is parallel with the posterior canal on the other side of the head, and these canals then function as an opposing pair. More specifically, as endolymph moves in one direction on one side of the head stimulating the hair cells and resulting in depolarization, hyperpolarization is occurring in the paired canal on the opposite side. The same phenomenon is observed in the horizontal canals. The precise manner in which the hair cells in the semicircular canals are stimulated is currently being investigated.

For many years it has been accepted that as the head turns, endolymph in the membranous semicircular canals lags behind the movement of the ducts and attached cupulae. Thus, as the cupulae move through the endolymph, stereocilia embedded in the cupulae and attached to hair cells on the cristae are bent. This bending results in depolarization or hyperpolarization of the receptor cell, depending on the direction of endolymphatic flow against the cupulae. Eventually, the endolymph gains momentum and matches the velocity of head movement, and a resulting loss of mechanical stimulation to the hair cells occurs. If head rotation diminishes, endolymph continues to move past the cupulae and the response of the hair cells is reversed as the cupulae pivots in the opposite direction.

Recently, these concepts of vestibular stimulation have been challenged. Dohlman [5] argues that direct fluid displacement of the stereocilia may occur in subcupular space with force sufficient for transduction. Although many aspects of this theory remain to be tested, convincing supporting evidence has been presented by Valli and Zucca [17], Hudspeth and Cory [9], and Orman and Flock [14].

The utriculi and sacculi maculae are oriented at right angles to each other as mentioned, but perhaps equally important is the observation that the hair cells on the maculae are oriented in relationship to curvature of the striolae. Thus, a multi-directional pattern of hair cell polarization occurs as the head moves through different positions. Either static tilts or linear acceleration causes shifts in the otoconia above the otolithic membrane hair cells of the maculae.

CENTRAL NERVOUS SYSTEM CONNECTIONS

The vestibular (Scarpa's) ganglion, located at the bottom of the internal auditory meatus, comprises approximately 20,000 primary bipolar afferent vestibular nerve cell bodies and is divided anatomically into superior and inferior divisions (see Fig. 17-2). As the superior division extends peripherally, four branches emerge to the superior and horizontal canal crista, the utricular macula, and the anterosuperior part of the saccular macula. The inferior division projects to innervate the main portion of the saccular macula and the posterior canal crista by way of the singulari nerve. Large and small nerve fibers have been identified in the superior division of the vestibular nerve [6]. The large fibers make contact with type I hair cells located primarily in the crests of the superior and horizontal cristae and the striolae of the maculae, and to a lesser amount in the sacculus. Small fibers end at type II hair cells peripherally to the type I hair cell regions. The functional significance of this relationship is not clear; however, the large nerve fibers terminate on large neurons in the brain stem and small fibers connect with small neurons. Medial to the vestibular ganglion, the now undivided vestibular nerve continues with the auditory portion of the

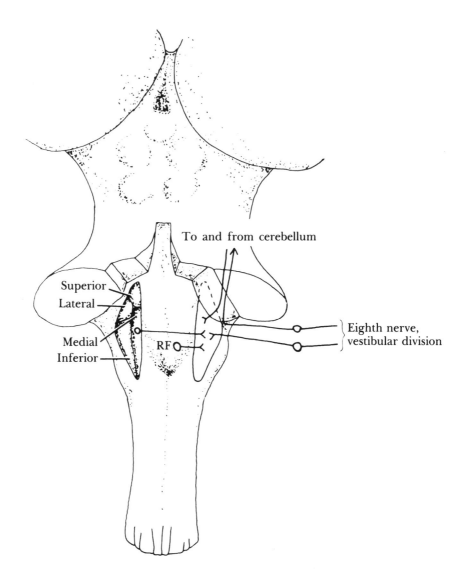

Figure 17-6. Location of right vestibular nerve terminations in the brain stem. Principal commissural connections to the right vestibular nuclei are also depicted; however, not all contacts between vestibular nuclei occur in the medial vestibular nuclei but are simplified for this drawing. RF = reticular formation. (Courtesy of J. Nolte, The Human Brain. St. Louis: Mosby, 1981.)

eighth cranial nerve. On exiting the internal auditory meatus they enter the brain stem near the cerebellopontile angle at the pontomedullary junction (Fig. 17-6).

Four vestibular nuclei are located in this region of the brain stem and are named for their relative cytoarchitecture: the superior (Bekhterevi), lateral (Deiters'), medial (Schwalbe's), and inferior (or spiral of descending) (see Fig. 17-6). All vestibular ganglion fibers bifurcate into ascending and descending branches as they enter the brain stem, and the majority of these primary neurons from each cristae and maculae then terminate in particular regions of the vestibular nuclei specific to that end organ. A small number of collateral fibers

from the semicircular canal cristae terminate in the interstitial nucleus just prior to the vestibular nuclei, while ascending branches continue beyond the vestibular nuclei to the cerebellum. Similarly, a few collateral fibers from the main macula sacculi branch terminate in the "Y" nucleus before terminating in the vestibular nuclei. Such organization is beyond the scope

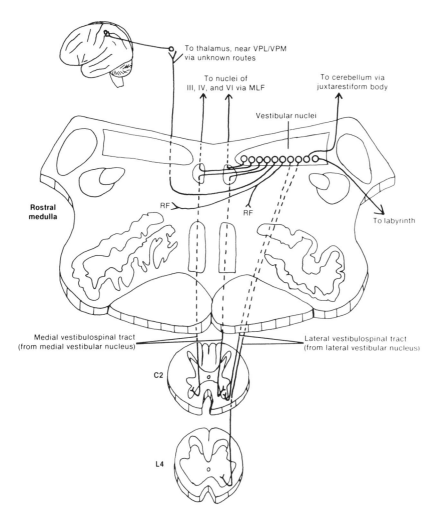

To thalamus, near VPL/VPM
via unknown routes

To nuclei of
III, IV, and VI via MLF

To cerebellum via
juxtarestiform body

Vestibular nuclei

Rostral
medulla

RF

RF

To labyrinth

Medial vestibulospinal tract
(from medial vestibular nucleus)

Lateral vestibulospinal tract
(from lateral vestibular nucleus)

C2

L4

Figure 17-7. Some projection routes for ascending and descending fibers from the vestibular nuclei. Projections to the contralateral vestibular nuclei are not shown. VPL = ventral posterolateral nucleus of thalamus; VPM = ventral posteromedial nucleus of thalamus; MLF = medial longitudinal fasciculus; RF = reticular formation. (Courtesy of J. Nolte, The Human Brain. St. Louis: Mosby, 1981.)

of this text; however, a thorough description is presented by Schuknecht [15], Gacek [8], and Nolte [13].

Vestibular nuclei likewise receive input from the cerebellum, the spinal cord, and the contralateral vestibular nuclei. These connections assist in integrating information from the peripheral vestibular system regarding posture, movement, tilt, and coordinated eye and head movements.

Secondary fibers from the vestibular nuclei also project to the cerebellum, the spinal cord, the contralateral vestibular nuclei,

the extraocular nuclei, the reticular formation, the peripheral vestibular end organs, and the thalamus (Fig. 17-7). Neuroanatomic investigations by Brodal and associates [3], Carpenter [4], and Gacek [7] indicate that secondary fibers from each vestibular nuclei follow specific pathways to terminate in regions of the central nervous system relevant to regulation and maintenance of equilibrium. For example, ascending neurons from the medial and descending vestibular nuclei pass through the juxtarestiform body to terminate in the cerebellum. Other projections from the vestibular nuclei extend to the anterior horns of the spinal cord through two separate descending routes. Some fibers from the lateral vestibular nucleus follow a direct ipsilateral course in the vestibule spinal tract to innervate all levels of the spinal cord. However, other branches from the medial and descending vestibular nuclei communicate bilaterally through the descending medial longitudinal fasciculi (MLF), a tract of fibers communicating through the rostral part of the brain stem and thoracic regions of the spinal cord. Both of these tracts innervate trunk and limb reflexes.

The vestibulo-ocular reflex is also dependent on secondary vestibular nerve projects. This reflex permits visual fixation on objects during head movements, but should not be confused with visual tracking phenomenon because the reflex can occur in darkness [13]. Four sets of fibers from vestibular nuclei innervate the third (oculomotor), fourth (trochlear), and sixth (abducens) nerves. Two of these sets arise from the superior and medial vestibular nuclei, pass through the ipsilateral and contralateral MLF respectively, and innervate the third and fourth cranial nerves. These nerves supply extraocular muscles to the exclusion of the inferior rectus. The other two sets of fibers arise from the lateral and medial vestibular nuclei and bypass the MLF en route to the extraocular nuclei. Involuntary rhythmic eye movements resulting from stimulation of the vestibulo-ocular reflex are called nystagmus, and its diagnostic significance is discussed at length in Chapter 18.

Secondary vestibular nerve fibers from vestibular nuclei to the reticular formation that forms the central core of the brain stem have been identified as having efferent fibers leading peripherally through the eighth nerve to hair cells in the vestibular end organs. Their purpose is poorly defined. Furthermore, the neuroanatomic pathways from vestibular nuclei to the thalamus and cortex beyond remains speculative, as does their function.

REFERENCES

1. Anson, B. J., and Donaldson, J. A. *The Surgical Anatomy of the Temporal Bone and Ear*. Philadelphia: Saunders, 1967.
2. Asher, D., and Sando, I. Perilymphatic communication routes in the auditory and vestibular system. *Otolaryngol. Head Neck Surg.* 89:822, 1981.
3. Brodal, A., Pompeiano, O., and Walberg, F. The vestibular nuclei and their connections, anatomy and functional correlations. The Henderson Trust Lectures. Edinburgh, Scotland: Oliver and Boyd, 1962.
4. Carpenter, M. The Ascending Vestibular System and Its Relationship to Conjugate Horizontal Eye Movements. In R. Wolfson (Ed.), *The Vestibular System and Its Diseases*. Philadelphia: University of Pennsylvania Press, 1966.
5. Dohlman, G. F. Critical review of the concept of cupula function. *Acta Otolaryngol.* [Suppl.] 376:1, 1980.
6. Gacek, R. The course and central termination of first order neurons supplying vestibular end organs in the cat. *Acta Otolaryngolog.* [Suppl.] 254, 1969.
7. Gacek, R. Anatomical demonstration of the vestibulo-ocular projections in the cat. *Laryngoscope* 81:1559, 1971.
8. Gacek, R. Neuroanatomical correlates of vestibular function. *Ann. Otol. Rhinol. Laryngol.* 89:2, 1980.
9. Hudspeth, A. J. Extracellular current flow and the site of transduction by vertebrate hair cells. *J. Neurol. Sci.* 2:1, 1982.
10. Hudspeth, A. J., and Corey, D. P. Sensitivity, polarity, and conductance change in the response of vertebrate hair cells to controlled mechanical stimuli. *Proc. Natl. Acad. Sci. USA* 74:2407, 1977.
11. Jahnke, K. Electronenmikroskopische Untersuchungen uber die Permeabilitats barrieren des Innenhores. *Arch. Klin. Exp. Ohrennasenkehlkopfheilk* 204:199, 1973.
12. Lindeman, H. Regional differences in structure of the vestibular sensory region. *J. Laryngol. Otol.* 83:4, 1969.
13. Mira, E., and Negro, dal F. Die histochemischen und histoenzymologischen Eigenschaften des Epithels der Ubergangzone der Crista Ampullaris. *Arch. Ohr. Nas.-Kehlk-Heilk* 193:222, 1969.
14. Nolte, J. *The Human Brain*. St. Louis: Mosby, 1981.
15. Orman, S. S., and Flock, A. Micromechanics of the hair cell stereociliary bundles in the frog crista ampullaris. Paper presented at Association for Research in Otolaryngology. Winter, 1981.
16. Schuknecht, H. F. *Pathology of the Ear*. Cambridge, Mass.: Harvard University Press, 1974.
17. Smith, C., and Rasmussen, G. Nerve endings in the maculae and cristae of the chinchilla vestibule, with special reference to the efferents. Third Symposium on the Role of the Vestibular Organs in Space Exploration. NASA SP-152, 1967.
18. Sobatta, J. Blood Vessels-Nervous System-Sense Organs-Integument and Lymphatics. In E. Uhlenhuth (Ed.), *Atlas of Descriptive Human Anatomy*, Vol. III. New York: Hafner, 1957. P. 309.
19. Valli, P., and Zucca, G. The origin of slow potentials in semi-circular canals of the frog. *Acta Otolaryngol.* 81:395, 1976.

18
Electronystagmography

Thomas W. Norris

A dizzy patient is seldom able to describe his symptoms. He may commonly use words like *giddy, lightheaded,* or *fuzzy.* Yet it is essential to obtain as much information and as accurate a description of his symptoms as possible, because such a patient may have serious organic problems that can be corrected medically or surgically. Electronystagmography can provide much information and ultimately assist in diagnosis.

Equilibrium is controlled by the vestibular systems, which are part of the inner ear. These systems should be considered early in the examination of the dizzy patient. The most accurate method of evaluating the vestibular apparatus is electronystagmography (ENG), which has become an accepted, routine test in the otoneurologic office.

ENG is an electrical method of recording eye movements. Its greatest advantage is that eye movement, or nystagmus, can be recorded when the patient's eyes are closed. When the eyes are opened, nystagmus (particularly that resulting from vestibular dysfunction) is often suppressed with visual fixation. ENG thus permits inspection of nystagmus that may otherwise be missed owing to visual fixation. The test also provides objective records and precise quantitative values rather than merely an examiner's subjective impression of a patient's eye movements. Also, the method provides a permanent record of a patient's spontaneous or induced nystagmus. Recording of nystagmus, however, does not define specific pathology. Findings must always be judged as nonpathognomonic and combined with the record of the patient's symptoms and other diagnostic test data before the physician diagnoses a disease. Perhaps a common misconception of ENG is that the test conclusively and independently defines the wide variety of diseases associated with dizziness. This, of course, is not the case. With proper interpretation ENG results provide information supporting an organic basis for a patient's symptoms. The data either will support a finding of a peripheral or a central lesion, or will provide evidence of pathology without additional information regarding localization. With experience in reviewing ENG tracings, the examiner can relate the findings to specific diseases with greater confidence.

LABYRINTHINE ANATOMY AND PHYSIOLOGY

The body orientation of human beings is monitored by three sensory systems: the somatosensory, the visual, and the vestibular. The primary equilibrium sensory receptors are in the vestibular apparatus, in the petrous portion of the temporal bone. The two vestibular systems function synergistically to send the brain information regarding head and body position.

The vestibular apparatus is in a constant state of tonic activity. Each vestibular system exerts a steady discharge of action potentials to eye musculature. Neural pathways lead from the right vestibular nuclei to the rectus muscles on the left side of both eyes (Fig. 18-1). Pathways from the left vestibular nuclei lead to the rectus muscles on the right side of the eyes. Thus, each vestibular apparatus influences muscles that pull the eyes in the opposite direction. Consequently, normal equilibrium

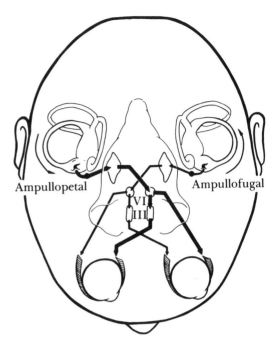

Ampullopetal   Ampullofugal

Figure 18-2. The head turns to the right, causing ampullopetal and ampullofugal displacement of the cristae in the right and left horizontal canals, respectively. III = oculomotor nuclei; VI = abducens nuclei.

Figure 18-1. Neural pathways from the cristae of the horizontal canals lead to the muscles that control eye movement in the horizontal plane. III = oculomotor nuclei; VI = abducens nuclei.

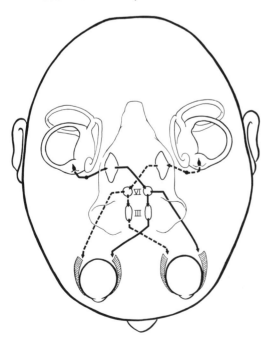

depends on equal and opposite contractions of the eye muscles.

The discharge rate of action potentials is increased when the endolymphatic flow within the horizontal canal is directed toward the cupula (ampullopetal motion). When the endolymphatic flow is away from the cupula (ampullofugal motion), it creates a decrease in the discharge rate of action potentials. The opposite is true for the vertical canals. When the head is turned to the right with the head erect and the lateral canal perpendicular to the plane of rotation, there is an ampullopetal displacement of the cupula in the right horizontal canal, and an ampullofugal displacement of the cupula in the left horizontal canal (Fig. 18-2). The complementing alterations of electrical discharge rates from the receptor organs, increased right and decreased left, signal the brain of the head movement. When the head movement stops, the endolymphatic flow in both lateral semicircular canals reverses in direction, causing an ampullofugal displacement of the cupula in the right horizontal semicircular canal and an ampullopetal displacement of the cupula in the left horizontal canal. Again, alterations in receptor systems alert the brain to the head movement. The eyes move in the direction of the endolymphatic flow and in the plane of the affected canal.

If one vestibular system becomes paretic, the opposite system becomes dominant and pulls the eyes slowly toward the paretic side. When the brain is alerted to the abnormal drift of the eyes, it pulls the eyes quickly back to the original point of gaze.

IDENTIFICATION OF NYSTAGMUS

Rhythmic movement of the eyes is termed nystagmus. Pendular movement with eyes opened, which is viewed or recorded as deflections right and left of equal intensity, is always of central origin. Vestibular nystagmus, referred to as jerk nystagmus eye movement, consists of a slow drift of the eyes in one direction with a quick recovery or jerk back to center line. Nystagmus is said to beat in the direction of the quick component. The direction of the beat is used to identify the direction of nystagmus. The slow phase of nystagmus is vestibular; the quick phase is central. Despite this fact, vestibular nystagmus is by convention defined by the direction of the quick component because the quick movement is the more evident to visual inspection. Figure 18-3 depicts an ENG recording of pendular or central nystagmus, vestibular right-beating nystagmus, and vestibular left-beating nystagmus.

CLASSIFICATION OF NYSTAGMUS

Nystagmus can be either spontaneous (produced within the patient) or induced (re-

Figure 18-3. A. Pendular nystagmus. B. Right-beating nystagmus. C. Left-beating nystagmus.

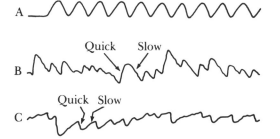

sulting from some form of stimulation provided by the examiner). Either type of nystagmus may occur with eyes opened or closed.

Coats [13] differentiates between spontaneous nystagmus and positional nystagmus occurring with eyes closed. He defines as spontaneous any nystagmus that occurs in a position previously determined as neutral (usually sitting or supine position), regardless of whether it appears in any of the other positions tested. Coats terms positional any nystagmus that does not occur in the neutral position but appears when the head is repositioned.

Nylen's [3] classification of positional nystagmus is generally accepted. Nylen's type I is directional-changing nystagmus beating in one direction when the head is in a given position but reversing direction when the head position is changed. Type II is directional-fixed nystagmus, in which the nystagmus always beats in the same direction, although it may be present only in some positions and may vary in intensity between positions. Type III is generally referred to as transient nystagmus, in which a positional nystagmus appears initially following a head movement and subsides within a few seconds. Type III also includes nystagmus that is influenced by posture but that cannot be categorized as either type I or type II.

Much has been written about the benign paroxysmal type of positional nystagmus described by Dix and Hallpike [17] in 1952. They concluded that a particular form of positional nystagmus elicited by bodily movement was indicative of a peripheral lesion. Dix and Hallpike attributed the occurrence of this type of nystagmus to utricular degeneration of the ear.

Nystagmus can be induced by various external stimuli, including electrical current, positive or negative angular acceleration, and application of heat or cold. The disadvantage of electrical current applied in the region of the ear is that the stimulation may not be limited to the vestibular apparatus but instead may reach the eighth nerve or its nuclei in the brain stem. Positive or negative acceleration in rotational testing has the disadvantage of subjecting both labyrinthine systems to a similar stimulation, making it difficult to interpret which system might be paretic.

The most widely used stimulation in vestibular testing today is the cold and warm water caloric. Caloric stimulation has the greatest clinical potential because it allows the examiner to assess each labyrinthine system independently of the other. Brown-Séquard first described the response of the vestibular apparatus to a syringe of cold water in the external auditory canal [22]. Bárány recognized the clinical importance of the response and first described the reasons for the action of the caloric stimulus [22]. The caloric test most commonly accepted today was originally developed by Fitzgerald and Hallpike [18].

A cold water caloric stimulus cools a section of the lateral canal and the endolymphatic fluid in that section. When the canal is positioned vertically, the cooled endolymph increases in density and falls. Conversely, a warm caloric stimulus heats a section of the lateral canal and the endolymph, causing the fluid to decrease in density and rise. Hence the cupula can be pushed in either an ampullofugal or an ampullopetal direction, depending on the temperature of the stimulus.

Caloric testing can also be done with hot and cold air. The air procedure has several advantages over the water method, as pointed out by Capps and associates [10] including greater convenience, improved patient tolerance and comfort, ease of applicability, and wide flexibility. With further development of equipment and research, air testing may become a more popular and accepted technique.

Both warm and cold stimuli should be used in the test. Jongkees [22] stressed that if only one is used a positive nystagmus response does not prove a viable labyrinth. It is possible for a dormant spontaneous nystagmus to be provoked by caloric stimuli, providing a false measure of sensitivity. Hart presents excellent rationale for using the warm caloric stimulus in preference to the cold for routine screening of patients for vestibular disorders. However, he states, "If any abnormality is detected, the case warrants a full Hallpike caloric test to clarify the situation" [20].

As discussed previously, a unilateral labyrinthine weakness causes the eyes to be pulled toward the side of the paresis (slow drift). This creates a directional preponderance away from the paretic side, and in acute peripheral dysfunction a spontaneous nystagmus also beats away from the paretic labyrinth. A warm caloric stimulus will cause a greater difference in responses between the two vestibular systems than will the cold caloric stimulus. For example, if a patient has a right labyrinthine paresis and left-beating spontaneous nystagmus, the warm caloric stimulus to the right will elicit right-beating nystagmus, but the reaction will be suppressed. This suppression will occur not only because of the paretic condition of the labyrinth but also because of the existing left-beating nystagmus that must be counteracted before an appropriate response is produced. The warm caloric stimulus to the left side is received by a normal labyrinth, and the response is enhanced by the already present left-beating spontaneous nystagmus. In the same example, the cold caloric stimulus presented to the right ear elicits a weak response (left-beating nystagmus) because of the paretic condition of this labyrinth. Yet the response will appear stronger because of the superimposed existing spontaneous nystagmus. The cold left caloric stimulus is presented to a normal labyrinthine system, yet the response (right-beating nystagmus) cannot be strong because of the counteracting left-beating spontaneous nystagmus. Consequently, the differences in the sensitivity measures are more pronounced when using a warm caloric than when using a cold. Testing with both water temperatures can help to minimize error.

TRACING EYE MOVEMENT

Eye movement can be recorded electrically because of the cornea-retina polarity differences. The cornea is electropositive and the retina is electronegative. This difference was discovered independently by Dewar and McKendrick in Edinburgh and by Holmgren in Upsala approximately 100 years ago [27].

The eye functions as a rotatable dipole. Skin electrodes properly placed at the outer canthus of each eye detect changes in the electrical potential. When the eyes deflect to the right, the positive voltage in

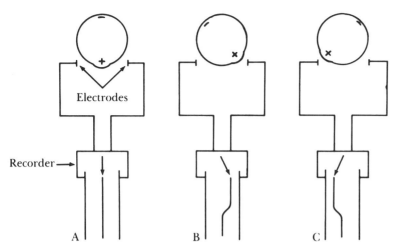

Figure 18-4. A. *ENG recording with the eye fixed at midline.* B. *When the eye deflects left, the tracing deflects downward.* C. *When the eye moves to the right, the pen deflects upward.*

the cornea moves nearer to the right electrode, and the negative voltage in the retina moves nearer to the left electrode. This change in the electrical potential (microvolt range) can be observed graphically using a galvanometer. Figure 18-4 illustrates the pen deflections of an ENG recording that coincide with eye movement. For horizontal nystagmus, a pen excursion upward always represents an eye movement to the right, and a pen deflection downward shows eye movement to the left.

Mechanics
ENG testing should be done in a darkened room with a washbasin. An adequately equipped laboratory requires several basic items of equipment [24].

A couch approximately 7 feet long with a headboard that can be raised to an angle of 30 degrees
A two-channel AC-coupler recorder
An optokinetic drum
A caloric irrigator containing a pump system

Other equipment that is helpful but not essential to ENG testing includes a commercially available calibrator, a computer to calculate the intensity of the slow phase of nystagmus, and an optokinetic stimu-lator in addition to the drum. This sort of stimulator is sometimes useful in dealing with children and patients who have visual problems.

Procedure
The ENG test procedure usually requires about one hour, with additional time for measurement and calibration. Initially, electrodes are placed at the outer canthus of each eye, providing a measurement of nystagmus in the horizontal plane. Electrodes are also placed above and below the eyes to trace vertical nystagmus. A fifth electrode, the ground, is attached to the forehead. It is important that the plane of the electrodes pasted at the outer canthi extends through the pupil when the patient is looking straight ahead. Similarly, the vertical electrodes should be placed on a plane that extends through the pupil. The area of electrode placement should be cleansed, and a small amount of contact paste applied to the skin. The electrode is then filled or covered with the same paste and attached to the skin with tape that can be removed easily.

In some instances, a patient may have a nonfunctional eye. If so, it is best to first place the electrodes at the outer canthi of both eyes and sample and record eye movement. Then, both electrodes are attached at the lateral canthi of the functional eye, and another sample tracing is recorded. The placement that produces the best tracing should be used.

To measure horizontal eye movement the electrodes must be placed so that eye movement to the right deflects the recording pen upward, and eye movement to the left deflects the pen downward. In recording vertical nystagmus, the electrodes must be placed so that upward eye movement produces an upward pen deflection and downward movement a downward deflection.

It is necessary that vertical nystagmus be evaluated because this response often predominates or occurs independently in certain test procedures.

Calibration. After the electrodes have been properly attached, the examiner must relate the amplitude of the recording pen excursion to a known eye movement, a process called calibration. Five dots are placed on the ceiling. The dots are arranged to form a diamond, with the fifth dot in the center. The center dot is located directly in front of the patient (lying supine) and on a line with the bridge of the nose. The dots are positioned so that by looking from the center point to any other dot, the eyes move 10 degrees. The distance between the eyes and the dots should be at least 3 feet to prevent convergent eye movement.

To determine exact placement of the dots, the distance from the bridge of the patient's nose to the center point is measured. That distance, in inches or centimeters, is then multiplied by the tangent of 10 degrees, or 0.176. The product is the distance that the horizontal and vertical dots should be placed from midpoint. Dots can be placed permanently on the ceiling so that all calibrations are done in the same way with all patients in the same position.

Calibration is accomplished by requesting that the patient look from the extreme left dot to the extreme right dot, an eye deflection of 20 degrees. The movement should be repeated approximately 10 times. The sensitivity of the ENG recorder should then be adjusted to obtain a pen deflection (amplitude) equivalent to approximately 20 mm. Similar calibration procedures are used for vertical eye displacement.

A calibrating device can also be obtained commercially, eliminating the need for use of the dot pattern.

The basic calibration measurements are used to determine the speed of the slow component of the nystagmus beat. Therefore, calibration is essential immediately prior to beginning the test and before each caloric stimulation later in the test sequence.

MEASUREMENT OF NYSTAGMUS RESPONSE

There are a variety of ways to analyze the caloric nystagmus response. Although measurements of latency and duration of the nystagmus response have been used, the speed of slow component has become the most popular method of assessing the magnitude of the nystagmus intensity. Aschan [1] and Henriksson [21] have reported that maximum speed of slow component correlates better with changes in stimulus intensity. Recently Dennis [16], investigating the reliability of several response parameters, reported that speed of the slow component, total beats, and the culmination of frequency are highly reliable and may be used with equal confidence. This chapter emphasizes the measurement of the speed of the slow component, but it is appropriate to define the other two parameters of latency and duration.

Latency is the time in seconds from the initiation of the caloric irrigation to the first nystagmus beat. *Duration* is the time in seconds from the beginning of the first nystagmus response to its termination. Prior to the development of ENG, duration was probably the most widely accepted parameter. After caloric stimulation, the examiner would require that the patient look straight ahead and time the duration of the nystagmus response with a stop-watch. Because vestibular nystagmus can be suppressed by visual fixation, Frenzel's glasses were used to magnify the eye for inspection and also to reduce the patient's ability to suppress nystagmus. These glasses are not completely effective, and cases have been recorded in which nystagmus was not observed with Frenzel's glasses but was detected by ENG.

Nystagmus duration can be measured by ENG with the eyes closed, but paper con-

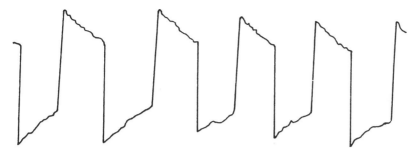

Figure 18-5. Tracing of a calibrated eye movement.

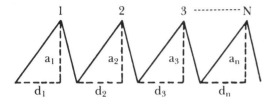

Figure 18-6. Example of the traditional method for determining the speed of the slow component. a = amplitude; d = duration.

sumption is a problem when recording a response that may last three to four minutes. Because few clinical programs use the parameters of latency or duration, it seems justifiable to depend on the measurement of speed of slow component.

Speed of slow component can be obtained by several measuring techniques that differ in terms of ease of application. An expedient measuring method is highly desirable in any ENG laboratory, providing there is no risk of increasing error. Currently, there are five methods by which the speed of slow component can be measured. They are

Traditional
Extended line
Protractor
Velocity
Computer

The traditional, extended line, and protractor methods require hand measurement of the raw nystagmus tracing, necessitating a two-step procedure. For these three hand measurement techniques, it is essential to first determine a calibration factor (CF) based on the tracing from a calibrated eye movement (Fig. 18-5). The calibration factor is obtained by averaging ten vertical pen deflections (mm) for 20 degrees for horizontal eye movements. (Adjust recorder gain as near as possible for 20-mm vertical pen deflections.)

$$average = \frac{sum\ vertical\ (mm)}{10}$$

Divide the average into 20 degrees for the vertical deflections factor (VDF) and multiply by paper speed (mm/sec.) For example, if average = 22 mm and paper speed = 10 mm/sec,

$$CF = VDF \times 10$$
$$VDF = \frac{20}{22}\ or\ .91°/mm$$
$$CF = .91°/mm \times 10\ mm/sec = 9.1°/sec$$

The calibration factor defines the number of degrees of eye arc movement per second per millimeter of vertical pen deflection. It is a measurement constant that must be derived for each patient.

The *traditional method* of determining the speed of the slow component requires that the average slope (AS) be defined for ten of the most intense consecutive nystagmus beats by summing their amplitude (mm) and dividing by the sum of their duration (mm) (Fig. 18-6). To obtain the speed of the slow component in degrees per second, average slope is multiplied by

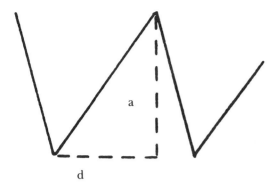

Figure 18-7. Velocity (°/sec) of any nystagmus beat equals calibration factor times amplitude (a) over duration (d).

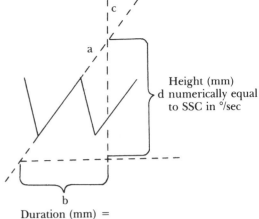

Duration (mm) =
calibration factor

Figure 18-8. a = Extended line representing the slow component; b = horizontal measurement of duration (mm) from the slow component, which is equal to the calibration factor; c = perpendicular extended line from the duration point representing the calibration factor limit to intersect with the slow component extension; d = the height of the line (mm) from duration to the point of intersection with the slow component, which is interpreted as SSC in °/sec.

the calibration factor. For example, if AS = 1.33 and CF = 9.1°/sec, speed of the slow component = 12.10°/sec.

The *extended line method* is based on the fact that velocity of any nystagmus beat in degrees per second equals the CF times amplitude (a) over duration (d), as shown in Figure 18-7.

$$\text{Velocity (°/sec)} = CF \times \frac{a}{d}$$

One or more nystagmus beats can be selected from the ten used in a typical traditional measurement. The slow component of this beat is extended to cover the duration, or rather the number of degrees of eye arc movement per second per millimeter per vertical pen deflection. Duration (mm) or the calibration factor is then horizontally measured and a perpendicular line is extended from the point representing the calibration factor limit to intersect with the slow component extension. The height of the perpendicular line in millimeters is the speed of the slow component in degrees per second (Fig. 18-8). When calibrating a patient's horizontal eye movement for an angle of 20 degrees, adjust recorder (pen excursion height) to equal 20 mm (1 mm/1°). The duration then can be made to numerically equal the calibration factor, canceling each other and allowing the velocity to become numerically equal to the amplitude of the slow component.

The *protractor technique* also uses several of the most intense consecutive nystagmus beats. The angle of these beats formed by the slow component and duration is measured by a protractor. The speed of the slow component is then calculated by multiplying the tangent of this angle by the calibration factor. Simmons, Gillam, and Mattox [29] report using a transparent template overlay to estimate the speed of slow component. The overlay has predetermined line slopes that can be matched to the slopes on the tracings, and the velocity can be read directly from the template's scale. Simmons and associates reason that the slow phase velocity varies by as much as 30% from beat to beat in some individuals, so they recommend taking an average of three measurements at 30-second intervals.

The *velocity method* uses the second (velocity) channel on an ENG recorder to display the differentiated nystagmus waveform. Proper calibration is essential and accomplished by applying a sawtooth waveform of known amplitude and convenient duration to yield a pen deflection of 20 mm. When this signal is differentiated and displayed on the second channel, the gain is adjusted to yield a vertical pen deflection of 20 mm. The speed of slow component can then be obtained from the second channel by multiplying the height of the vertical pen deflection by a gain factor that converts millimeters of pen deflection to degrees per second. The gain factor is specific to the type of recorder used.

The speed of slow component can be measured by *computer method*. This measurement is accomplished by coupling to the ENG recorder a computer-type instrument that will automatically calculate and display the speed of slow component. The computerized system obtains a series of scores, each based on ten beats. The examiner selects the highest score as representing the speed of the slow component for the final measurement of the caloric nystagmus intensity.

All of these methods were compared over the same tracings in a study by Norris, Pruitt, and Fennigkoh [25]. A mean difference occurred only with the velocity measurement. However, variance was increased in both the velocity and computer measurements. Based on the authors' findings, the speed of slow component scores obtained by either the extended line, protractor, or computer methods agreed with the traditional scores. The velocity method as defined did not agree with the traditional method. Of importance was the finding that greater variance exists for both the velocity and computer methods, increasing the possibility of inaccurate measurements when depending on these two methods. In conclusion, the authors stated that the extended line and the protractor methods can both be easily applied with confidence in terms of the findings agreeing with the traditional method. Either of these methods offers a quick measure, particularly if the calibrated horizontal eye movement for an angle of 20 degrees can be adjusted to show a pen deflection equal to 20 mm or 1 mm per 1 degree.

ENG TEST BATTERY
Currently seven separate tests are incorporated into the ENG test battery.

Ocular dysmetria
Gaze
Sinusoidal tracking
Optokinetic
Paroxysmal nystagmus
Positional
Bithermal caloric

Although some tests are often modified or deleted by particular laboratories, these procedures appear to be the most widely accepted in terms of performing a complete assessment of vestibular function. The test procedures are discussed in the sequence most appropriate for clinical application. Included in the discussion of each test are descriptions of normal and abnormal findings and the significance of the abnormal findings.

It is important to recognize that a clinical diagnosis is not to be attempted based entirely on ENG findings. ENG results provide evidence to support either a peripheral lesion, a central lesion, or the existence of pathology without defining its location. In instances where a specific diagnosis is suspected, ENG findings can help to confirm or to rule out that diagnosis.

Ocular Dysmetria Test
The test for ocular dysmetria is done during the calibration procedure. As previously stated, the patient is instructed to look back and forth between two points that are situated so the eye movement is 20 degrees.

For the normal patient the procedure results in tracings that are essentially rectangular (see Fig. 18-5). An abnormal finding results when either an overshoot or undershoot of the eyes occurs when fixating on a particular target. Figure 18-9 shows hypermetria (overshoot) and hypometria (undershoot) of the target. Because

Figure 18-9. Forms of ocular dysmetria obtained from horizontal calibration tracings. A. Overshoot. B. Undershoot.

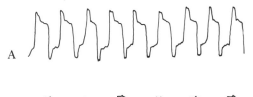

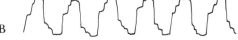

normal patients will occasionally reveal an overshoot during the ENG calibration, some liberty must be taken in interpreting a positive ocular dysmetria. Haring and Simmons [19] indicate that when 50% of the calibrations show an overshoot, ocular dysmetria is considered present. The final clinical decision is, however, arbitrary, as no data exist on which to base an estimate of occurrence in the normal population.

When a basis for ocular dysmetria is being defined, Coats [14] points out that in practical clinical application, such findings should be considered indicative of either cerebellar or brain stem pathology. One of the functions of the cerebellar hemispheres is to control smooth integration of body muscles. Diseases of the cerebellum or its neuroconnections in the brain stem cause a disruption of the smooth muscle movement resulting in ocular dysmetria.

Gaze Test
The gaze test is done while the patient is sitting. The patient is instructed to fixate on a point in the midline, points 20 and 30 degrees to the right and left of midline, and points 20 and 30 degrees above and below midline. It is important that eye deflections never exceed 30 degrees from midline. In extreme gaze, muscle strain often produces clonic jerks of the ocular muscles, which can be mistaken for nystagmus. During each fixation, eye movement should be recorded for approximately 20 seconds.

The purpose of the gaze test is to detect any existing nystagmus with eyes open and to determine whether a paretic ocular deviation is present. A patient without an organic problem will be able to fixate on the points with little or no eye movement. Nystagmus recorded at any of the fixation points is abnormal and an indicator of central nervous system (CNS) pathology. If present, horizontal nystagmus generally beats in the direction of the gaze and may be enhanced by ocular fixation. It may appear unilaterally, bilaterally equal, or bilaterally unequal. Gaze nystagmus indicates brain stem or cerebellar disease, unless a spontaneous nystagmus beating in the same direction is recorded with the patient's eyes closed or unless the patient

is sedated. In the latter case, gaze nystagmus indicates the presence of pathology but not its location.

Vertical nystagmus is quite common with eyes closed. However, with eyes open, vertical gaze nystagmus indicates a CNS pathology that is probably associated with the brain stem. When vertical gaze nystagmus appears without a horizontal nystagmus, either a midline or a bilateral lesion in the upper pons or midbrain should be suspected [14, 23].

Interpretation also depends on the recognition of various types of gaze nystagmus in terms of equating bilateral intensity. When the nystagmus is equal bilaterally, as stated previously, CNS pathology probably involves the brain stem. However, the effects of drugs, particularly barbiturates and alcohol, may exaggerate this nystagmus [2, 7]. When an unequal horizontal gaze nystagmus is present, drug toxicity is unlikely. Therefore, this type of gaze nystagmus adds further support to an organic CNS pathology. Finally, a peripheral vestibular dysfunction resulting in spontaneous nystagmus can also be responsible for a unilateral horizontal gaze nystagmus. This possibility can be ruled out by asking the patient to close his eyes. If a spontaneous nystagmus appears in the same direction as the gaze nystagmus with the slow phase speed greater than 8 degrees per second, then the gaze nystagmus should not be considered a sign of central pathology.

Gaze nystagmus can best be identified by visual inspection of the eyes rather than through ENG recording. The examiner's eye is a better detector of gaze nystagmus than a recorder, particularly when the patient's eyes are open and visual fixation suppresses spontaneous nystagmus. An existing nystagmus resulting from CNS pathology may be horizontal or vertical, yet it also may be oblique or rotatory. ENG recording systems do not record oblique nor rotatory eye movements. Moreover, the nystagmus often varies considerably in amplitude and may decline in intensity over time.

There are exceptions to the persistent nystagmus with eyes open and closed with various types of pathologic origins. Barber and Stockwell [6] have an excellent discussion of the gaze nystagmus and associated pathologies.

Sinusoidal Tracking Test

The sinusoidal tracking test is accomplished by having the patient fixate on a spot that is moving in a sinusoidal pattern. Typically an orange tennis ball attached to a string from the ceiling is used. The tennis ball simply swings back and forth and the patient is instructed to track its movements. Coats [14] specifies frequency of movement and indicates that the horizontal pattern should subtend an angle that approximates 20 degrees from center gaze. Coats also suggests that vertical tracking be used.

A person should be able to perform a smooth tracking pattern with few interruptions. Abnormal sinusoidal tracking patterns will show saccadic eye jerks, generally in the direction of the target movement. These eye jerks are referred to as break-up of the smooth sinusoidal pattern and classified as abnormal. Positive findings associated with the sinusoidal tracking test result from central ocular motor lesions generally associated with the brain stem. Generally, the break-up of the smooth pattern is associated with a gaze nystagmus and a bilateral optokinetic weakness. Finally, it is important to note that sedation may contribute to the break-up of a sinusoidal pattern.

Optokinetic Testing

The optokinetic nystagmus (OKN) test consists of having the patient look at an optokinetic drum held approximately 18 inches from the eyes. The drum's vertical white stripes are 1½ inches wide, the black stripes ⅜ inch wide. The diameter of the drum is 6¼ inches [13]. The drum is held vertically and rotated first from right to left with a speed approximating one revolution every 10 seconds for 20 seconds. Then it is turned left to right at the same speed again for 20 seconds. The test is repeated in both directions at a speed of one revolution every 4 seconds. The OKN test sequence is also to be performed by rotating the drum at the same two speeds horizontally in front of the patient's eyes.

When the drum is held vertically, horizontal nystagmus is elicited. Holding the drum horizontally produces vertical nystagmus. The OKN will show the slow phase in the direction of rotation of the drum. Manual rotation may cause the speed of the drum to vary; however, with practice acceptable tracings can be obtained.

There are a variety of methods by which to elicit OKN. Perhaps one of the major requirements is that the stimulus fill the patient's visual field. As a consequence, some laboratories use a lighted cylinder that can be lowered over the patient's head to fill the lateral visual fields. Moving targets can also be shown on the wall of the test room with a filmstrip projector. This particular system can be used to stimulate vertical as well as horizontal OKN.

OKN results are interpreted by evaluating the symmetry between left- and right-beating nystagmus and the formation of the nystagmus beats. Normal tracings appear symmetric between left and right, and the beats are well shaped and consistent. Asymmetry and poorly formed nystagmus are abnormal. Asymmetry exists when the intensity of the nystagmus is stronger in one direction than the other. If asymmetry occurs, the direction of the predominant nystagmus should be identified. The nystagmus may be poorly formed in one direction but equally intense in both. Questionable asymmetry is accepted as normal.

Central pathology is suggested by either vertical or horizontal OKN asymmetry. However, when asymmetry exists and intense spontaneous nystagmus with eyes closed is present in the direction of the predominant OKN, this suggests pathology but does not provide evidence of its location. In this instance, labyrinthine dysfunction could be responsible for both the spontaneous nystagmus and the OKN asymmetry.

In vertical OKN asymmetry, brain stem lesions should be strongly suspected. A bilaterally absent or weak OKN is also indicative of midline brain stem lesion. Coats [12] has cited OKN abnormality associated with a gaze nystagmus (eyes open) or gaze paresis as evidence of a cerebellar or brain stem lesion. In brain stem or cerebellar lesions, the lateralizing value of OKN asymmetry is poor [15]. An OKN abnormality with normal gaze suggests a cerebral hemisphere lesion with the fast phase of the asymmetric OKN response directed toward the side of the lesion.

Paroxysmal Test

The test for paroxysmal vertigo was described by Dix and Hallpike [17] in 1952 and consists of a violent maneuver to determine the type of nystagmus elicited. In patients with certain types of vestibular system disorders, the maneuver elicits an intense but transient response. (This test should not be interpreted as an assessment of positional-type nystagmus as described by Nylen [26], whereby the patient assumes different head positions but with very slow movements.) The Hallpike test is performed with patient's eyes closed. First the patient is moved rapidly from the sitting position to a point where the head is lower than the body and turned to the right. The patient is held in this position for 90 seconds. Then the patient is allowed to rest for two to three minutes and the maneuver is repeated with the head turned to the left.

Many times a patient will attempt to sit up before the recording can be completed. Because a complete recording is necessary, the patient should be restrained. When the Hallpike test is performed, it is important to obtain recordings of vertical eye movements. Often only vertical nystagmus occurs in response to the Hallpike test, and if only horizontal nystagmus is being traced, a positive response may be completely overlooked.

A classic finding in the Hallpike test points toward a benign peripheral lesion. The classic, or positive, response includes the following:

1. A latent period before the patient reports being dizzy. The ENG recording will also show a latent period before nystagmus begins.
2. Nystagmus of limited duration, generally less than 90 seconds.
3. Nystagmus that fatigues or disappears with repeated tests.

Any response that does not meet these criteria is considered negative and yields no useful information.

This test frequently gives positive results in patients older than 55 years and in patients who have dizziness following head trauma [4]. Middle ear pathology can create episodic dizziness and the patient can have a classical paroxysmal nystagmus, which is also occasionally found after stapes surgery [4, 28].

Positional Test

For positional testing the patient is placed in a series of seven positions with eyes closed, and eye movement is recorded from 60 to 90 seconds in each position. If nystagmus is present in any of the positions, a longer sample of the recording should be made to determine such factors as fatigue, change in intensity, or change in direction. Care should be taken to move the patient slowly from one position to the next to avoid the effects of motion.

The seven positions are as follows:

1. Sitting. The patient sits erect with the chin lowered slightly to place the lateral canals in the horizontal plane.
2. Supine. The head is elevated approximately 30 degrees to place the lateral canals in the vertical position.
3. Head right. The patient remains in the supine position but turns his head to the right.
4. Right lateral. The patient turns the body to lie on his right side. The lateral position is included to eliminate the possibility of nystagmus resulting from a vascular insult.
5. Head left. The patient returns to the supine position and turns his head to the left.
6. Left lateral. The patient turns his body to lie on his left side.
7. Head hanging. The patient is moved to the top or side of the couch and his head is dropped below the level of his body.

Patients who have prolonged symptoms of dizziness develop the ability to suppress nystagmus. Therefore, throughout positional testing, the examiner should ask the patient to perform various mental tasks, such as stating female names in alphabetical order, counting backward from 100, or subtracting 3 from 100 and subsequent numbers. The task should be adapted to the individual's capabilities—neither too difficult nor too easy.

The positional test is used to confirm the existence of spontaneous or positional nystagmus. If nystagmus is present with eyes closed in the neutral position (sitting or supine), then it is classified as spontaneous whether or not it is observed in any other position. On the other hand, if nystagmus does not appear in the neutral position, yet occurs when the patient is repositioned, it is labeled positional.

Coats [14] has suggested that nystagmus intensity greater than 7.5 degrees per second in any position is a sign of pathology. Barber [5], however, considers nystagmus intensity of 9 degrees per second or a single beat of 14 degrees per second clearly pathologic. Barber has also concluded that nystagmus in three fourths of the positions tested is probably pathologic. He regards directional-changing nystagmus in a single position with eyes open or closed as always pathologic and diagnostic of central nervous system disease.

ENG testing of positional nystagmus can yield useful information. However, positional nystagmus is quite common in asymptomatic patients and has been recorded in 26% of a sample of test pilots [8]. Both spontaneous and positional nystagmus are commonly seen in dizzy patients who have no other evidence of pathology. Bruner and Norris [9] reported the incidence of spontaneous (33%) and positional (26%) nystagmus in a group of 293 patients who had no additional positive clinical evidence of pathology. Coats [11] reported similar findings—36% spontaneous and 35% positional—for a group of similar patients. Therefore, in positional test records, findings often support rather than confirm pathology. Excessive spontaneous or positional nystagmus can support a finding of an organic basis for a patient's symptoms but viewed alone cannot provide evidence for the site of lesion.

Caloric Test

Today's most widely accepted caloric procedure was originally described by Fitzgerald and Hallpike [18]. Their test consisted of syringing each ear for 40 seconds with water at 7° C above and 7° C below body temperature. The test was intended to be used with eyes open and fixed. With the eyes open, the water temperatures were thought to be a minimal stimulus. However, ENG testing with eyes closed has shown that the stimulus is quite strong. The effect of stimulation depends on the temperature of the water, the quantity of water, and the duration of irrigation. However, small quantities of water result in highly variable responses, and large quantities often cause weak responses, the latter because the caloric reaction extends beyond the lateral canal. To reduce the reaction, it is more appropriate to irrigate for 40 seconds at water temperatures 6° C below and above the body temperature [13]. This method appears to be not only adequate, but more acceptable to the patient.

The patient is placed in the supine position with the head elevated 30 degrees, placing the lateral canal in a vertical position, the optimum position for stimulation. The examiner should position the irrigating tube so that the syringing covers the entire eardrum. Most commercial irrigators have a controlled pump system and ensure the proper quantity of water, generally approximately 250 ml. It is also acceptable to use gravitational flow if a pump system is not available.

The test sequence consists of right cold, left cold, left warm, and right warm irrigations. This procedure is recommended so that successive nystagmus responses are in opposite directions. Normally there is a rest period of five minutes between left and right irrigations, with a ten-minute rest period between cold and warm irrigations. These rest intervals should be measured from the end of the last nystagmus response to the beginning of the next syringing. Immediately prior to each irrigation, it is necessary that calibration be performed by having the patient look between two dots on the ceiling.

The nystagmus response to caloric stimulation generally begins approximately 30 seconds after the initiation of the syringing and becomes most intense within 60 seconds. If duration measures are used in the analysis of vestibular sensitivity, it is essential that the entire nystagmus response be recorded. If duration is not used, the recording can be terminated after approximately two minutes to save paper. The recorder may be turned on again within 30 to 90 seconds to ensure that the nystagmus response has ended.

It is important that the patient's head position be maintained between and during each caloric syringing and the recording of the response. Head repositioning can vary the nystagmus response and produce erroneous data. It is equally important for the patient to maintain a high level of alertness. Often the patient becomes adept at controlling the nystagmus response, and if efforts are not made to distract the patient, he may suppress the total response by the third irrigation. The alertness tasks mentioned earlier in connection with positional testing are equally adaptable for the caloric response. The patient can be asked to answer aloud to assure the examiner that the tasks are being performed.

The test for fixation suppression is introduced during at least two of the caloric nystagmus responses. The patient is asked to open his eyes and fixate on a point on the ceiling. This fixation should be done immediately after an intense part of the response, and should continue for 15 to 20 seconds.

The caloric test provides the examiner with information related to labyrinthine sensitivity, revealing unilateral or bilateral weakness and the directional preponderance of the nystagmus.

To compare the sensitivity of the two ears or to check for unilateral weakness, the total responses for all four caloric irrigations are added. Then the two right responses are added separately from the two left responses. The formula for comparing relative sensitivity between the right and left ears is as follows:

$$\left(\frac{\text{right cold} + \text{right warm}}{\text{total responses}}\right) \times 100$$
$$- \left(\frac{\text{left cold} \times \text{left warm}}{\text{total responses}}\right) \times 100$$
$$= \text{unilateral weakness}$$

To determine directional preponderance, this formula is applied.

$$\left(\frac{\text{right warm} + \text{left cold}}{\text{total responses}}\right) \times 100$$
$$- \left(\frac{\text{right cold} + \text{left warm}}{\text{total responses}}\right) \times 100$$
$$= \text{directional preponderance}$$

To determine whether bilateral weakness is present, add the speed of the slow component scores from all four irrigations (same as the total responses figure used in the unilateral weakness formula).

Unilateral weakness is a difference of 20% between the nystagmus responses to stimulations of the right ear and the left ear. Directional preponderance is a 30% difference in the intensity of right-beating and left-beating nystagmus elicited from the caloric stimuli. Bilateral weakness is a total response of less than 30 degrees per second.

Unilateral or bilateral weakness occurring without any additional findings is generally compatible with peripheral pathology. Directional preponderance frequently occurs with or without unilateral or bilateral weakness. Directional preponderance, when observed alone, does not define site of lesion nor even provide sufficient evidence to confirm pathology. In the acute phase of labyrinthine dysfunction, a loss in sensitivity may suggest that the preponderance is directed away from the paretic side, but this is not always the case. There seems to be no set pattern that establishes the direction of preponderance in either peripheral or central lesions. However, directional preponderance may be related to hearing loss, as reported by Bruner and Norris [8]. Their study suggested that the direction of preponderance is toward the ear with the greater high-frequency hearing loss.

Failure of Fixation Suppression. As mentioned earlier, the patient should be tested for fixation suppression during at least two of the caloric responses. Failure of fixation suppression is a sign of central nervous system pathology.

A summary of abnormal findings and their significance pertaining to all sections of the ENG test is given in Table 18-1.

Table 18-1. ENG Results and Site of Lesion

Abnormal ENG findings	Possible site of lesion	Comments
OCULAR DYSMETRIA TEST		
Overshoot or undershoot	Cerebellar or brain stem	
GAZE TEST (EYES OPEN)		
Nystagmus recorded at any fixation point	CNS (brain stem or cellebellar)	Spontaneous nystagmus greater than 8°/sec in the same direction with eyes closed. Findings could be related to peripheral or vestibular pathology
Vertical nystagmus (generally beating up)	Brain stem	
Vertical nystagmus without horizontal nystagmus	Midline or bilateral, involving upper pons or midbrain	
Horizontal nystagmus equal bilaterally	Brain stem	Watch for barbiturates or alcohol, which may contribute
Horizontal nystagmus unequal	CNS	If unequal, not likely associated with drug toxicity
Oblique or rotatory nystagmus (nonrecordable)	CNS	
SINUSOIDAL TRACKING TEST		
Break-up of smooth sinusoidal tracking	Brain stem	
OPTOKINETIC TEST		
Poorly formed or asymmetric vertical and/or horizontal nystagmus	CNS	Existence of intense spontaneous nystagmus can contribute to OKN asymmetry related to a peripheral ocular pathology
Vertical OKN asymmetry	Brain stem	
Bilaterally absent or weak horizontal OKN	Midline brain stem	
Abnormal OKN plus gaze nystagmus or gaze paresis	Brain stem or cerebellar	
Abnormal OKN plus normal gaze	Cerebral hemisphere	In cerebral hemisphere lesions, the predominant OKN beats toward the side of the lesion
PAROXYSMAL TEST (POSITIVE DIX-HALLPIKE TEST)		
Latent period before dizziness and nystagmus — Nystagmus of limited duration — Nystagmus fatigues with repeated maneuvers	Vestibular system (peripheral)	
POSITIONAL TEST		
Excessive or spontaneous nystagmus with eyes closed	When viewed singly cannot provide site of lesion	

Table 18-1. (Continued)

Abnormal ENG findings	Possible site of lesion	Comments
CALORIC TEST		
Unilateral weakness equals 20% difference in the nystagmus response between the right- and left-ear irrigations	Vestibular	
Bilateral weakness results when nystagmus responses less than 7.5°/sec for each ear	Possibly peripheral	
Directional preponderance results when a 30% difference in intensity of right- and left-beating nystagmus exists	Nonlocalizing information	
Failure of fixation suppression	CNS	

ENG FINDINGS IN SPECIFIC DISEASE ENTITIES

Frequently, a physician requests ENG testing to confirm or to support a particular impression regarding a patient's probable disorder. The ENG examination assists the physician in making an anatomic, not a pathologic diagnosis; therefore any ENG findings are to be regarded as typically present in specific diseases, but not pathognomonic.

Vestibular Neuronitis

Vestibular neuronitis tends to occur in relatively young persons and can be related to an antecedent infection such as an upper respiratory infection, strep throat, or bacterial infection. Vertigo frequently occurs with a sudden onset and without an associated auditory problem. In such instances, ENG findings show a unilateral caloric weakness with an intense spontaneous nystagmus beating away from the weak side.

Viral Labyrinthitis

Viral labyrinthitis probably is a condition secondary to a viral infection. It appears almost identical to vestibular neuronitis, except that in viral labyrinthitis, there frequently is an associated auditory deficit. The ENG results reveal a unilateral weakness and an intense spontaneous nystagmus beating away from the weak side.

Idiopathic Sudden Deafness

Idiopathic sudden deafness can frequently be related to a latent diabetic condition or a viral infection. The patient experiences a severe unilateral sensorineural hearing loss. ENG findings may reveal a unilateral caloric weakness. Vertigo may or may not be present. Recovery from the auditory deficit is questionable.

Meniere's Disease

In Meniere's disease, a sensorineural hearing deficit fluctuates, showing an audiogram that is characteristically flat or ascending. The patient generally reports a sensation of tinnitus or fullness in the involved ear. The ENG test results show no distinctive pattern. There may be a unilateral caloric weakness and spontaneous nystagmus that may beat either toward or away from the involved side. In many instances patients have completely normal ENG test results.

Ototoxicity

Patients who have overwhelming infections or who are at risk of serious infection are frequently treated with aminoglycoside antibiotics, such as streptomycin, kanamycin, or vancomycin. The patient frequently develops an ototoxic reaction resulting in hearing loss and dizziness. ENG findings reveal bilateral caloric weakness with perhaps very weak spontaneous or positional nystagmus.

Cervical Vertigo

In cervical vertigo, the patient often reports vertigo associated with a particular head position. The resultant nystagmus is related to the twisting of the neck. Confirmation can be determined by recording eye movement when the head is turned either to the right or to the left with the neck twisted. Nystagmus is absent when the patient assumes the right or left lateral position without twisting the neck.

Benign Paroxysmal Nystagmus
Benign paroxysmal nystagmus is often associated with trauma, middle ear pathology, or the degenerative processes of aging. ENG findings yield a classic Hallpike response.

Acoustic Neuroma
ENG findings may reveal a unilateral caloric weakness on the involved side, although this is not present in every case. The spontaneous or positional nystagmus may be related to the size of the tumor; with a small tumor, no spontaneous nystagmus is present, while large tumors produce ENG findings consistent with central lesions.

REFERENCES

1. Aschan, G. The caloric test. *Acta Soc. Med. Upsalionsis* 60:99, 1955.
2. Aschan, G. Different types of alcohol nystagmus. *Acta Otolaryngol.* Suppl. 140, 1958.
3. Aschan, G., Bergstedt, M., and Stahle, J. Nystagmography: Recording of nystagmus in clinical neuro-otological examinations. *Acta Otolaryngol.* Suppl. 129, 1956.
4. Barber, H. O. Positional nystagmus: Testing and interpretation. *Ann. Otol. Rhinol. Laryngol.* 73:838, 1964.
5. Barber, H. O. Positional vertigo and nystagmus. In R. J. Wolfson (Ed.), *The Otolaryngologic Clinics of North America Symposium on Vertigo.* Philadelphia: Saunders, 1973.
6. Barber, H. O., and Stockwell, C. W. *Manual of Electronystagmography.* St. Louis: Mosby, 1976.
7. Bergman, P. S., Nathanson, M., and Bender, M. B. *Transactions of the American Neurological Association*, Richmond, Va.: William Bird Press, 1951.
8. Bruner, A., and Norris, T. W. Lateralization of hearing loss and vestibular nystagmus in test pilots. *Aerosp. Med.* 41:684, 1970.
9. Bruner, A., and Norris, T. W. Age-related changes in caloric nystagmus. *Acta Otolaryngol.* [Suppl.] 282, 1971.
10. Capps, M. J., et al. Evaluation of the air caloric test as a routine examination procedure. *Laryngoscope* 83:1013, 1973.
11. Coats, A. C. Directional preponderance and spontaneous nystagmus as observed in the electronystagmographic examination. *Ann. Otol. Rhinol. Laryngol.* 75:1135, 1966.
12. Coats, A. C. Central electronystagmographic abnormalities. *Arch. Otolaryngol.* 92:43, 1970.
13. Coats, A. C. *Electronystagmography: A Compendium.* Houston: Baylor College of Medicine, 1972.
14. Coats, A. C. Electronystagmography. In L. J. Bradford (Ed.), *Physiological Measures of the Audio-vestibular System.* New York: Academic, 1975.
15. Daroff, R. B., and Hoyt, W. F. Supranuclear Disorder of Ocular Control Systems in Man: Clinical, Anatomical, and Physiological Correlations—1969. In P. Bach-Y-Rita, C. C. Collins, and J. E. Hyde (Eds.), *The Control of Eye Movements.* New York: Academic, 1971.
16. Dennis, J. M., Moran, W. B., and Studebaker, G. A. Absolute and relative reliability of several response parameters used in vestibular assessment. *J. Otolaryngol.* 7:5, 1978.
17. Dix, M. R., and Hallpike, C. S. The pathology, symptomatology and diagnosis of certain common disorders of the vestibular system. *Proc. R. Soc. Lond.* 45:341, 1952.
18. Fitzgerald, G., and Hallpike, C. S. Studies in human vestibular function: I. Observations on the directional preponderance ("Nystagmusbereitschaft") of caloric nystagmus resulting from cerebral lesions. *Brain* 65:115, 1942.
19. Haring, R. D., and Simmons, F. B. Cerebellar defects detectable by electronystagmography calibration. *Arch. Otolaryngol.* 98:14, 1973.
20. Hart, C. W. J. The value of the hot caloric test. *Laryngoscope* 75:302, 1965.
21. Henriksson, N. G. Speed of slow component and duration in caloric nystagmus. *Acta Otolaryngol.* Suppl. 125, 1956.
22. Jongkees, L. B. W. The Caloric Test and Its Value in Evaluation of the Patient with Vertigo. In R. J. Wolfson (Ed.), *The Otolaryngologic Clinics of North America Symposium on Vertigo.* Philadelphia: Saunders, 1973.
23. Kestenbaum, A. *Clinical Methods of Neuro-Ophthalmologic Examination* (2d ed.). New York: Grune & Stratton, 1961.

24. Norris, T. W. *Electronystagmography*. New York: MEDCOM, 1974.
25. Norris, T. W., Pruitt, M., and Fennigkoh, L. Slow component nystagmus measuring techniques. Presented at the American Speech-Language-Hearing Association, Annual Convention, November 21–24, 1980.
26. Nylen, C. O. The posture test. *Acta Otolaryngol*. Suppl. 109, 1953.
27. Rubin, W. Electronystagmography and its value in the diagnosis of vertigo. In R. J. Wolfson (Ed.), *The Otolaryngologic Clinics of North America Symposium on Vertigo*. Philadelphia: Saunders, 1973.
28. Schuknecht, H. F. Cupulolithiasis. *Arch. Otolaryngol*. 90:113, 1969.
29. Simmons, F. B., Gillam, S. F., and Mattox, D. E. *An Atlas of Electronystagmography*. New York: Grune & Stratton, 1979.

19

Diagnosis and Medical Treatment of Dizziness

Donald W. Goin

Spatial orientation depends on the proper function and central integration of impulses from several organ systems, including the eyes, statokinetic or vestibular system (vestibular labyrinth, eighth nerve, and vestibular nuclei in the brain stem), central pathways from vestibular nuclei to the cerebral cortex, cerebellum, and proprioceptive system [5]. Because each system may be affected by many different disease states, the number of diagnostic possibilities in a patient complaining of dizziness is great. To sort through this tangle, the clinician must use a systematic scheme, eliminating some diagnoses by a thorough history, others with a careful neurologic examination, and still others with special studies such as electronystagmography (ENG). Taken in total, these inquiries constitute the otoneurologic evaluation. In addition to reviewing the relevant aspects of such an evaluation, this chapter summarizes the diagnostic features and medical management of common disorders that cause dizziness.

THE OTONEUROLOGIC EVALUATION

Although space limitations preclude a description of all syndromes involving dizziness, consideration of those signposts that direct diagnostic attention down one path or another will clarify thinking and provide a framework on which to base specific diagnoses.

History

Throughout the assessment, the clinician keeps two major questions in mind: (1) Is the vestibular system involved? (2) Is the problem peripheral or central? A detailed, probing history provides tentative answers to these questions and directs the remainder of the evaluation. The following information is sought:

1. Does the patient experience a sensation of motion? Vertigo refers to a spinning sensation and reflects disease of the vestibular system. The patient either finds himself in a tight spin or experiences the room whirling about him. Nonvestibular dizziness, on the other hand, is described as unsteadi-

ness, queasiness, giddiness, light-headedness, or a blacking-out sensation.

2. What is the nature of the attacks? Vestibular disease, especially if peripheral in origin, causes episodic vertigo with normal equilibrium between attacks. The spells last from seconds, as in the case of benign paroxysmal postural dizziness, to hours, as in the case of Meniere's disease. Central, nonvestibular disease begins insidiously and lasts for days to months.

3. Are there associated cochlear symptoms; such as hearing impairment, tinnitus, or a sensation of fullness? Are they exaggerated when the dizziness is worse? These symptoms, especially if unilateral, suggest peripheral (end organ) or eighth nerve pathology.

4. Does head motion incite or aggravate the dizziness? If so, peripheral vestibular disease is likely.

5. Are there other symptoms suggesting central nervous system disease, such as altered consciousness, double vision, slurred speech, difficulty swallowing, numbness of the face or extremities, or loss of memory?

6. Were there antecedent head injury, flulike symptoms, or upper respiratory infection? Thinking of a perilymph fistula, the examiner asks about unusual activities, such as heavy lifting or straining, scuba diving, or air travel. What is the status of the patient's general health, life-style, and family status? Does he use alcohol, medications, or other drugs?

Physical Examination
Complete head and neck and neurologic examinations are performed, with special attention being paid to external or middle ear disease and the presence or absence of spontaneous or positional nystagmus. The problem may be found when the outer and middle ear are examined as some degree of dizziness may result from cerumen impaction, middle ear effusion, perforation, or cholesteatoma. A fistula test is indicated in any patient with evidence of chronic otitis media (tympanic membrane perforation with or without otorrhea or cholesteatoma) and consists of applying positive pressure to the middle ear space with a pneumatic

otoscope or Politzer's bag. If a fistula is present, this maneuver induces a sharp deviation of the eyes and a sense of transient vertigo.

The word *nystagmus* stems from the Greek *nystazein,* which means to nod, especially in sleep. Clinically, it refers to an involuntary, rapidly alternating movement of the eyes. If carefully sought and thoroughly evaluated, nystagmus helps determine whether the disease process lies centrally or peripherally.

Vestibular or jerk nystagmus, the type associated with vestibular disorders, has quick and slow components; that is, the eyes jerk either horizontally, vertically, or around the visual axis and drift slowly in the opposite direction. The direction of the quick component dictates nomenclature. For example, if the eyes jerk right and drift left, the nystagmus is called *right-beating, horizontal;* if they jerk to the left around the visual axis, *left rotary;* if upward, *up-beating vertical.* Vestibular nystagmus should not be confused with ocular nystagmus, which has no quick and slow components and is not associated with dizziness as a rule (see Chap. 18 for further detail).

Vestibular nystagmus is further divided into spontaneous and induced [4]. When being tested for spontaneous nystagmus, the patient observes the examiner's index finger, which is first held 18 to 24 inches from the patient's eyes in their primary position, then moved slowly to the right and left until the eyes have deviated 30 degrees in either direction. Deviation beyond this point results in stretch nystagmus in normal patients. Finally, gaze is directed up and down to detect vertical nystagmus. Visual fixation suppresses spontaneous nystagmus of peripheral (labyrinthine) origin, a problem that can be circumvented with either 20 diopter lenses on the patient's eyes or ENG. Table 19-1 summarizes the difference between spontaneous nystagmus resulting from peripheral and central diseases.

Nystagmus may be induced by electrical current, caloric stimulation, angular acceleration, or placing the patient's head in various positions. For practical reasons, most clinicians rely on ENG for positional testing; however, it is often possible to

Table 19-1. Spontaneous Nystagmus

PERIPHERAL
Visually suppressed
Often with auditory symptoms
Associated with vertigo
Horizontal or horizontorotary
Beats toward irritated or hyperactive laby-
rinth, away from paretic labyrinth

CENTRAL
Not visually suppressed; may be accentuated
with visual fixation
Auditory symptoms unusual
May or may not occur with vertigo
Any direction, often vertical
Beats toward side of lesion

reach an early diagnosis by including positional tests in the physical examination, especially if the history suggests postural dizziness. The Hallpike test is the easiest to
perform and the most productive [6]. From
a sitting position with head turned to the
right, legs outstretched, and the support of
the examiner, the patient assumes a supine
position and hangs (extends) his head over
the edge of the table. The eyes are examined for 30 seconds for the presence of
nystagmus. The patient then returns to the
sitting position, and after a rest period, the
test is repeated with the head turned to
the left. If nystagmus is present, it is important to determine if it beats in the same
direction with each head position, if it
comes on immediately or after a period of
latency, and if it abates (fatigues) after repeatedly returning to the position in which
it was observed. Table 19-2 summarizes the
characteristics of positional nystagmus as
they relate to peripheral and central disease.

Table 19-2. Positional Nystagmus

PERIPHERAL
Occurs after latent period
Fades out within 60 seconds
Fatigue: weaker and of shorter duration when
offending position is repeatedly assumed
Direction fixed: beats in same direction in
different positions

CENTRAL
Occurs instantly
Lasts longer than 60 seconds
Does not fatigue
Direction changing

The neurologic examination includes
station and gait testing, cranial nerve testing, and cerebellar tests. The audiologic
assessment includes air, bone, speech, and
impedance audiometry. These tests are performed whether cochlear symptoms are
present or not.

After the evaluation, which must be routine in every dizzy patient, the clinician
has sufficiently narrowed the diagnostic
range to direct further testing along more
individually tailored pathways. Depending
on the case in question, any or all of the
following studies may be indicated:

1. Audiology: site-of-lesion testing, central
   auditory tests, and brain stem and cortical evoked response audiometry
2. Visual and somatosensory evoked potential evaluation
3. ENG: considered by many a routine
   test in evaluating the dizzy patient
4. Rotation test: computerized rotary chair
   systems are gaining popularity as an
   adjunct to ENG
5. X-rays: tomograms, computed tomography (CT scan), arteriography, and my-
   elography
6. Neurologic and ophthalmologic consultation
7. Allergic testing
8. Blood studies: hemoglobin and hemato-
   crit (for anemia), fluorescent treponemal
   antibody absorption test (FTA-ABS; for
   syphilis), five-hour glucose tolerance test
   (for diabetes or hypoglycemia), thyroid
   profile, and lipid profile

MEDICAL MANAGEMENT OF
THE DIZZY PATIENT
It is appropriate to discuss diagnosis and
medical management together because a
thorough evaluation forms the cornerstone
of successful therapy. The sudden loss of
spatial orientation is a frightening experience for the patient. Complicating this
fear are both the patient's certainty that he
has either a brain tumor or a stroke and
his concern of being mistaken for an ine-
briate during attacks. The typical patient
has seen several physicians and received
medications ranging from vitamins to thyroid hormones. Often, he has been told to
learn to live with his disease. Nothing dis-

pels these anxieties more than a detailed history, thorough physical examination, and a discussion of the problem in understandable terms. Only then will the patient hear the clinician's reassurance that the odds are against life-threatening disease and that the symptoms can in all likelihood be controlled or eliminated.

Following are brief diagnostic profiles and comments on medical management of common disorders encountered in a neuro-otologic practice. Most are peripheral vestibular diseases and, although not all-inclusive, the list affords an opportunity to discuss most of the nonsurgical modalities used in the management of dizziness.

Meniere's Disease

Patients with classic Meniere's disease complain of intermittent spinning vertigo associated with fluctuating hearing impairment, tinnitus, and a sensation of pressure or fullness in the involved ear. It is a capricious disease with variations in this classic constellation of symptoms being the rule rather than the exception (see Chap. 11).

Medical Management. The myriad of medications employed in the management of Meniere's disease (and vestibular disorders in general) bespeaks the shaky foundation on which their rationale for use stands. Although some forestall or control the vertigo, none prevent the gradual and irreversible corrosion of hearing that typifies this disease. Many of the following drugs are employed in other conditions besides Meniere's disease.

General Measures. During the acute attack, the patient is kept at bed rest and sedated. If vomiting is protracted, hospitalization with administration of intravenous fluids is necessary.

Diuretics. Furstenberg [7] first employed ammonium chloride in conjunction with a low-sodium diet in patients with Meniere's disease. Since that time, numerous other diuretics have been tried. These drugs restore fluid and electrolyte balance and, because one of the theories of Meniere's disease postulates an electrolyte imbalance as causative, they have enjoyed

sustained popularity in long-term management. Recently, carbonic anhydrase inhibitors (acetazolamide; Diamox) and thiazide diuretics have been popular, their use being supplemented with restriction of salt.

Vasodilator Therapy. Many drugs that alter circulation have been tried on patients with Meniere's disease [11]. Focusing on the longitudinal-flow theory of endolymph production and absorption, some investigators [11] see increased capillary permeability in the stria vascularis, where endolymph is produced, as the problem, yet others are certain that either mechanical obstruction along the endolymphatic duct or ischemia in the sac, where absorption takes place, causes the hydrops [9]. Theoretically, vasodilators can reverse pathophysiologic processes at either end of the system. For example, if autonomic dysfunction causes capillary vasospasm that in turn leads to increased capillary permeability or decreased absorption, then drugs that relieve the spasm would be beneficial. The use of many medications, including histamine, papaverine, and nylidrin (Arlidin) are based on this ischemic theory. On the other hand, if the increased capillary permeability is due to sensitivity to histamine in the stria vascularis, as suggested by Williams [18], then desensitization by repeatedly administering small doses of histamine may be beneficial.

Snow and Suga [16] studied the effect on the guinea pig of numerous drugs and found several, including papaverine, to effectively increase circulation to the ear. Neither did they imply, nor should their results be interpreted to mean, that these agents reduce the hydrops of Meniere's disease, for which purpose they are so commonly used.

Vestibular Suppressing Drugs. Sekitani and associates [15] have demonstrated that diazepam (Valium) decreases the physiologic activity of the medial vestibular nucleus in the cat. Their observations are supported by experience with patients, in whom diazepam effectively controls acute attacks of Meniere's disease. Some of the antihistamines (dimenhydrinate [Dramamine], meclizine [Bonine]) that are widely used are also believed to act, at least in part, on the vestibular nuclei. These drugs are often used in combination with anticholinergic agents, which inhibit transmission of nerve impulses both peripherally and centrally. Examples are atropine and scopolamine.

Vitamins. Many of the vitamin B complexes have been tried. Niacin is especially popular. The bioflavinoids (vitamin P) are believed to be effective because they decrease permeability in capillary beds.

Ototoxic Antibiotics. Some authors have reported ablating the vestibular labyrinth with either streptomycin [12] or gentamicin [8].

Miscellaneous. Arslan [1] relied on osmotic induction to relieve hydrops when he elevated tympanomeatal flaps and placed sodium chloride crystals in the round window niche in patients with Meniere's disease.

Inciting spinal fluid pressure changes and altering ambient pressure as forms of therapy have their proponents. Some clinicians instruct their patients to lie head down on a slant board for 15 to 30 minutes every day. Others alter pressure in the external auditory canal, usually with an impedance audiometer, as a means of inducing changes in perilymph and endolymph pressure dynamics. Tjernstrom and Casselbrant [17] improved hearing in 40% of their patients with Meniere's disease by exposing them to underpressure in a pressure chamber.

Vestibular Neuritis

As the name implies, vestibular neuritis (epidemic vertigo, vestibular paralysis, acute labyrinthitis) is caused by an inflammatory reaction of the vestibular division of the eighth cranial nerve. The diagnosis is based on a single, severe, prolonged episode of vertigo, often with vomiting and complete debilitation. Unlike Meniere's disease, there is no involvement of the auditory system. After the acute episode, which usually lasts three or four days, the patient may experience residual unsteadiness or postural dizziness for a prolonged period but usually recovers completely within six months. A small percentage of patients develop a chronic form of the disease [14]. Caloric testing demonstrates a unilateral canal paresis.

The key to diagnosis is a finding of reduced vestibular response to caloric testing in a patient who has a single episode of violent dizziness with no auditory symptoms. Because of the paretic vestibular nerve, it is important to rule out a small acoustic tumor by ordering x-rays, brain stem–evoked response audiometry, and tests for acoustic reflex decay or latency.

Treatment. Because the course is usually one of gradual improvement, treatment is supportive during the acute attack. Bed rest, sedation, and intravenous fluids are supplemented with vestibular suppressing drugs such as diazepam or dimenhydrinate. Positional dizziness may persist after the acute attack and, if bothersome, Cawthorne positional exercises may be instituted to hasten resolution. In performing these exercises, which are designed to promote vestibular compensation, the patient assumes various head and body positions several times a day.

Benign Paroxysmal Postural Dizziness

The vertigo caused by this condition, which was first described by Bárány in 1921 [2], occurs only in certain positions. The spinning sensation lasts less than 30 seconds, a fact helping to differentiate this from other peripheral vestibular disorders. The spinning typically occurs when the affected ear is in the dependent position, although sometimes the problem develops after the head is turned sharply to the right or left or by looking upward.

Schuknecht attributed this condition to inorganic deposits on the cupula of the posterior semicircular canal, the sensitivity of their mass to gravitational force being the proposed mechanism of stimulation. He designated the condition *cupulolithiasis* [13]. Benign postural dizziness may occur without other evidence of labyrinthine or central nervous system disease, or it may be a symptom of vestibular neuritis, acoustic tumor, perilymph fistula, or otitis media. It is commonly seen following head injuries and rarely seen after stapedectomy.

On examination, nystagmus and vertigo are induced when the head is extended over the edge of the table and turned to the involved side (Hallpike maneuver). The nystagmus is horizontal, vertical, or rotary, delayed in onset, and fatigues when the head position is assumed repeatedly, all findings suggestive of peripheral labyrinthine disease.

Treatment. Medications are usually ineffective. The most obvious treatment is to avoid the offending positions. A few persistent and severe cases require vestibular nerve section.

Otosclerosis
Dizziness may complicate otosclerosis in the following several ways:

1. Endolymphatic hydrops. There is no clear-cut evidence that otosclerosis per se causes endolymphatic hydrops, and the association of the two is probably incidental.
2. Otosclerotic inner ear syndrome. The patient complains of intermittent vague unsteadiness or mild sensations of motion but not severe vertigo [10]. Spells last from minutes to several hours and are not associated with a sensorineural hearing impairment more pronounced than one would expect from the otosclerosis. The condition disappears after stapedectomy.
3. Dizziness following stapes surgery may be due to a postoperative middle ear granuloma or a perilymph fistula. Treatment is surgical. Prolonged positional dizziness may rarely complicate stapes surgery.

Labyrinthitis
The majority of cases referred to as acute labyrinthitis, inner ear infection, epidemic vertigo, and toxic labyrinthitis are probably examples of vestibular neuritis. However, there are conditions that result in inner ear inflammatory change that are properly referred to as labyrinthitis. Varieties include viral (mumps), circumscribed (associated with cholesteatoma eroding one of the semicircular canals), serous (following stapedectomy), and suppurative (associated with meningitis) [11]. Treatment depends on cause.

Trauma
Dizziness secondary to head trauma varies from violent vertigo compounding the pro-

found hearing impairment of a transverse temporal bone fracture to the vague, ill-defined unsteadiness of the malingerer who has been injured on the job. Barber observed positional dizziness in 47% of patients with longitudinal temporal bone fractures and in approximately 25% of patients who had sustained head injuries without temporal bone fractures [3]. Pathophysiologic mechanisms include trauma to the eighth cranial nerve and brain stem nuclei, inner ear concussion, endolymphatic hydrops, and perilymph fistula.

In the majority, symptoms can be expected to resolve over a 12- to 18-month period. In a small percentage, either surgical closure of a perilymph fistula, vestibular nerve section, or endolymphatic shunt may be necessary.

Acoustic Neuroma
Acoustic tumors usually cause unsteadiness rather than violent vertigo. The dizziness is not episodic and improves with time because as the paralysis of the vestibular nerve becomes complete the opposite vestibular system compensates. Exceptions exist, however, and in their incipient stages neuromas may mimic Meniere's disease or paroxysmal postural dizziness. If they occlude the internal auditory artery, the presenting symptoms are violent dizziness and profound hearing impairment.

Central Causes of Dizziness
The etiology of dizziness lies beyond the scope of this discussion. However, it should be emphasized that the investigator must not direct his attention too strongly to the inner ear, even if the dizziness is rotational because other parts of the vestibular system (vestibular nuclei, cerebellum, and cortical projections) may produce identical symptoms. Examples are multiple sclerosis, vestibular migraine, brain stem and cerebellar tumors, impaired circulation to the vestibular nuclei as occurs in atherosclerosis and posterior inferior cerebellar artery syndrome, and vestibular epilepsy.

Finally, nonrotational dizziness can be caused by a great many conditions, including anemia, cervical spine problems, metabolic disorders, cardiac arrhythmias, and psychoneurosis.

REFERENCES

1. Arslan, M. Treatment of Meniere's disease by opposition of sodium chloride crystals on the round window. *Laryngoscope* 82:1736, 1972.
2. Bárány, R. Diagnose von Krankheitsercheinungen im Bereiche des Otolithenapparates. *Acta Otolaryngol.* 2:434, 1921.
3. Barber, H. Positional nystagmus: Testing and interpretation. *Ann. Otol. Rhinol. Laryngol.* 73:838, 1964.
4. Coats, A. C. *Electronystagmography: A Compendium.* Houston: Baylor College of Medicine, 1972.
5. DeWeese, D. D., and Saunders, W. H. *Textbook of Otolaryngology.* St. Louis: Mosby, 1964.
6. Dix, M. R., and Hallpike, C. S. The pathology, symptomatology and diagnosis of certain common disorders of the vestibular system. *Ann. Otol. Rhinol. Laryngol.* 61: 987, 1952.
7. Furstenberg, A. C., Lashmet, F. H., and Lathrop, F. Meniere's symptom complex: Medical treatment. *Ann. Otol. Rhinol. Laryngol.* 43:1035, 1934.
8. Lange, G. Transtympanic treatment for Meniere's disease with gentamicin sulfate. In K. H. Volsteen, et al. (Eds.), *Meniere's Disease.* New York: Thieme-Stratton, 1981.
9. Lawrence, M. Theories of the cause of hydrops. In J. Pulec (Ed.), *Meniere's Disease.* Philadelphia: Saunders, 1968.
10. McCabe, B. F. Otosclerosis and vertigo. *Trans. Pac. Coast Otoophthalmol. Soc.* 47: 37, 1966.
11. Paparella, M. M. Labyrinthitis. In M. M. Paparella and D. A. Shumrick (Eds.), *Otolaryngology, Volume 2: The Ear.* Philadelphia: Saunders, 1980.
12. Schuknecht, H. F. Ablation therapy in the management of Meniere's disease. *Acta Otolaryngol.* [Suppl.] 132:14, 1957.
13. Schuknecht, H. F. Cupulolithiasis. *Arch. Otolaryngol.* 90:765, 1969.
14. Schuknecht, H. F. *Pathology of the Ear.* Cambridge: Harvard University Press, 1974.
15. Sekitani, R., McCabe, B. F., and Ryu, J. H. Drug effects on the medial vestibular nucleus. *Arch. Otolaryngol.* 93:581, 1971.
16. Snow, J. B., and Suga, F. Labyrinthine vasodilators. *Arch. Otolaryngol.* 97:365, 1973.
17. Tjernstrom, O., et al. Current status of pressure chamber treatment. *Otolaryngol. Clin. North Am.* 13:723, 1980.
18. Williams, H. L., Jr. A review of the literature as to the physiologic dysfunction of Meniere's disease: A new hypothesis as to its fundamental cause. *Laryngoscope* 75: 1661, 1965.

20

Surgical Management of Vertigo and Fluctuant Hearing Loss

Robert E. Mischke

The most accurate otologic diagnosis is made by in-depth history review, careful physical examination, and complete laboratory and audiologic testing. In most cases requiring surgical treatment of vertigo or fluctuating hearing loss, careful documentation of hearing sensitivity, hearing fluctuation, and hearing loss progression is of paramount importance in arriving at the best decision for the patient. The audiologic record is often the key determining factor in the diagnosis of pathology and selection of a surgical procedure.

A patient who is faced with a decision regarding surgery to control his vertigo or fluctuating or progressive hearing loss has probably already undergone thorough audiologic and medical evaluation as well as had an adequate trial of medical therapy. Initial trial of medical treatment is crucial as some patients have medically treatable problems that precipitate the vertigo or hearing loss, and these patients will often respond dramatically to medical management.

When it is apparent that medical management will not suffice, there is growing recognition that timely surgical treatment of vertigo will preserve hearing in some cases. Therefore, if undertaken early in the course of the disease, surgery for uncontrollable dizziness or vertigo may save useful hearing specifically in cases of Meniere's disease, Mondini deformity, or inner ear fistulas.

Portmann [9] described the endolymphatic sac operation for the relief of vertigo in 1927. Since that time, many varied procedures have been tried to control the vertigo in patients with Meniere's disease including ultrasound and cryosurgery of the labyrinth or cochlea, decompressing or draining the endolymphatic sac, draining or creating a fistula into the saccule in the vestibule, and destroying vestibular function. All recent advances are variations of these principles, but the actual prognosis for the vertiginous patient has not been dramatically altered, with the possible exception that preservation of hearing is now more common than in the past.

Surgical management of vertigo must be considered not only for Meniere's disease and inner ear fistulas, but also for intracta-

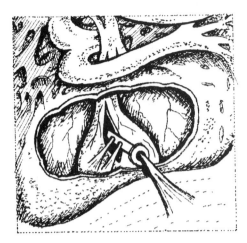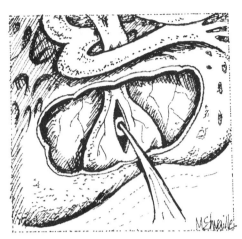

Figure 20-1. Endolymphatic sac is opened and shunt placed into cerebellopontile angle resulting in endolymph flow through shunt. A. Flanged, perforated tube introduced into subarachnoid space through opening in inner sac wall. B. Tube fully inserted with flange inside sac.

ble dizziness from positional vertigo, posttraumatic vertigo, labyrinthitis, prior surgery, positional etiology, ototoxicity, sudden vascular occlusion, and acoustic neuroma.

MANAGEMENT OF SPECIFIC PROBLEMS
Meniere's Disease
Surgery for Meniere's disease is classified into two major categories: surgery that preserves hearing and surgery that sacrifices any remaining hearing. Surgical operations that generally preserve hearing include the insertion of a shunt, vestibulotomy, and middle fossa nerve section. Surgical procedures that sacrifice remaining hearing in the involved ear include transcanal approach, labyrinthectomy, and translabyrinthine section.

After surgery, the patient must remain in the hospital a week or more to accommodate severe disequilibrium caused by the destruction of the diseased labyrinth. Full recovery may require weeks, or even months, depending on the individual. There may be a permanent disequilibrium in approximately 10% of patients who undergo destructive labyrinthine procedures.

Shunt. The shunt operation is currently done in either of two major ways. One method developed by House [6] drains the

endolymphatic sac into the cerebellopontile angle so that the endolymph can communicate with the spinal fluid (Fig. 20-1). The other major method is to drain the sac into the mastoid by plastic valves or tubes (Fig. 20-2). In a few patients the sac is not opened but simply decompressed by removing the surrounding bone. The operation is done with general anesthesia, takes one to two hours, and requires approximately two days in the hospital.

The results generally quoted are that the patient has a 65 to 75% chance of obtaining relief of vertigo and preservation of hearing [1, 10, 12]. Hearing may actually be improved in some patients. There is growing concern that shunt-type procedures are too often subject to failure after a 6-month to 1-year "shock" effect when the surgery wears off. However, there is definitely a place for shunt surgery in the control of Meniere's disease, with carefully selected patients who have realistic expectations.

The risks of shunt-type surgery include loss of hearing, increased dizziness, infection, spinal fluid leak, and facial nerve

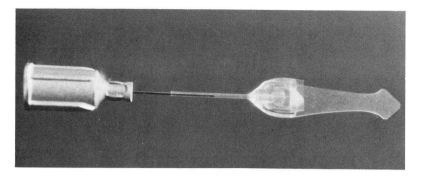

Figure 20-2. One type of shunt device (Denver valve) is placed into mastoid to drain endolymph. Needle is inserted to show hollow portion of valve.

paralysis. Complications are uncommon, so the morbidity of the procedure itself is not a great factor in the decision to institute surgical treatment.

Vestibulotomy. There are various procedures that are aimed at creating a fistula in the saccule by entering the vestibule (vestibulotomy). The concept is the same as the Cody tack procedure [3]. There is no evidence to date to show this surgical procedure gives better long-term relief than the shunt procedure.

Middle Fossa Nerve Section. The most definitive procedure to relieve attacks of vertigo is to cut the vestibular nerves. The hearing is preserved in approximately 75% of cases if the middle fossa approach is used (Fig. 20-3). Permanent relief of vertigo is more than 90% if both superior and inferior vestibular nerves are cut. Some surgeons prefer to cut only the superior vestibular nerve, owing to the technical difficulty of cutting the inferior division and the slightly greater risk of loss in hearing.

This procedure has gained increasing popularity in recent years as otologic surgeons become comfortable with the craniotomy approach to the vestibular nerves. It may be used as the first procedure in a patient severely incapacitated by vertigo for maximum chance of relief of symptoms. This operation may be used after a more "conservative" procedure (such as the shunt technique) has failed to relieve symptoms. Risks with the middle fossa

nerve section are uncommon and may include spinal fluid leak, facial paralysis, hearing loss, infection, and, rarely, brain injury causing paralysis of speech or movement of the opposite arm or leg. Hospitalization time is approximately 1 week.

If the hearing in the involved ear is already poor and if there is no evidence of Meniere's disease in the opposite ear, a surgical procedure may be considered that sacrifices the remaining hearing. The old guidelines that a "poor" ear has hearing loss greater than 50 dB with poorer than 50% speech discrimination is no longer useful because bilateral disease is believed to be more common than was originally thought. Nearly 40% of such patients have bilateral problems instead of only 20%, as previously considered. Therefore, any decision to sacrifice remaining hearing must be made cautiously. The current trend is to be conservative and sacrifice hearing only when no other alternative exists.

Transcanal Surgery (Cawthorne Procedure). Another technique that may be used when preservation of hearing is not possible is transcanal ablation of the saccule and utricle in the vestibule and destruction of the crista of the ampullated ends of the semicircular canals. Cawthorne [2] described this technique in 1951. The vestibule may be packed with Gelfoam soaked with an ototoxic drug such as neomycin to ensure complete ablation. The approach is relatively simple, the morbidity low, and therefore this procedure is useful in elderly or debilitated patients. This surgical procedure, when conducted properly, is only slightly less effective than the labyrinthectomy or vestibular nerve section.

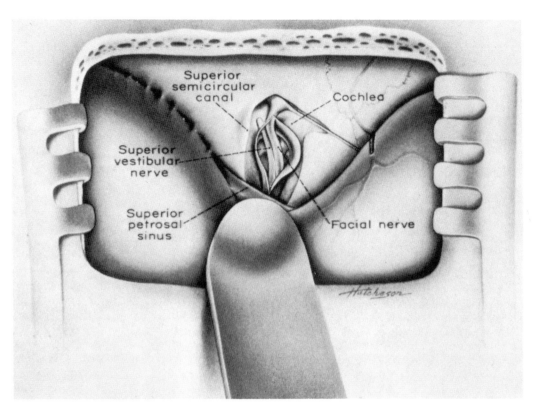

Figure 20-3. Middle fossa approach to vestibular nerves by retracting temporal lobe and drilling away bone over internal auditory canal.

Labyrinthectomy. The vestibular labyrinth may also be destroyed by drilling out the semicircular canals through a mastoidectomy surgical approach [11] (Fig. 20-4). This procedure is very effective and carries little more risk than the Cawthorne technique. The major considerations are increased surgical time with greater exposure of the facial nerve.

Translabyrinthine Nerve Section. The vestibular nerves may be severed with the translabyrinthine approach. A high percentage of patients experience relief of vertigo with this technique although residual hearing must be sacrificed. The increased risk of this surgical procedure is that of entering the cerobellopontile area, which may cause complications including spinal fluid leak, infection, or facial nerve paralysis.

Mondini Deformity
Special mention should be made of the Mondini deformity as the shunt operation is used for this problem of hydrops of the

inner ear although vertigo is not the primary problem.

The Mondini deformity is diagnosed by radiologic confirmation of an incompletely formed cochlea showing only one or 1½ turns. The vestibule may be enlarged with shortened or widened semicircular canals (Fig. 20-5). The vestibular aqueduct and endolymphatic sac area may be enlarged. The audiologic pattern may be a step-by-step decrease in hearing, which begins in early childhood. The patient may have episodic vertigo [8].

The shunt operation is controversial in view of these fluctuating decreases in hearing sensitivity. The endolymphatic sac is often found to be huge relative to normal standards. The surgical theory is to shunt these grossly enlarged sacs into the spinal fluid space so that a large volume of endolymph can be drained. The current trend is to perform surgery as soon as the diagnosis is made, especially if it is apparent

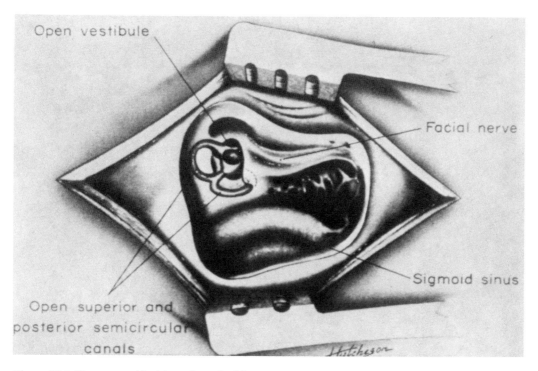

Figure 20-4. Transmastoid approach to the laby-rinth. Labyrinthectomy is done by drilling away semicircular canals.

that the hearing loss is progressing. The alternative of postponing surgery may result in permitting the progressive hearing loss to continue until profound deafness is reached. More experience and research are required for better management of this difficult problem.

Intractable Labyrinthine Disease
The procedures previously described to ablate the vestibular labyrinth in various ways are used for surgical treatment of persistent vertigo because of peripheral pathology from various causes [14]. These include damage to the labyrinth from sudden vascular insult, temporal bone fracture, injury from previous ear surgery, chronic otitis media, labyrinthitis, and even intractable symptoms of "benign" positional vertigo. In addition to the previously described operations, there is a procedure to selectively cut the singular nerve for patients with positional vertigo [5], as the symptoms often originate primarily from pathology in the posterior semicircular canal (Fig. 20-6).

Diagnostic care must be taken to differentiate central from peripheral causes of dizziness [4]. Total ablation of the peripheral labyrinthine function in a presumably diseased ear will result in disappointingly incomplete relief of symptoms if there is a significant central component creating the dizziness. Examples in which central and peripheral pathology coexist are vertigo persisting after head trauma and vascular insult (stroke).

Labyrinthine Fistula
This otologic emergency must be immediately diagnosed and treated if the outcome is to be enhanced by surgery [13]. A fistula, or opening, in the round or oval window membrane may occur as a result of barotrauma from forceful blowing of the nose; situations in which atmospheric pressure changes such as scuba diving, flying, or skydiving; or vigorous physical exertion. In some cases of confirmed fistula, however, no specific associated incident can be elicited from the patient's history. Therefore, it is possible that some fistulas may be spontaneous. It is important to have a high index of suspicion for fistula in any

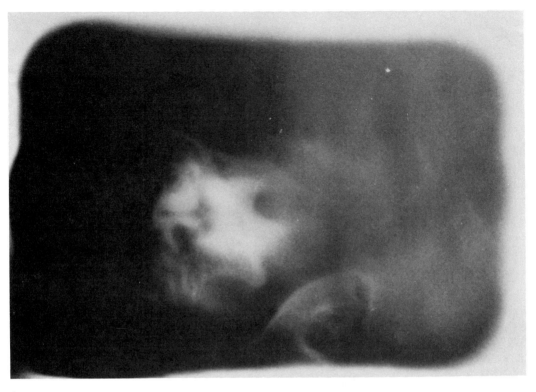

A

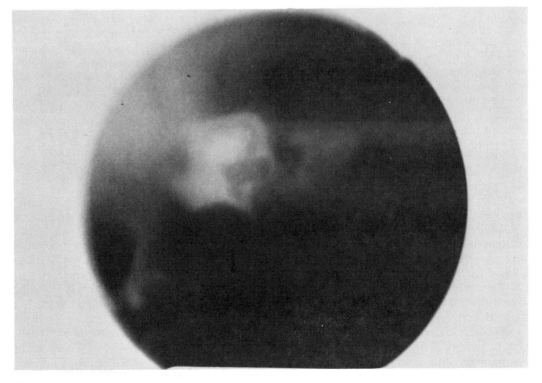

B

Figure 20-5. A. Normal superior and lateral semicircular canals showing sized and shaped vestibule. B. Mondini deformity with dilated, short lateral semicircular canal dilated vestibule.

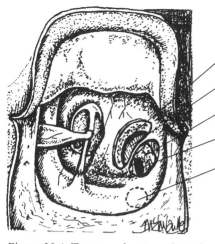

Superior lip of round window niche removed

Round window membrane

Inferior lip of round window niche "saucerized"

Posterior ampullary (singular) nerve

Underlying ampulla of posterior semicircular canal

Figure 20-6. Transcanal approach to the singular nerve, viewed through operating microscope.

patient who has sudden onset of hearing loss or dizziness.

A fistula test is conducted for diagnostic purposes. Positive air pressure is created in the external ear canal, which pushes the tympanic membrane and middle ear mechanism medially. The positive pressure, in presence of a fistula, creates sensations of dizziness in the patient. In approximately 50% of the confirmed fistula cases, the fistula test is positive, with subjective or objective vertigo resulting from positive pressure introduced into the affected ear canal.

Bed rest and conservative management are often recommended for the initial days of symptoms. Many fistulas are thought to heal spontaneously. Pure-tone auditory thresholds should be closely monitored during this time. Any continued hearing fluctuation or progressive hearing loss, with or without associated symptoms of dizziness, should provoke consideration of immediate surgical exploration of the ear. The round and oval windows are inspected through a transcanal tympanotomy, which is usually conducted under local anesthesia. Any inner ear fluid leak may be repaired by placing a tissue graft (such as perichondrium or fat) over the fistula.

Acoustic Neuroma
Acoustic neuroma is a relatively uncommon, but notable, cause of dizziness [7]. The character of the symptoms is unsteadiness rather than true vertigo. Unilateral hearing loss is present in 98% of these patients. It is the responsibility of the otology-audiology team to rule out a retrocochlear lesion in the face of these symptoms. Not all acoustic tumors need to be surgically removed. Very small size, slow growth, advanced patient age, or limited patient life expectancy may justify simple observation rather than surgical intervention.

The diagnosis and selection of the surgical approach is elucidated in Chapter 15. Subtotal or complete removal of the acoustic neuroma will often result in complete relief of the unsteadiness or vertigo. However, residual positional dizziness may persist indefinitely. Because the superior and inferior vestibular nerves are routinely sacrificed in the affected ear with the removal of the acoustic nerve tumor, further surgical management of persistent balance problems is not possible.

REFERENCES
1. Arenberg, I. R. Meniere's disease. *Otolaryngol. Clin. North Am.* 13:4, 1980.
2. Cawthorne, T. Membranous labyrinthectomy via the oval window for Meniere's disease. *J. Laryngol. Otol.* 1:524, 1951.
3. Cody, D. T. R. Automatic repetitive saccelotomy in endolymphatic hydrops. *Otolaryngol. Clin. North Am.* 1:637, 1968.
4. Frederic, M. W. Central vertigo. *Otolaryngol. Clin. North Am.* 6:26, 1973.
5. Gacek, R. R. Transection of the posterior ampullary nerve for the relief of benign positional vertigo. *Am. Otol. Laryngol.* 83:596, 1974.

6. House, W. F. Subarachnoid shunt for drainage of endolymphatic hydrops. *Laryngoscope* 2:713, 1962.

7. House, W. F. *Acoustic Tumors, Vols. I and II.* Baltimore, Md.: University Park Press, 1979.

8. Maniglia, A. J. Phylogeny and its clinical significance. *Otolaryngol. Clin. North Am.* 14:45, 1981.

9. Portmann, G. The saccus endolymphaticus and an operation for draining the same for the relief of vertigo. *J. Laryngol. Otol.* 42: 809, 1927.

10. Pulec, J. L. Meniere's disease. *Otolaryngol. Clin. North Am.* 6:25, 1973.

11. Pulec, J. L. Labyrinthectomy: Indications, technique and results. *Laryngoscope* 84: 1552, 1974.

12. Shea, J. J. (Ed.) Fluctuant hearing loss. *Otolaryngol. Clin. North Am.* Vol. 8, 1975.

13. Simmons, F. B. Theory of membrane breaks in sudden hearing loss. *Arch. Otolaryngol.* 88:41, 1968.

14. Wolfson, L. J. (Ed.). Vertigo. *Otolaryngol. Clin. North Am.* Vol. 6, 1973.

IV

Contemporary Aspects of Hearing

21

Mechanisms of the Middle Ear

David M. Lipscomb

The middle ear contains several mechanisms that allow us to hear sounds with extremely small pressures. These mechanisms provide for a number of interrelated functions, which together meet the primary purpose of transmitting acoustically derived vibrations to the inner ear with remarkable effectiveness. Breakdown of function or structure in this portion of the ear will cause conductive impairments that can greatly reduce hearing sensitivity.

Sound undergoes three energy transformations during the process of hearing. First, the acoustic energy striking the eardrum is converted to mechanical energy and carried across the middle ear by the transmitting mechanism. At the junction between the middle ear and inner ear regions, a second transformation occurs when the mechanical vibrations become hydraulic energy in the fluid of the vestibular and cochlear structures. Third, the hydraulic motion is converted by the tiny and complex sensory cells of the inner ear into neuroelectric events, which are carried to the brain for perceptual analysis. Thus, there are four forms of energy handled by the ear and three energy transformations. All but the latter form and transformation involve the middle ear.

STRUCTURES OF THE MIDDLE EAR

Located just medial to the end of the external canal, the middle ear is an irregularly shaped space that contains air and mechanically important components. The cavity in its anterior-posterior dimension measures 15 mm at most. In the vertical dimension, the greatest distance across the cavity is also 15 mm. The transverse diameter of the middle ear ranges between 2 and 6 mm. This small opening in the skull has an overall capacity of between 1 and 2 cc.

Although the middle ear cavity (also called the tympanic cavity) is irregularly shaped, it is helpful to consider it as a simple cube to understand the orientation of the middle ear structures and landmarks (Fig. 21-1). The predominant structure in the tympanic or lateral wall is the tympanic membrane (eardrum). The eustachian tube opening comprises most of the

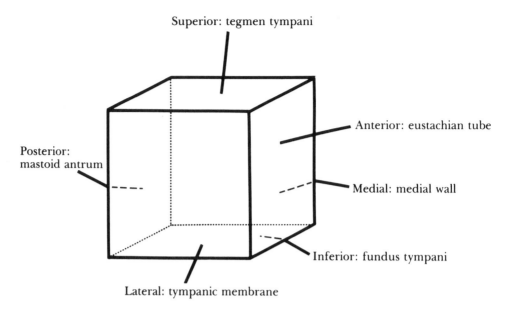

Superior: tegmen tympani

Anterior: eustachian tube

Posterior:
mastoid antrum

Medial: medial wall

Inferior: fundus tympani

Lateral: tympanic membrane

Figure 21-1. Schematic view of middle ear boundaries and landmarks.

anterior or pharyngeal wall. On or near the medial (membranous) wall of the middle ear (also the lateral wall of the inner ear) are a number of structures or landmarks such as the oval window, round window niche, promontory, pyramidal eminence of the stapedius muscle, the canal for the tensor tympani muscle, and the prominence of the facial canal. On the posterior surface of the middle ear is the mastoid antrum. This entrance to the labyrinth of mastoid cavities is a system of pneumatic cells, which apparently contributes to the acoustic resonance characteristics of the middle ear. The upper surface of the cavity is termed the tegmen tympani, a thin shelf of bone that separates the cranial (brain cavity) from the tympanic regions. The floor or jugular wall lies immediately superior to the jugular bulb and is separated from that important cardiovascular reservoir by a thin plate of bone, the fundus tympani. The entire middle ear cavity is lined with mucous membrane.

In addition to the boundaries of the middle ear cavity, there are important structures that are contained within the middle ear, each of which plays a significant role in hearing function. The ossicular chain (Fig. 21-2) consists of the three hardest and smallest bones in the body:

the malleus, incus, and stapes. Two very small muscles are attached, one at each end of the ossicular chain. The tendon of the tensor tympani muscle extends from its canal immediately superior to the eustachian tube to attach at the region of the neck of the malleus. The tendon of the stapedius muscle arises from a cone-shaped enclosure and attaches at the neck of the stapes. In both cases, the muscles themselves are housed within their bony enclosures and only their tendons are exposed. The tensor tympani muscle is primarily innervated by a branch of the trigeminal nerve (fifth cranial nerve), and the stapedius muscle is served by the facial nerve (seventh cranial nerve). Mastoid cells are a pneumatic region immediately posterior to the middle ear cavity providing drainage in the event of infection and resonance for the acoustic energy impinging on the ear. The eustachian tube is a funnel-shaped opening in the anterior wall of the middle ear. The larger, patent portion of the eustachian tube, lined by bone, is at the front edge of the middle ear. At the other end of the tube, there is a partially collapsed cartilaginous opening into the posterior wall of the nasopharynx. The tympanic membrane at the lateral wall of the middle ear is a

AUDITORY OSSICLES - Ligaments and Muscles

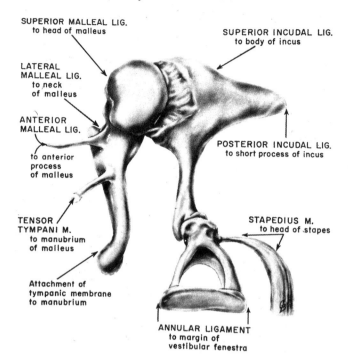

SUPERIOR MALLEAL LIG.
to head of malleus

SUPERIOR INCUDAL LIG.
to body of incus

LATERAL
MALLEAL LIG.
to neck
of malleus

ANTERIOR
MALLEAL LIG.

to anterior
process
of malleus

POSTERIOR INCUDAL LIG.
to short process of incus

TENSOR
TYMPANI M.
to manubrium
of malleus

STAPEDIUS M.
to head of stapes

Attachment of
tympanic membrane
to manubrium

ANNULAR LIGAMENT
to margin of
vestibular fenestra

Figure 21-2. The auditory ossicles, ligaments, and muscles. (From B. J. Anson and J. A. Donaldson, Surgical Anatomy of the Temporal Bone and Ear *[2nd ed.].* Philadelphia: Saunders, 1973.)

compound structure that consists of three layers: epithelium on the lateral side, radial and circular fibers in the middle, and mucous membrane on the medial surface. A small segment of the upper portion of the tympanic membrane contains only epithelial and mucous tissue and is void of fibrous material. This region, called Shrapnell's membrane, is a sort of "blow-out valve" in the event that extreme pressure is directed against the membrane, providing protection against total destruction of the tympanic membrane.

FUNCTION OF THE MIDDLE EAR MECHANISMS

For the most part, the various functions of the structures previously discussed can be considered to be independent, but all the functions blend to provide adequate operation of the total auditory response system.

Tympanic Membrane

The tympanic membrane is the receiver and collector of acoustic pressure directed against the ear by vibratory energy in the air around us. This thin (0.07 mm), delicate, elastic, and somewhat tense portion of the ear is extremely sensitive to pressure changes, so that very minute forces acting on the membrane are sufficient to elicit action of the entire auditory mechanism. The tympanic membrane is conical, pointing medialward so that more surface area of the membrane can be available without having a larger opening for a canal. The angle of the membrane to the general course of the external canal is about 55 degrees from perpendicular with an obtuse angle at the junction of the superior margin (attic) of about 150 degrees, making it less round but somewhat elliptical. The average human tympanic membrane has an area of approximately 63 mm². Because its attachments are firmer at the superior margin, movement of the membrane is not pistonlike. It has considerably more lateral mobility at the inferior margin than at the

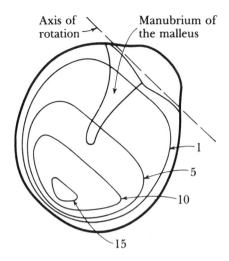

Axis of rotation

Manubrium of the malleus

1
5
10
15

Figure 21-3. Isocontours of membrane movement, showing equal-amplitude curves for eardrum vibrations at frequencies less than 2000 Hz. 1, 5, 10, and 15 are relative differences in the equal-amplitude vibrations of the tympanic membrane. (From G. von Bekesy [trans. and ed. by E. G. Wever], Experiments in Hearing. New York: McGraw-Hill, 1960.)

top, thus its movement is swinglike. This type of mobility partially accounts for the sensitivity of the tympanic membrane to sounds of very small magnitude. In fact, sound pressures no greater than 0.0002 millionths of average barometric pressure are sufficient to produce an auditory sensation. This amount of pressure causes the tympanic membrane to move only about 1/100,-000,000 inch, which is less than 1/100 the thickness of a hydrogen molecule. These statistics are significant because they indicate that the sensitivity of the ear is molecular in magnitude of function at hearing threshold levels. As the pressure of the sound increases, however, the pattern of tympanic membrane movement changes so that it becomes more like the total motion of a loudspeaker when intense sound is directed against it.

In the last century, Helmholtz (*On the Sensations of Tone*) thought that the tympanic membrane was a conical lever that collected the sound force, magnified it, and directed it against the malleus, setting the ossicular chain in motion. He attributed most of the middle ear sensitivity to that physical concept. More recent work has contradicted Helmholtz, however. Bekesy

[6] and others have undertaken experimental investigations to discover the relative motion of the surface regions of the tympanic membrane. In an illustration taken from Bekesy (Fig. 21-3), the isocontours of membrane movement can be seen. These show that the surface of the membrane moves considerably more in the inferior aspect than elsewhere. This observation caused Bekesy to estimate that the effective movement of the tympanic membrane is confined to only about two thirds of its surface.

It is apparent that the first contributing structure to much of our hearing sensitivity is the tympanic membrane. When it becomes too flaccid or too tense, sound pressure will be either absorbed or reflected. This will stop vibratory motion from being directed along the ossicular chain. When the suspension of and tension on the tympanic membrane is appropriate, its ability to convert acoustic energy to mechanical motion is enhanced.

Ossicular Chain

The ossicles (see Fig. 21-2) consist of three bones, each with some dense and heavy regions along with other areas that are thin and relatively fragile. Of considerable importance to the function of the chain is the complex suspension system consisting of attachments to lateral and medial borders, ligaments, articulations, and muscle attachments. As was the case with the tympanic membrane, too much or too little tension will impede the ability of the ossicular chain to transmit vibrations collected by the tympanic membrane. The importance of the suspension system is underscored when it is realized that the ossicles are allowed to move around finely aligned axes, which cause them to transmit the vibrations with utmost efficiency. Comparative anatomic studies have shown that lower animals have slightly different structures. Birds, reptiles, and amphibians have a columella, which is a single straight bone connecting the tympanic membrane with the inner ear. In their case, no lever action of the ossicles is provided. Rodents and some primates have markedly different suspension systems, which doubtless somewhat alters the transmission characteristics of the ossicular chain.

The size, mass, and interconnections of the three ossicles are quite varied. The malleus of the human being averages approximately 25 mg. Its configuration is such that it resembles a club with the thin and delicate handle (manubrium) attached to the tympanic membrane. The head of the malleus articulates at a true joint with the head of the incus. Although shaped very differently, the incus weighs the same as the malleus. Its head and body make up most of the mass. There is a small extension from the body called the long crus (leg), which terminates with an angled tip called the lenticular process. This process articulates with the head of the tiny stapes, which is shaped very much like a saddle stirrup. The mass of the stapes is only one tenth that of the other ossicles (2.5 mg). Because it is so small, the stapes requires much less support. In fact, it is anchored in place by only the annular ligament that radiates from the footplate of the stapes to the surrounding wall of the oval window into which the stapes vibrates in the presence of sound energy. The attachment of the stapedius muscle to the stapes is not thought to provide any supportive function. Although the legs (crura) of the stapes are hollow and extremely fragile, the configuration of the crura is reminiscent of a gothic arch, known by architects to be one of the strongest support structures. Thus, the extreme delicacy of the stapes superstructure is compensated by its well-engineered shape. The reduction in stapes mass coupled with the retention of its strength allows for better response to high-frequency sounds because it is known that mass loading of a structure reduces its ability to respond to the higher frequencies. It is far more important for the mass of the stapes to be low than it is for the mass of the malleus and incus to be low. They are suspended and revolve around an axis of rotation. The suspension system of the first two ossicles negates their contribution of mass loading to the system.

Ossicular motion is schematized in Figure 21-4. When positive pressure is exerted against the tympanic membrane, the manubrium of the malleus is moved medially and the head of the malleus swings laterally, pulling the head of the incus with it. This movement causes the lenticular pro-

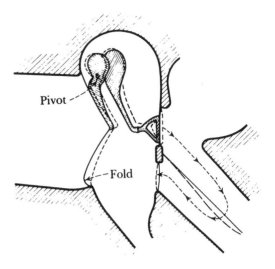

Figure 21-4. Schematic view of ossicles showing movement when positive pressure is exerted against the tympanic membrane. ([3] Adapted from G. Stevens and H. Davis, Hearing: Its Psychology and Physiology. Wiley: New York, 1938.)

cess to move across the region of the head of the stapes, causing the tiny innermost bone to displace some of the fluid immediately behind the oval window. In Figure 21-4, the stapes is shown to be at right angles to its normal placement for illustrative purposes. Because the fluid in the inner ear is practically incompressible, it is necessary to provide for fluid movement. This is the function of the round window membrane. It is basically a relief valve that moves in opposite directions to the motion of the footplate of the stapes. In the diagram, positive pressure at the tympanic membrane causes the footplate of the stapes to enter the oval window, and the displaced fluid of the inner ear forces the round window membrane laterally. In the event of negative pressure on the tympanic membrane, all the motion shown in Figure 21-4 will be reversed. This oscillatory movement creates alternate positive and negative pressure waves in the inner ear, the results of which are discussed in Chapter 22 of this book.

Vibratory motion of the footplate of the stapes is not of a simple pistonlike character. The attachment of the stapedius muscle impedes this type of motion. Also, the presence of slightly thicker annular ligament tissue in the posterior portion of the oval window accounts for the motion, and more movement is allowed at the anterior portion of the footplate because of a small series of folds in the annular ligament of that region. Because the lenticular process of the incus is located slightly anterior to the center of the head of the stapes, motion of that process will have a tendency to force the anterior edge of the stapes footplate farther into the oval window than would be the case for the posterior portion. These factors combine to cause the stapes to rock in and out of the oval window with the hinged portion located at the posterior margin of the footplate.

Bekesy [6] has observed that stapes vibratory motion changes with sound pressure levels of approximately 70 dB and higher. As the sound pressure continues to increase until very high levels are reached, the mode of vibration of the stapes changes radically so that at one moment the top half of the stapes moves into the oval window as the bottom half is pulling out. This reduces the amount of pressure transferred into the inner ear. Fluids inside the cochlear region are not set in motion as effectively because of the equalization of fluid pressure at the stapes footplate by a form of compensatory shunt when half the footplate moves in contradistinction to the other half. In this case, the relief of pressure is not at the round window membrane; rather, it is at the other half of the stapes footplate. Possibly, this is a protective function of the middle ear in that extremely high sound levels are not allowed to create concomitant high pressures in the cochlear region. If this were not the case, high-level noise might well cause more cochlear damage than is already the case.

For sound pressure levels of low and medium amplitude, the ossicular chain provides efficient transport of the vibrations across the middle ear. For high level sounds, the efficiency is reduced, partially because of the alteration in vibratory mode of the stapes and the slight protective function of the middle ear muscles.

Middle Ear Muscles

The tensor tympanum muscle attaches to the malleus in such a way that contraction of the muscle pulls the manubrium and the tympanic membrane medially. This has the effect of tensing both the structures and can reduce the response of the middle ear to sound stimulation. This muscle is the larger of the two middle ear muscles, being approximately 25 mm long with a cross-section area of 5 mm². In the uncontracted state, the tendon of the tensor muscle exerts a slight pull against the malleus of approximately 0.5 gm. In this context, it serves as a very slight tensing agent to the tympanic membrane.

In opposition to the direction of stress provided by the tensor tympani muscle, the smaller stapedius muscle is oriented to pull the stapes footplate away from the oval window. This smaller muscle is only 6 to 7 mm long with a cross-section area of 5 mm². But the effectiveness of its reduction of transmission of energy across the middle ear exceeds that of the tensor muscle because the stapedius muscle directly affects the stapes itself.

It is possible to observe on the surface of the tympanic membrane whether either of the middle ear muscles have contracted. When the tensor muscle fires, the tympanic membrane can be distinctly seen to move in a medial direction. With the contraction of the stapedius muscle, a slight lateral motion of the tympanic membrane can be seen. Seldom, however, do the two muscles contract independently. When one contracts, the other will do likewise, which stiffens the middle ear transmitting mechanism and makes it slightly less sensitive to sound stimulation.

Middle ear muscle contractions can be voluntarily initiated by some persons. Tensor contractions can be caused by tickling the face or external canal or by blowing a jet of air into the ear canal. Some persons can cause the tensor muscle to fire by closing their eyelids firmly or by wincing. Firm pressure on the eyeballs can also initiate a contraction of the tensor muscle. The most consistent means of causing the reflex, however, is to present high-level sound to the ear. A complex neurologic mechanism (reflex arc) allows for the contraction of the stapedius muscle in response to sound stimulation. When the cochlea sends nerve impulses to the brain after intense sound stimulation, there is a neurologic crossover between the ascending sensory nerves and descending motor fibers of the facial nerve. The facial nerve, then, activates the stapedium muscle, causing it to contract. Because there is no known acoustically initiated reflex arc for the tensor muscle, it is thought that the tensor reacts to the contraction of the stapedius muscle because the two muscles are antagonistic.

An interesting discussion of the effect of middle ear muscles on perceptual activity has been given by Simmons [5]. In essence, Simmons postulates that changes in muscle tone modulate amplitude and frequency components of the sound environment. He feels these changes are a function of the level of alertness of the organism. This provides a means whereby a specific desired sound can be separated from the mélange of background sounds allowing for better maintenance of attention to ongoing sound stimulation. He also considers the possibility that modulations of muscle tone may eliminate middle ear resonances without sacrificing transmission efficiency. Muscle activity, especially the initial "twitch," may provide a means for quickly identifying the environmental or internal origin of an unknown sound. Simmons offers the possibility that middle ear muscle contractions that occur with such activities as vocalization and chewing considerably reduce the low-frequency noise of those activities. This preserves the sensitivity for higher frequency external sounds. These thoughts argue for an altogether new dimension of thinking regarding middle ear muscle function. It is hoped that additional information will be forthcoming to allow adequate consideration of these factors.

Four theories have been advanced to account for the presence and function of the middle ear muscles.

1. Intensity-control theory. The muscles are seen as reducing inordinately high sound pressure stimulation of the inner ear, thereby protecting the cochlear structures from damage that could result from excessive sound levels. This principle is most effective for the low frequencies and seems to be of little or no importance for sounds the frequency of which exceeds 2000 Hz.

2. Frequency-selection theory. This idea advances the notion that the muscles can be caused to contract differentially to favor the transmission of some frequencies more efficiently than others.

3. Fixation theory. This theory asserts that the presence, attachments, and varying contraction of the muscles can cause the suspension system of the ossicular chain to reach its maximally sensitive degree of tension to facilitate transmission of sound.

4. Labyrinthine pressure theory. This concept holds that the muscles can vary the inner ear fluid pressure by the degree to which the stapes is pressed into or pulled out of the oval window to alter the mechanical performance of the inner ear.

The only theory to receive strong experimental support has been the intensity-control or protective theory. The others attribute too much capability to the muscles and their innervation than is apparently the case. It must be noted, however, that the protective function of the muscles is also limited. Maximum contraction of the muscles reduces the transmission of sound between 10 and 20 dB primarily for the lower frequencies, an inadequate amount for total protection from some of the high-level sounds encountered in many environments.

A second limiting factor for the protective characteristics of the muscles is the latency of response. It takes approximately 63 msec for the stapedius and 132 msec for the tensor to reach maximum contraction. If the sound is of brief duration, such as a gunshot, the muscles contract too slowly to combat the transmission of acoustic energy across the middle ear.

Eustachian Tube
Although it does not contribute directly to the transmission of sound across the middle ear into the cochlear region, the absence of proper eustachian tube function signals its importance in maintaining proper conditions in the middle ear. The middle ear cavity is filled with air that can only be vented through the eustachian tube. If the tube is occluded, a gradual vacuum will build up creating an inward pull on the tympanic membrane, which

can be painful and overly tense the membrane. This condition can give rise to the secretion of a clear serum into the middle ear cavity, further reducing the effectiveness of the transmission system. Not only does the eustachian tube allow long-term passage of air into and out of the middle ear, but momentary changes in air pressure outside the head necessitate equalization of that air pressure in the middle ear. When the ears "pop" on changing altitude rapidly, the eustachian tube has allowed air in the middle ear to equalize with the pressure outside the head. Failure to do so will result in considerable discomfort if not corrected quickly.

The eustachian tube performs another vital function. It acts as a drainage conduit for any fluid that has collected in the middle ear. As a side effect of a head cold, one often has inflammation of the mucous membrane that lines the mouth, throat, nasal cavity, eustachian tube, and the entire middle ear including pneumatic cells of the mastoid region. This inflammation can cause the mucous membrane to secrete serum, which will collect in the middle ear cavity. As the fluid accumulates and the secretion continues, there can be several undesirable side effects. Fluid pressure can build up, causing discomfort from pressure on the tympanic membrane. This pressure tenses and irritates the membrane, reducing its sensitivity. The ossicles, when immersed in fluid, partially lose their ability to vibrate, further cutting down on the efficiency of the middle ear transmission system. If the fluid is allowed to remain in the middle ear cavity, the potential for bacterial development becomes a problem. Adequate eustachian tube drainage function will abate these problems and allow the middle ear to carry on its normal and important task.

Two reasons children suffer more middle ear problems than adults are swollen adenoids and the course of the eustachian tube. In children the direction of the eustachian tube between the middle ear and the posterior nasopharynx is nearly horizontal, which works against the gravitational effect for drainage of accumulating fluid. In the adult, owing to slight changes in configuration of the head during growth to adulthood, the course of the eustachian tube changes from horizontal to downward, allowing the forces of gravity to act more fully on any fluid in the middle ear, facilitating drainage. These anatomic concepts can be readily observed by holding a ruler on a line between the opening of the ear canal and the opening of the nasal cavity, using an adult and a child. One can note considerably more downward slant of the ruler for adult heads.

In effect, this 1½-inch tube, formally called the pharyngotympanic tube of eustachius, contributes immensely to the normal function of the middle ear mechanisms. Fortunately, however, the opening of the tube at the posterior nasopharynx is not conventionally open. For, if that were the case, encroachment of bacteria-laden mucus, food particles, and other foreign substances into the middle ear cavity would constitute a serious problem. This opening, which is lined with sphincter-ring muscles, the torus tubarius, can usually be made functional by yawning or by chewing gum unless there is some serious obstruction of the opening caused by swollen adenoid tissues or by generalized inflammation of the tissues of the posterior nasopharynx.

Pneumatic Cavities

Located immediately posterior to the middle ear cavity is a system of air cells in the mastoid process of the temporal bone. The air cells are all interconnected and lined with mucous tissue. Apart from making the skull lighter and more balanced (as opposed to the region being solid bone), the pneumatic spaces probably have a resonance function that adds to the resonating characteristics of the middle ear cavity itself. The size of the total area of these regions conceivably could make the cavity resonate to certain frequencies, which would play at least a small role in facilitating auditory response to those frequencies. At best, however, this is a minor characteristic of middle ear function.

CONTRIBUTION OF THE MIDDLE EAR MECHANISMS TO HEARING SENSITIVITY

The mammalian ear is almost unbelievably sensitive to those small pressure changes in the atmosphere we call *sound*. In effect, there are two major contributors to that extreme sensitivity: (1) the shearing motion of the sensory region of the organ of Corti in the inner ear (discussed in Chapter 22); and (2) the middle ear transformer mechanism.

Sound energy is not equally transferable from one medium of sound propagation to another. Waterborne sound vibrations not only travel more rapidly than do airborne sound vibrations, but they are far more capable of inducing sympathetic vibration on a fluid-filled area such as the inner ear. When airborne vibrations impinge on a fluid, more than 99.9% of the sound energy is reflected from the surface of the fluid. This leaves a transmission loss of approximately 35 dB. Therefore, if it were left to the sound coming into the ear canal directly to stimulate the fluid in the inner ear, we would have a considerable loss of hearing. But the middle ear mechanisms combine to match transmission characteristics of the air with transmission characteristics of the fluid in the inner ear to allow much more effective conductivity of vibrations than would be the case without middle ear function. In effect, the middle ear performs a transformer function for sound conduction much the same as a matching transformer is used between a microphone amplifier for a public address system to get the output impedance of the microphone equivalent to the input impedance of the amplifier. Any impedance mismatch would result in serious loss of sound quality and amplitude.

Impedance
The previous description of the stapes superstructure included a discussion of the importance of reducing mass to transmit higher frequencies, a consideration bearing upon impedance theory. Impedance can be described as the total responsiveness (or lack of responsiveness) of a mechanism being driven by some force. For the ear, the impedance of the air, measured to be approximately 41.5 ohms, is mismatched to the impedance of the fluid of the inner ear, which is about 143,000 ohms. Therefore, sound borne by a transmitting medium with very little impedance will have considerable difficulty creating sympathetic vibrations in a medium with quite high

impedance. Something must be placed between these two media to allow better sound transmission into the fluid of the inner ear. The middle ear structure accomplishes this task.

It is not appropriate in this context to enter into some of the complicated and complex mathematical and physical computations necessary to understand fully the impedance characteristics of middle ear function. Impedance of any physical phenomena (e.g., electronic, mechanical, or acoustic) is an admixture of three components. In acoustic terms, these components are acoustic resistance, acoustic mass, and acoustic compliance.

Acoustic Resistance. Opposition posed by the resistance of a responding mechanism will reduce the amount of sound conducted from one transmitting medium to another. Analogous to mechanical friction, acoustic friction is not frequency-dependent. That is, when it acts to impede sound transmission, it acts with equal opposition to all sound frequencies.

Acoustic Mass. The size and weight of an object, such as the mass of an ossicle or the mass of the tissues in the cochlea, will offer inertial opposition to the *change* from silence to the presence of sound and back to the silence state. These opposition forces to *changes* in acoustic energy pose a barrier to the adequate transmission of sound from one medium to another. This component, mass, is more significant for high-frequency sounds than for low-frequency ones. This can be demonstrated by holding a pencil between the thumb and forefinger of one hand. By slowly moving the pencil back and forth in an oscillatory motion, there is relatively little pressure against the fingers. As the speed of the oscillatory motion is increased, however, one becomes much aware of additional pressure against the fingers. This practical demonstration is suggested to instill the important concept that mass loading is a high-frequency phenomenon. Thus, when an impedance mismatch occurs, the mass component reduces the transmission of high-frequency energy.

Acoustic Compliance (Stiffness). This third component has to do with the ability a structure has to comply with a driving force. A very stiff or noncompliant structure will offer more opposition to the changes from silence to the presence of sound and back to silence in addition to the effect already mentioned in the discussion of mass. In the case of compliance, however, the effect is maximized for the low-frequency energy portion of the sound. Thus, it can be said that acoustic compliance is a low-frequency component in the impedance characteristics of a responding mechanism. Another simple example can be described. If one were to affix a rubber band to a weight and lift the weight with the rubber band, slow up-and-down movements of the hand will cause the weight to bounce up and down quite noticeably. But, when the hand motion is increased in speed, the weight does not move with the hand nearly as much because the "springiness" of the rubber band's compliance characteristics absorb the more rapid motion, causing commensurately less force on the weight. Again, this simple example is intended to etch firmly in the mind that acoustic compliance or stiffness is basically a low-frequency component.

These three factors are combined to create the total impedance of a certain structure or mechanism. In the case of the middle ear, resistance in the middle ear structures, mass of the moving parts of the middle ear, and compliant features of the middle ear add together to generate total impedance for that region of the ear. All these characteristics are taken into account when the impedance characteristics of the ear are measured. If the middle ear is too stiff (e.g., otosclerosis) or too compliant (e.g., ossicular discontinuity), the effect will be noted in its ability to transmit low-frequency sounds. Increased mass in the structures would reduce the transmission of high-frequency sounds. When the resistance is increased, the effect will not be frequency-specific.

Acoustic compliance and acoustic mass act on opposite ends of the frequency spectrum. In addition, they operate to some degree in phase opposition. Therefore, when certain frequencies are transmitted, acoustic mass and acoustic compliance act against each other partially to cancel each other out. In this condition, for that fre-

quency, the only remaining opposition to signal transmission is acoustic resistance. Therefore, the sound energy at that frequency will be transmitted more readily across the middle ear. This point, at which mass and compliance cancel, is regarded as the natural frequency, which for the normal ear is approximately 800 to 1000 Hz. In the development of the middle ear, mass and compliance factors were designed to interact at the middle frequencies to allow for less impedance and therefore better transmission for the purpose of hearing sensitivity at the middle frequency region.

Middle Ear Transformer Function

The acoustic impedance of air is 41.5 ohms, and the impedance of inner ear fluid is 143,000 ohms. The middle ear mechanisms provide a means whereby airborne sounds more effectively stimulate the inner ear fluid with the aid of the middle ear to overcome the potential transmission loss of 35 dB. Two factors should be considered in this matching activity: the areal relationship between the tympanic membrane and footplate of the stapes and ossicular lever action.

Areal Relationship. The tympanic membrane is approximately 21 times greater in total area than is the footplate of the stapes. But because Bekesy's measures [6] indicate that only about two thirds of the tympanic membrane moved effectively, it is necessary to reduce the total 21 : 1 ratio of areas by one third yielding an effective size ratio of 14 : 1 between the tympanic membrane and the stapes footplate. This relationship can be calculated to be 22.9 dB. In effect, the greater size of the collecting surface of the tympanic membrane results in nearly a 23 dB increase in the effectiveness of the sound transmission system to the inner ear.

Ossicular Lever Action. There is some slight improvement in sound transmission characteristics from the lever action of the ossicular chain. Using the calculations and measurements of Dahmann [2] in 1929, we can suggest that the lever action gives an improvement ratio of 1.32 : 1 or 2.5 dB. When the effects of both factors are combined (adding 22.9 dB and 2.5 dB) we find that the middle ear transformer is responsible for overcoming 25.4 dB of the 35 dB, which would have been lost by attempting to stimulate the inner ear fluid directly with airborne sound energy. Although this is not a perfect match, it is far better than if the middle ear were not present.

The historic significance of the development of this mechanism is that without it, human beings in their present form might never have emerged. When sea-dwelling creatures first came on land, they had primitive auditory structures that were built for receiving waterborne sounds. There was no need for any matching transformer. But in the atmosphere they doubtless had a considerable hearing deficiency that would have made it quite easy for lumbering predators to sneak up on their prey. With the development of the middle ear and the accompanying increased hearing sensitivity, the smaller animals could hear their attackers coming from behind and take flight. It was this factor that caused Dr. El-Mofty [4] of Egypt to comment that the birth of the middle ear was one of the most remarkable scenes in the theater of evolution.

Two conditions must be obtained for normal and effective middle ear function: (1) barometric pressure must be equal on both sides of the tympanic membrane, a function of the eustachian tube; and (2) the mobility of the moving parts in the middle ear must be preserved. The stapes must be free to move unhindered by adhesions, calcium deposits, or accumulated fluid, and the round window membrane must be mobile to allow free incursion and excursion of the footplate of the stapes.

Interestingly, modifications to improve this system would result in lessening of some effects we now consider to be benefits. If the tympanic membrane were increased in area, our hearing would not be as omnidirectional, and if it were smaller, the response to low frequencies would be diminished. If the resistance of the structures were decreased and the suspension system made less rigid, our ears would ring, causing one sound to blend into another, as happens with the use of a "sustain" setting on an organ. Alteration in the location of ossicles could cause them to be more easily disarticulated in the event of an intense sound. It can be said that the structure of the middle ear evolved into an organ of total function, developing into the most useful and definitive sound vibration system possible.

REFERENCES

1. Anson, B. J., and Donaldson, J. A. *Surgical Anatomy of the Temporal Bone and Ear* (2nd ed.). Philadelphia: Saunders, 1973.
2. Dahmann, H. Zur Physiologie des Hörens. *Z. Hals-Nasen-Ohrenheilk* 24:462, 1929.
3. Davis, H., and Silverman, S. *Hearing and Deafness* (2nd ed.). New York: Holt, Rinehart & Winston, 1970.
4. El-Mofty, A., and El-Serafy, S. The ossicular chain in mammals. *Ann. Otol. Rhinol. Laryngol.* 76:903, 1967.
5. Simmons, F. B. Perceptual theories of middle ear muscle function. *Ann. Otol. Rhinol. Laryngol.* 73:724, 1964.
6. von Bekesy, G. (trans. and ed. by E. G. Wever). *Experiments in Hearing.* New York: McGraw-Hill, 1960.

SUGGESTED READINGS

De Reuck, A. V. S., and Knight, J. (Eds.). *Hearing Mechanisms in Vertebrates.* London: Churchill, 1968.

Donaldson, J. A. *Surgical Anatomy of the Temporal Bone and Ear* (3rd ed.). Philadelphia: Saunders, 1981.

Fletcher, J. L. (Ed.). *Middle Ear Function Seminar,* Report No. 576, U.S. Army Medical Research and Development Command, 1963.

Harris, J. D. *Anatomy and Physiology of the Peripheral Hearing Mechanism.* Indianapolis: Bobbs-Merrill, 1974.

Helmholtz, H. L. F. *On the Sensations of Tone.* New York: Dover, 1954.

Jepsen, O. Middle-ear muscle reflexes in man. In J. Jerger (Ed.), *Modern Developments in Audiology.* New York: Academic Press, 1963.

Lipscomb, D. M. Anatomy and Physiology of the Hearing Mechanism. In N. J. Lass, et al. (Eds.), *Speech, Language and Hearing.* Philadelphia: Saunders, 1982.

Lilly, D. Measurement of acoustic impedance at the tympanic membrane. In J. Jerger (Ed.), *Modern Developments in Audiology* (2nd ed.). New York: Academic Press, 1973.

Polyak, S. L., McHugh, G., and Judd, D. K. *The Human Ear in Anatomical Transparencies.* New York: Sonotone, 1946.

Wever, E. G., and Lawrence, M. *Physiological Acoustics.* Princeton, N.J.: Princeton University Press, 1954.

22

Physiology of
the Cochlea

Allen F. Ryan
Peter Dallos

The cochlea translates the mechanical stimulus of sound, delivered from the tympanic membrane via the ossicular chain, into the sequence of electrical discharges that is the language of the nervous system. This exquisitely engineered sense organ accomplishes the translation in several stages (Fig. 22-1). The mechanical vibrations of the stapes are delivered to the cochlear fluids, where they are manifested as a hydromechanical disturbance, or wave. This wave, in traveling through the membranous structures of the inner ear, acts to displace cilia, which project from the cochlea's specialized sensory cells. These hair cells convert the deformation into an electrochemical event which, in turn, promotes synaptic transmission between the cells and the neurons of the auditory portion of the eighth nerve. Finally, the resultant electrical potentials in the eighth nerve dendrites initiate impulses that are transmitted to the central nervous system. All these functional steps, and the additional analysis of stimulus frequency, intensity, and phase, are performed by an organ considerably less than 1 ml in volume. The details of this intricate mechanism are the subject of one of the most fascinating stories in sensory biology.

ANATOMY

Structurally, the mammalian cochlea is an elongated, fluid-filled cavity in the temporal bone of the cranium. This cavity is coiled into a tight spiral that resembles the shell of a snail (Fig. 22-2). The broad end of the spiral, which lies close to the middle ear, is called the base. The narrow end is known as the apex. The cochlea is divided lengthwise into three channels by the basilar membrane and Reissner's membrane (Fig. 22-3). The channel that lies between Reissner's membrane and the upper bony wall of the cochlea is known as the scala vestibuli. The channel between the basilar membrane and the opposite wall is called the scala tympani. The remaining channel, which lies between the two membranes, is called the cochlear duct. One of the most important characteristics of the cochlear duct is its elasticity. Because it is bound on two sides by tissue membranes,

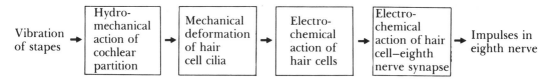

Figure 22-1. Schematic representation of the cochlea.

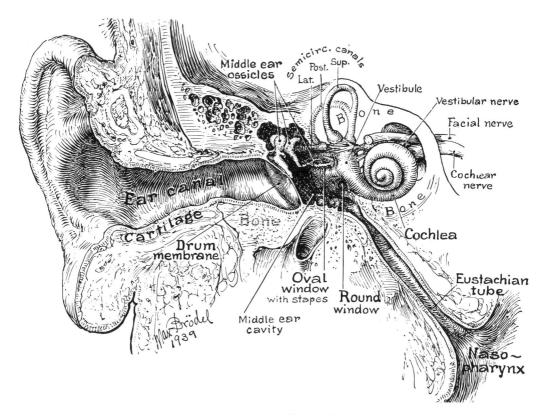

Figure 22-2. A cross-section of the human ear. (From M. Brodel, Three Unpublished Drawings of the Anatomy of the Human Ear. Philadelphia: Saunders, 1946.)

it responds to pressure from either side by moving in the appropriate direction.

The scala vestibuli and scala tympani are separated by the cochlear duct throughout the length of the cochlea, except at the apical end, farthest from the middle ear. Here the cochlear duct ends blindly, and the two canals communicate through an opening called the helicotrema.

The outer chambers, scala vestibuli and tympani, are filled with a fluid called perilymph. This fluid has a high sodium content and is low in potassium. The cochlear duct contains a different fluid known as endolymph, which is low in sodium and

high in potassium, the reverse of perilymph [24]. The fluid-filled spaces are separated from the air spaces of the middle ear by the bony wall of the cochlea. However, there are two openings in the bone. One leads from the middle ear into the scala vestibuli. It is sealed by the innermost of the ossicles, the stapes. The flat end, or footplate, of the stapes fits loosely into the opening, known as the oval window. It is held in place by the flexible an-

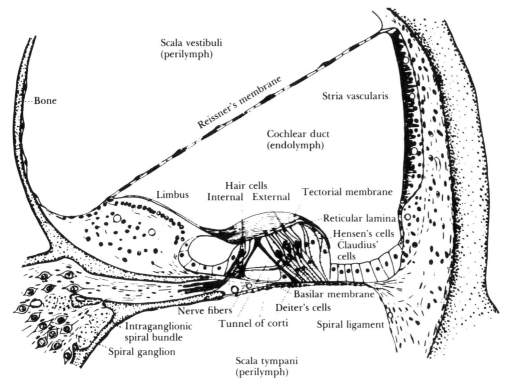

Figure 22-3. A cross-section of the central portion of the cochlear cavity. (From H. Davis et al., Acoustic trauma in the guinea pig. J. Acoust. Soc. Am. 25:1180, 1953.)

nular ligament, which seals the perilymph into the scala vestibuli and yet allows the stapes to move within the oval window. Therefore, movement of the stapes is transferred through the oval window to the molecules of the perilymph. The other opening between the cochlea and the middle ear is known as the round window. This opening leads into the scala tympani, on the other side of the cochlear duct from the oval window. It is covered by a thin, flexible membrane. When pressure is applied to the cochlear fluids through the oval window, this membrane compensates by bulging outward. From these characteristics, it can be appreciated that the cochlea is a complex hydraulic system.

The basilar membrane, which separates the cochlear duct from scala tympani, supports the structures that are directly responsible for sensory function in the cochlea. These include the organ of Corti and the tectorial membrane. With the bas-

ilar membrane, these structures make up the cochlear partition. Because this composite structure is so important to cochlear function, we will discuss its anatomic features in some detail.

The cochlear partition changes in character as it progresses from the base of the cochlea to the apex in three ways that are especially important to its function. First, the width of the partition increases, base to apex, approximately tenfold. Second, its mass increases with the width, primarily owing to an increase in the size and number of supporting cells in the organ of Corti. Third, the flexibility of the partition changes drastically. Largely because of the structural properties of the basilar membrane, it is quite stiff at the base and becomes progressively more elastic toward the apex. The change in elasticity is more than one hundredfold [47].

Figure 22-4 provides a cross-sectional view of the cochlear partition. The organ of Corti rests directly on the basilar membrane. It consists of sensory cells that are embedded in a matrix of supporting cells. The supporting cells make up the bulk of

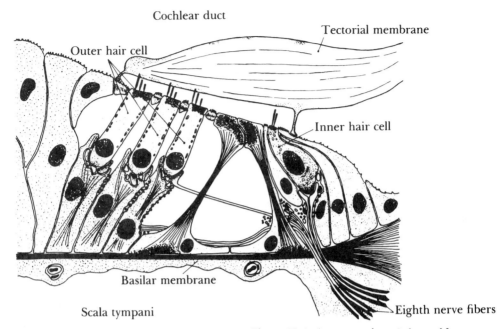

Figure 22-4. A cross-section of the cochlear partition.

the organ, and they anchor it and the embedded sensory cells firmly to the basilar membrane. Thus, if the membrane moves, the sensory cells follow its motion closely. The sensory cells occur in rows that run along the organ throughout the length of the cochlea (Fig. 22-5). The top of each sensory cell forms part of the upper surface of the organ of Corti and bears a cluster of stiff cilia, or hairs. For this reason, they are known as hair cells. The sensory hairs project above the surface of the organ.

Two types of hair cells are found in the mammalian cochlea. The inner hair cells lie in a single row close to the inside of the cochlear spiral. They are flask-shaped, and completely surrounded by supporting cells except for the hairbearing surface. The outer hair cells form three or four rows that lie more toward the outer edge of the cochlea. These cells are in contact with the supporting cells only at their very top and bottom. The bulk of the elongated, cylindric cell body is suspended in the fluid spaces that occur inside the organ of Corti. These spaces are filled with a fluid occasionally called cortilymph, which is similar to perilymph in its chemical composition [17].

Lying directly above the organ of Corti, but separated from it by a narrower space, is the tectorial membrane. This noncellu-

lar, gelatinous structure is attached at its inner edge to the lining of the bony cochlear wall. Otherwise, it is only loosely coupled to the organ of Corti by slender processes. The tallest of the hairs of the outer hair cells are in firm contact with the underside of the tectorial membrane [30, 39]. This contact facilitates the transmission of movement from the membrane to the outer hair cells. Alternatively, if outer hair cells are themselves mechanically active as has recently been suggested (see following discussion), then this contact permits the modification of cochlear micromechanics by their action. The fluid underneath the tectorial membrane, which bathes the hairbearing surfaces of the hair cells, is endolymph [35].

The fibers of the eighth (auditory) nerve enter the cochlea through the center of the cochlear spiral. They emerge from tiny openings in the inner edge of the bony cochlear wall and enter the organ of Corti. The vast majority (95%) of these afferent, or ascending, fibers approach the nearest inner hair cell and form one-to-one connections, about 20 per hair cell. The remaining 5% travel across the organ of Corti, turn down the cochlea toward the base, and contact groups of outer hair

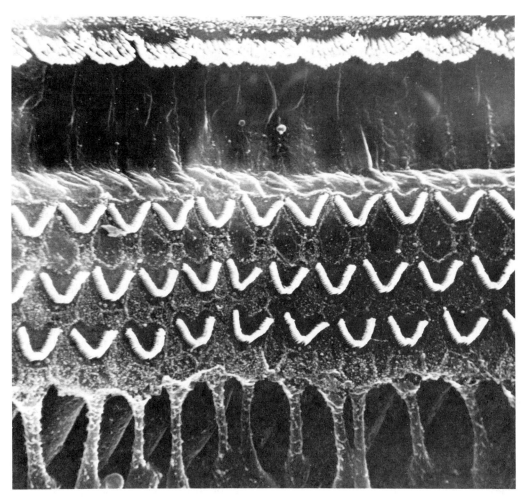

Figure 22-5. The organ of Corti as viewed from the cochlear duct, with the tectorial membrane removed, in a scanning electron microgram. Note the sensory hairs of the single row of inner hair cells and of the three rows of outer hair cells. (From G. Bredberg, H. Ades, and H. Engstrom, Scanning electron microscopy of the normal and pathologically altered organ of Corti. Acta Otolaryngol. [Suppl.] 301:3, 1972.)

cells. Each such fiber can be connected to approximately 20 sensory cells, and each outer hair cell may receive processes from approximately 20 afferent fibers [40]. Obviously, the innervation pattern of the two types of hair cells is quite different. The nerve fibers contact both types of hair cells at the bottom at the end farthest from the sensory hairs. Under great magnification, this end of the hair cell is seen to contain the presynaptic structures that are neces-

sary for chemically transmitting signals to the afferent nerve endings [38]. The cell bodies of the eighth nerve cells are located in the spiral ganglion, just inside the bone of the modiolus from the organ of Corti. There are two types of spiral ganglion neurons [25, 34], which correspond to the two types of afferent nerve fibers that independently innervate the two populations of hair cells [29].

A small number of the fibers in the eighth nerve are efferent, that is, they transmit impulses from higher auditory centers to the cochlea. These fibers arise from neurons whose cell bodies are located in the brain stem, mostly on the side opposite from the ear to which they travel. Two populations of efferent nerve fibers have been identified in the cochlea. Each population originates from a distinct cell group in the brain stem [48], and they also differ biochemically [37]. Once they reach the cochlea, the efferent fibers branch out to form a large number of nerve endings. One group contacts the afferent fibers beneath the inner hair cells [32, 37, 39]. The other group terminates primarily on the outer hair cells themselves, but also supplies some endings that contact the afferent fibers under the inner hair cells [37, 39].

The cochlea consumes a great deal of energy and consequently possesses an extensive network of blood vessels that supply its oxygen and nutrient requirements. The cochlear artery enters the inner ear alongside the eighth nerve and then divides into two major pathways. One of these is an extensive network of capillaries that occupies the outer wall of the cochlear duct and supplies the stria vascularis, spiral prominence, and spiral ligament (see Fig. 22-3). These structures consume large quantities of energy even when the inner ear is at rest [34]. The outer wall structures and especially the stria vascularis are thought to be responsible for generation of the endocochlear potential, a resting potential that is critical to the function of the inner ear and for the secretion of endolymph [42, 43]. The other source of arterial blood is the spiral vessels that run longitudinally just beneath the basilar membrane and probably supply most of the nutrition for the organ of Corti.

THE TRAVELING WAVE

As we have seen, the cochlea can be described as a hydromechanical system. The stimuli that activate this system are delivered to the cochlear fluids by the stapes footplate. Inward motion of the footplate produces an increase in pressure in the perilymph adjacent to the oval window. Outward motion results in lowered pressure in the same region. Because the bony cochlea is inflexible, this pressure must be compensated for by an outward or inward bulging of the round window membrane. However, to reach the membrane, the pressure must be absorbed and transmitted across the cochlear partition. Because the partition is flexible, it can be displaced in both directions, thus transferring the pressure change to the fluids in the region of the round window. The resulting energy exchange between the surrounding fluids and the moving partition initiates a characteristic wave pattern that progresses along the partition from base to apex. Because of its progression along the cochlea, this phenomenon is known as a traveling wave.

Because of the structural characteristics of the partition and the properties of the adjacent fluid layer, the traveling wave does not maintain a uniform amplitude throughout the cochlea. From its origin at the base, it increases in amplitude while progressing toward the apex until it reaches a maximum, beyond which it declines rapidly. Moreover, the location along the cochlea at which the traveling wave reaches its largest amplitude changes with the frequency of the stimulating signal. High-frequency stimuli generate the maximum wave amplitude at the base of the cochlea. For low frequencies, the maximum amplitude of displacement is toward the apex [44].

Figure 22-6 illustrates some basic features of the traveling wave. Positions of the cochlear partition are drawn for four successive instants. The stimulus is a continuous sinusoid, a pure tone. For purposes of illustration, the cochlea has been "uncoiled" into a straight tube. The base lies on the left side of the figure. The amplitude of displacement of the partition has been greatly enlarged. The dotted lines represent the displacement envelope, within which all vibrations are confined for a given stimulus. The envelope rises slowly to a maximum and then falls rapidly

Figure 22-6. Diagram of the traveling wave produced by a 200 Hz tone at four successive instants in time. Amplitude is greatly enlarged. Dotted lines represent displacement. (From G. von Bekesy [trans. and ed. by E. G. Wever], Experiments in Hearing. New York: McGraw-Hill, 1960.)

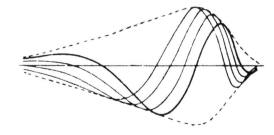

Base   Apex

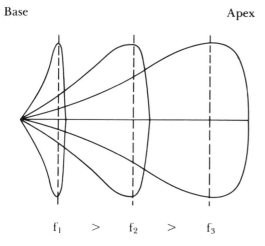

f_1 > f_2 > f_3

Figure 22-7. Diagram of traveling wave envelopes for three frequencies. Amplitude of displacement has been greatly exaggerated.

thereafter. The waveforms illustrate the progression, or travel, of the wave from the base toward the apex.

Except for the lowest, the vibrations of all audible frequencies do not travel the entire length of the cochlear partition. Instead, they die down before reaching the helicotrema. High-frequency stimuli are extinguished quite close to the base, whereas low-frequency stimuli are propagated further toward the apex (Fig. 22-7). This difference in the behavior of the partition to different frequencies of stimulation is due to its peculiar structure. Because of its base-to-apex increases in width, mass, and especially compliance, the ability of the partition to absorb energy from high-frequency changes in fluid pressure decreases toward the apex. Thus, high-frequency energy excites only the basal region whereas low-frequency energy is allowed to travel further along the cochlea [44, 47]. The end result of this characteristic of the cochlear partition is that different frequencies of stimulation produce displacement envelope maxima at different locations along the cochlea. Different locations are therefore tuned to different stimulus frequencies. The hydromechanic wave action of the cochlea maps the frequency of a given stimulus in the spatial extent and maximum amplitude of the traveling waves that that stimulus produces.

FINE MOTION PATTERNS

What happens when a particular region of the cochlear partition is set into motion? It has been fairly well established that the effective stimulus to the cochlear hair cells is the displacement of its sensory hairs from their resting position [47]. This displacement is thought to occur in the following fashion: The principal points of attachment of the basilar and tectorial membranes, the points about which they rotate during the displacement of the cochlear partition, are different (see Fig. 22-3). Also, the outer edge of the tectorial membrane has no firm attachment. The effect of this structural arrangement on the outer hair cells is shown schematically in Figure 22-8. Vertical displacement of the cochlear partition produces a radial shearing force on the longest row of sensory hairs whose tips are embedded in the tectorial membrane [13, 47]. Because the hairs of a given hair cell appear to be interconnected by

Figure 22-8. Probable pattern of shearing action between the tectorial membrane and the spiral organ. The hairs of the inner hair cells, which are not attached to the tectorial membrane, are thought to be displaced by fluid movement. Bottom: organ at rest. Top: during displacement toward scala vestibuli.

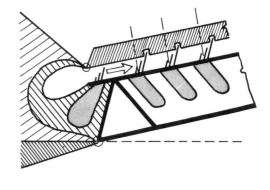

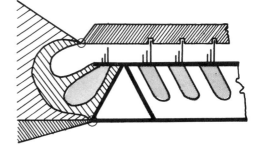

mucopolysaccharide filaments, all the hairs probably bend with this shearing force [39].

The inner hair cells, which do not appear to be connected to the tectorial membrane, are thought to be stimulated by fluid streaming between the two membranes and through the sensory hairs. The fluid is set in motion by the movements of the partition, more specifically by the relative movement between the tectorial membrane and the organ of Corti [1, 12]. It has been suggested [6] that outer hair cells may change their mechanical characteristics, either in response to stimulation or efferent input. This change could involve variation in stiffness of the hair cell cilia, which have been shown to contain actin [21]. A change in outer hair cell mechanical response could modify the relative motion between the organ of Corti and tectorial membrane and, thus, the input to the inner hair cells.

TRANSDUCTION

It is generally accepted that the cochlear hair cells are responsible for the actual translation of mechanical vibrations into electrochemical phenomena that precede the generation of nerve impulses, a process known as transduction. In short, displacement of the sensory hairs produces a response in these cells, which in turn causes transmitter release from the presynaptic area at the base of the hair cell. The transmitter ultimately generates nerve impulses in the fibers of the eighth nerve. The exact nature of the intracellular response, the intermediate step between sensory hair movement and transmitter release, is not known. However, it is thought that electrical events must be involved. To understand what evidence is available regarding the nature of the transduction process, it is necessary to understand the electrical environment of the cochlea.

If an electrode is inserted into the cochlear duct it registers a positive potential, or voltage difference from the rest of the body, of approximately 80 mv [43]. This endocochlear potential is maintained by an active ionic pump located in the border cells of the stria vascularis. Either this or a separate ionic pump is also responsible for the unique chemical composition of the endolymph [24, 43].

Extremely fine electrodes penetrating the organ of Corti record negative potentials. These resting potentials are obtained from the inside of individual cells, both supporting cells and hair cells. Outer hair cells have resting potentials of approximately −80 mv [7], whereas those of inner hair cells are approximately −40 mv [33]. This means that between the inside of the hair cell and the endolymph above its upper surface there exists a potential difference, or gradient, of approximately 120 or 160 mv depending on cell type, which is a very high gradient for a biologic system. It is likely that this potential difference initiates a continuous flow of positively charged potassium ions into the hair cells from the endolymph. These ions would quickly diffuse into the low potassium fluid that fills the spaces within the organ of Corti.

When a stimulus is delivered to the cochlea, the balance of electrical potentials is disturbed. To examine these events, we can place electrodes on either side of the cochlear duct (one in the scala tympani and one in the scala vestibuli) and observe the electrical activity in the region of the cochlear partition between the electrodes. Two principal responses to stimulation that can be recorded from the cochlea are shown in Figure 22-9.

At the top of the figure is the stimulus applied to the eardrum, a short tone burst. The lower portions show the response recorded from the cochlea. Two features of this response are apparent. First, the frequency of the stimulus is reproduced by the cochlea as a pattern of voltage fluctuation. This electrical reproduction is known as the cochlear microphonic (or potential) [46]. Second, a sizeable shift in the baseline voltage level is produced. This shift is called the summating potential [15, 45]. The two potentials are recorded simultaneously, as a mixture. In the figure they have been electrically separated for purposes of illustration.

Both the cochlear microphonic and the summating potential at a particular cochlear location vary greatly with changes in

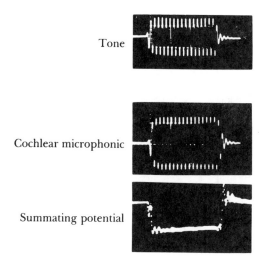

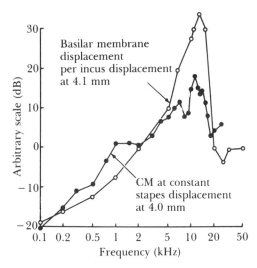

Figure 22-9. The cochlear microphonic and summating potential response to a pure-tone stimulus. The two potentials, normally recorded simultaneously, have been electrically separated.

Figure 22-10. Comparison of the basilar membrane displacement and cochlear microphonic produced at various frequencies of stimulation and recorded at a cochlear location close to the base. CM = cochlear microphonic. (From P. Dallos, M. A. Cheatham, and J. Ferraro. Cochlear mechanics, nonlinearities and cochlear potentials. J. Acoust. Soc. Am. 55:597, 1973.)

Figure 22-11. Schematic diagram of the relationship between the traveling wave envelope (shaded area) and the differential (DIF) and average (AVE) summating potential. The apex is to the right. (From P. Dallos, The Summating Potentials of the Cochlea. In M. Sachs [Ed.], Physiology of the Auditory System. Baltimore: National Education Consultants, 1971.)

stimulus frequency. This maximum corresponds to the displacement peak of the traveling wave envelope (Fig. 22-10). Below the best frequency the microphonic declines slowly, whereas above it exhibits a rapid decrease in amplitude [42].

The behavior of the summating potential is somewhat more complex. It may be observed as a local phenomenon by examining the potential difference between the scala tympani and vestibuli electrodes. This limits the region of the cochlea that the electrodes "see" to a small segment. In this case (Fig. 22-11), the differential summating potential is positive at low frequencies and rises to a peak slightly below the cochlear microphonic best frequency. Then it declines rapidly, changing polarity and reaching a negative peak. This corresponds to the steep, leading edge of the traveling wave envelope. The summating potential may also be recorded from a much larger segment of the cochlea by taking the average of the voltage recorded from the two electrodes. This average summating potential (see Fig. 22-11) is negative at all frequencies except for a narrow band that corresponds, again, to the leading edge of the traveling wave envelope. Here it rises sharply to a positive peak [10, 23].

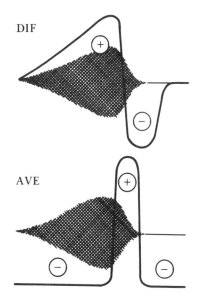

The cochlear microphonic and summating potential have been shown to be largely the product of outer hair cells. If these cells are destroyed while the inner hair cells remain intact, both potentials are very much reduced (30–40 dB) and altered [11]. For example, the cochlear microphonic produced by the inner hair cells appears to be related to the velocity of cochlear partition movement rather than to its displacement [12]. This is consistent with the proposed stimulation of the inner hair cell by fluid movement rather than by actual partition displacement.

The cochlear microphonic and summating potential reflect the activity of vast numbers of sensory cells. It is also possible to record from individual hair cells during stimulation of the cochlea with sound. Such recordings suggest that both types of hair cells respond to sound with a fluctuation of the intracellular potential reminiscent of the cochlear microphonic, and with a large decrease in the negative resting potential, which is in some ways similar to the summating potential. These changes in the intracellular potential primarily occur for a limited range of frequencies and are greatest for a very narrow band of frequencies that corresponds to the maximum amplitude of mechanical response of the basilar membrane at that cochlear location. The individual inner hair cells are thus quite sharply tuned to a specific frequency region [33]. An inner hair cell tuning curve is illustrated in Figure 22-12. The tuning of the inner hair cells appears to be as sharp as that of single auditory nerve fibers indicating that frequency selectivity is fully established at the level of these hair cells. The relationship between the frequency tuning of inner hair cells and of the frequency specificity of the basilar membrane is not yet clear. Most observations of mechanical motion of the membrane suggest that inner hair cell and auditory nerve fiber tuning is somewhat sharper than the mechanical tuning of the basilar membrane. These observations have led to the hypothesis of a "second filter," which provides further sharpening by some biologic process that requires metabolic energy [20]. However, recent measurements suggest that mechanical tuning may be as sharp as that ob-

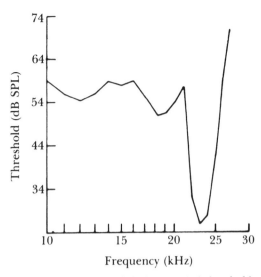

Figure 22-12. Intracellularly recorded thresholds of a cochlear inner hair cell to stimulation with pure tones at various frequencies. Note the narrowly tuned region of greatest sensitivity of the cell. (Adapted from I. J. Russell and P. M. Sellick, The Tuning Properties of Cochlear Hair Cells. In E. F. Evans and J. P. Wilson [Eds.], Psychophysics and Physiology of Hearing. London: Academic, 1977.)

served in hair cells and nerve fibers, eliminating the need for a second filter [27].

The intracellular potentials recorded from individual hair cells are quite different from the cochlear microphonics and summating potentials because the latter reflect the combined activity of many individual hair cells. It is difficult to assess the role that these extracellular and intracellular potentials play, if indeed they play a role, in the transduction process. However, two possibilities are frequently discussed.

The first possibility is that the intracellular potentials themselves mediate the release of a chemical transmitter from the presynaptic zone at the lower end of the hair cell. The transmitter, in turn, stimulates the afferent endings of the eighth nerve neurons. This idea is attractive, as the receptive area of the hair cell, the hair-bearing surface, is separated from the presynaptic zone by a relatively great distance. The potentials may provide the link between the two locations. In this scheme, displacement of the sensory hairs would cause a potential change in the receptive area, perhaps by modulation of a steady flow of potassium ions from the endolymph into the cell. This change would then be conducted by passive current flow to the presynaptic region, where it would cause the release of transmitter. This corresponds to current neurophysiologic theory, because it is thought that the release of transmitter chemicals in the nerve cell is caused by a change in voltage in the presynaptic area.

The second possibility is that the potentials are merely an incidental product of the transducer process. That is, the movement of the sensory hairs causes some yet unidentified process, which in turn initiates the release of transmitter. As a by-product of this process (or perhaps of transmitter release), the intracellular potentials, cochlear microphonics and summating potentials are produced. If this possibility is the correct one, the potentials are indicators of receptor function but do not play a causal role in the transduction process.

As yet, there is no conclusive evidence that confirms either of these two possibilities. It is perhaps more conservative to assume that the cochlear potentials are actually involved in the transduction process, the position taken by most authorities.

The role that the two groups of cochlear hair cells have in the transduction process is also unclear. It should be remembered that approximately 95% of the afferent fibers of the eighth nerve originate on inner hair cells, whereas the extracellular cochlear microphonics and summating potentials are largely produced by the outer hair cells. The large extracellular response of the outer hair cells seems out of proportion to the 5% contribution of their afferent neurons to the eighth nerve. Also, the loss of outer hair cells has a large effect on inner ear function. Because of these considerations, it has been suggested [19, 31, 50] that the outer and inner hair cells interact in some unknown fashion. In this case, nerve fibers from inner hair cells may also carry information derived from the stimulation of outer hair cells. It has recently been observed [26] that active mechanical processes can originate in the cochlea, suggesting that such interaction may be mechanical. It is thus possible that outer hair cells alter the micromechanical environment of inner hair cells in response to acoustic stimulation or efferent activation.

The final stage of transduction is the release of a chemical transmitter from the hair cell base, which stimulates the afferent endings of the fibers of the auditory nerve. Small vesicles that presumably contain transmitter have been identified in the hair cells [38]. The identity of the transmitter substance is unknown.

THE EIGHTH NERVE
The end product of transduction is transmitted to the brain stem via the eighth cranial nerve. The activity in the 30,000 auditory afferent fibers is normally examined in one of two ways.

If a relatively large electrode is placed anywhere near the cochlea (the round window is a common recording site), and a temporally distinct stimulus such as a click or the leading edge of a tone burst is applied to the ear, a potential is observed (Fig. 22-13), which is known as the compound action potential [14] and is produced by the synchronous discharge of hundreds of neurons. The compound ac-

Figure 22-13. Compound action potential response at the onset of a pure-tone stimulus of 8000 Hz. (From P. Dallos, The Auditory Periphery: Biophysics and Physiology. *New York: Academic, 1973.)*

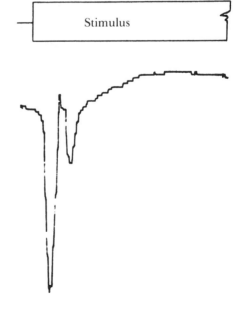

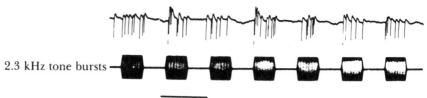

2.3 kHz tone bursts

$\overline{\text{100 msec}}$

Figure 22-14. Discharges of a single eighth nerve fiber in response to repetitive tone bursts. (From N. Y.-S. Kiang et al., Discharge Patterns of Single Fibers in the Cat's Auditory Nerve. Cambridge, Mass.: M.I.T. Press, 1965. © M.I.T. Press, 1965.)

tion potential is the basis of electrocochleography and can serve as a useful index of eighth nerve and cochlear function. Through the use of masking, it can also provide information about the manner in which small groups of single fibers carry information to the brain stem [8, 22].

If a fine microelectrode is inserted into the nerve itself, single-fiber responses can be recorded. Such fibers are found invariably to be spontaneously active; that is, they discharge even in the absence of sound stimulation to the ear. Because the amplitude of nerve impulses cannot change, the fiber can convey information only by varying the rate or timing or both of its impulses. An example of a single-fiber response to tone stimulation is shown in Figure 22-14.

Each fiber will respond only to a limited range of stimulus frequencies. This range includes the characteristic frequency, that frequency to which the fiber is most sensitive. This frequency selectivity can be demonstrated graphically by charting the intensity necessary to produce a response from a given fiber at various frequencies. Several such "tuning curves" are shown in Figure 22-15. Their similarity to the frequency selectivity of inner hair cells can be seen by comparison with Figure 22-12.

Predictably, the characteristic frequency of a fiber reflects its point of origin along the cochlea: high-frequency fibers originate in the base, low-frequency fibers at the apex. Moreover, the spatial frequency organization of the inner ear is preserved in the eighth nerve and passed on to the higher centers of the brain. High-frequency fibers run along the outside of the nerve. Progressively lower-frequency fibers are found toward the center [28]. Thus, information about the frequency content of a stimulating acoustic signal can be transmitted to

the brain in terms of which nerve fibers are activated.

Another type of frequency information may also be seen in the discharge of eighth nerve fibers. At certain frequencies, a fiber will discharge in synchrony with the stimulus. For example, it might produce an impulse for every cycle of a sinusoidal stimulus, or perhaps an impulse every few cycles,

Figure 22-15. Tuning curves of single eighth nerve fibers. Each point represents the lowest intensity that would produce a response from the fiber at that frequency. Note the similarity to the inner hair cell potential function of Figure 22-12. (From E. F. Evans, Narrow tuning of cochlear nerve fibre responses in the guinea pig. J. Physiol. 206:14, 1970.)

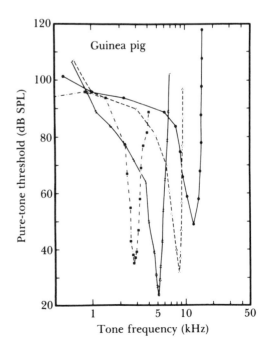

but always in phase (in the same region of the waveform). Because the fibers rarely discharge at rates of more than 200 impulses per second, frequency information could be carried in this manner by a single fiber only at frequencies up to 200 Hz. By sampling the rates of several fibers that discharge on different cycles, the brain might be able to process such information at higher frequencies. However, it is generally agreed that such stimulus-locked discharge is not measurable at frequencies of more than 3000 to 4000 Hz [28].

All eighth nerve fibers will respond to a click stimulus with a single discharge or a burst of discharges. Fibers with a low characteristic frequency of less than 5000 Hz produce a burst of impulses in which the interval between discharges is related to the characteristic frequency. The interval is a multiple of the period of that frequency. The latency of response to the click also varies with characteristic frequency. This reflects the distribution of fibers along the cochlea. Because the disturbance of the cochlear partition must travel from the base to the apex, high-frequency fibers respond more rapidly after delivery of the stimulus than low-frequency fibers [28].

The afferent fibers of the eighth nerve appear to constitute a single group. That is, there is no clear-cut criterion by which the observed fibers may be reliably divided into two groups that could correspond to the fibers that innervate the two populations of hair cells [28]. Whether this indicates an interaction between the two types of hair cells or merely our inability to sample the fiber population effectively is not clear.

In summary, as noted in Chapter 21, the actions of the middle ear and the vibration pattern of the stapes are well understood. Of the various stages of cochlear function, only the hydromechanic action of the cochlear partition and the traveling wave have been clearly documented. We have only promising theories and limited evidence about the deformation of the hair cell cilia, and the electrochemical action of the hair cell and its synaptic connection to the eighth nerve is at best poorly understood. Also, there are many unanswered questions about the coding of auditory information in the eighth nerve.

REFERENCES

1. Billone, M., and Raynor, S. Transmission of radial forces to cochlear hair cells. *J. Acoust. Soc. Am.* 54:1143, 1973.
2. Bredberg, G., Ades, H., and Engstrom, H. Scanning electron microscopy of the normal and pathologically altered organ of Corti. *Acta Otolaryngol.* [Suppl.] 301:3, 1972.
3. Brodel, M. *Three Unpublished Drawings of the Anatomy of the Human Ear.* Philadelphia: Saunders, 1946.
4. Dallos, P. The Summating Potentials of the Cochlea. In M. Sachs (Ed.), *Physiology of the Auditory System.* Baltimore: National Educational Consultants, 1971.
5. Dallos, P. *The Auditory Periphery: Biophysics and Physiology.* New York: Academic, 1973.
6. Dallos, P. Cochlear physiology. *Ann. Rev. Psychol.* 32:153, 1981.
7. Dallos, P. Unpublished observations, 1980.
8. Dallos, P., and Cheatham, M. A. Compound action potential (AP) tuning curves. *J. Acoust. Soc. Amer.* 59:591, 1976.
9. Dallos, P., Cheatham, M. A., and Ferraro, J. Cochlear mechanics, nonlinearities and cochlear potentials. *J. Acoust. Soc. Am.* 55:597, 1973.
10. Dallos, P., Schoeny, Z., and Cheatham, M. A. Cochlear summating potentials: Descriptive aspects. *Acta Otolaryngol.* [Suppl.] 302:1, 1972.
11. Dallos, P., and Wang, C.-Y. Bioelectric correlates of kanamycin intoxication. *Audiology* 13:277, 1974.
12. Dallos, P., et al. Cochlear inner and outer hair cells: Functional differences. *Science* 177:356, 1972.
13. Davis, H. Transmission and transduction in the cochlea. *Laryngoscope* 68:359, 1958.
14. Davis, H. Peripheral Coding of Auditory Information. In W. A. Rosenblith (Ed.), *Sensory Communication.* New York: Wiley, 1961. P. 119.
15. Davis, H., Fernandez, C., and McAuliffe, D. The excitatory process in the cochlea. *Proc. Natl. Acad. Sci. USA* 36:580, 1950.
16. Davis, H., et al. Acoustic trauma in the guinea pig. *J. Acoust. Soc. Am.* 25:1180, 1953.
17. Engstrom, H. The cortilymph, the third lymph of the inner ear. *Acta Morphol. Neerl. Scand.* 3:192, 1960.
18. Evans, E. F. Narrow tuning of cochlear nerve fibre responses in the guinea pig. *J. Physiol.* 206:14, 1970.
19. Evans, E. F. Auditory Frequency Selectivity and the Cochlear Nerve. In E. Zwicker and E. Terhardt (Eds.), *Psychophysical Models*

and Physiological Facts in Hearing. Berlin: Springer-Verlag, 1974. P. 118.

20. Evans, E. F. The sharpening of cochlear frequency selectivity in the normal and abnormal cochlea. *Audiology* 14:419, 1975.

21. Flock, A., and Cheung, H. C. Actin filaments in sensory hairs of inner ear receptor cells. *J. Cell Biol.* 75:339, 1977.

22. Harris, D. Action potential suppression, tuning curves and thresholds: Comparison with single fiber data. *Hear. Res.* 1:133, 1979.

23. Honrubia, V., and Ward, P. H. Properties of the summating potential of guinea pig's cochlea. *J. Acoust. Soc. Am.* 45:1443, 1969.

24. Johnstone, B. M., and Sellick, P. M. The peripheral auditory apparatus. *Q. Rev. Biophys.* 5:1, 1972.

25. Kellerhals, B. Die Morphologies des Ganglion spiral cochleae. *Acta Otolaryngol.* Suppl. 226, 1967.

26. Kemp, D. T. Evidence of mechanical nonlinearity and frequency selective wave amplification in the cochlea. *Arch. Otorhinolaryngol.* 224:37, 1979.

27. Khanna, S. M., and Leonard, D. G. B. Interferometric measurement of basilar membrane vibrations in cats using a round window approach. *J. Acoust. Soc. Amer.* 68: S43, 1980.

28. Kiang, N. Y.-S., et al. *Discharge Patterns of Single Fibers in the Cat's Auditory Nerve*. Cambridge, Mass.: M.I.T. Press, 1965.

29. Kiang, N. Y.-S., et al. Hair cell innervation by spiral ganglion cells in adult cats. *Science* 217:175, 1982.

30. Kimura, R. S. Hairs of the cochlear sensory cells and their attachment to the tectorial membrane. *Acta Otolaryngol.* 61:55, 1966.

31. Lynn, P. A., and Sayers, B. McA. Cochlear innervation, signal processing and their relation to auditory time-intensity effects. *J. Acoust. Soc. Am.* 47:525, 1969.

32. Rossi, G. The Control Mechanism at the Hair Cell/Nerve Junction, of the Central Auditory Pathways and Centers, and the Pathways of the Cerebral Coordination. In J. Tonndorf (Ed.), *Morphology and Function of Auditory Input Control*. Chicago: Translations of Beltone Institute for Hearing Research, 1967.

33. Russell, I. J., and Sellick, P. M. The Tuning Properties of Cochlear Hair Cells. In E. F. Evans and J. P. Wilson (Eds.), *Psychophysics and Physiology of Hearing*. New York: Academic, 1977.

34. Ryan, A. F., and Schwartz, I. R. A biochemically distinct subpopulation of neurons in the spiral ganglion identified by preferential amino acid uptake. *Hear. Res.* 9:173, 1983.

35. Ryan, A. F., Wickham, M. G., and Bone, R. C. Studies of ion distribution in the inner ear: Scanning electron microscopy and x-ray microanalysis of freeze-dried cochlear specimens. *Hear. Res.* 2:1, 1980.

36. Ryan, A. F., et al. Auditory stimulation alters the pattern of 2-deoxyglucose uptake in the inner ear. *Brain Res.* 234:213, 1982.

37. Schwartz, I. R., and Ryan, A. F. Differential labeling of sensory cell and neural populations in the organ of Corti following amino acid incubations. *Hear. Res.* 9:185, 1983.

38. Smith, C. A., and Sjostrand, F. S. Structure of the nerve endings on the external hair cells of the guinea pig cochlea as studied by serial sections. *J. Ultrastruct. Res.* 5:523, 1961.

39. Spoendlin, H. *The Organization of the Cochlear Receptor*. Basel: Karger, 1966. P. 277.

40. Spoendlin, H. The innervation of the cochlear receptors. In A. Moller (Ed.), *Basic Mechanisms in Hearing*. New York: Academic, 1973. P. 185.

41. Spoendlin, H. Neural connections of the outer haircell system. *Acta Otolaryngol.* 79: 381, 1979.

42. Tasaki, I., Davis, H., and Eldredge, D. H. Exploration of cochlear potentials with a microelectrode. *J. Acoust. Soc. Am.* 26:765, 1954.

43. Tasaki, I., and Spiropoulos, C. S. Stria vascularis as a source of endocochlear potential. *J. Neurophysiol.* 22:149, 1959.

44. von Bekesy, G. The vibration of the cochlear partition in anatomical preparation and in models of the inner ear. *J. Acoust. Soc. Am.* 21:233, 1949.

45. von Bekesy, G. DC potentials and energy balance of the cochlear partition. *J. Acoust. Soc. Am.* 22:576, 1950.

46. von Bekesy, G. Gross localization of the place of origin of the cochlear microphonics. *J. Acoust. Soc. Am.* 24:399, 1952.

47. von Bekesy, G. *Experiments in Hearing* (trans. and ed. by E. G. Wever). New York: McGraw-Hill, 1960.

48. Warr, W. B., and Guinan, J. J. Efferent innervation of the organ of Corti: Two separate systems. *Brain Res.* 173:152, 1979.

49. Wever, E. G., and Bray, C. Action currents in the auditory nerve in response to acoustic stimulation. *Proc. Natl. Acad. Sci. USA* 16:344, 1930.

50. Zwislocki, J., and Sokolich, W. Neuromechanical frequency analysis in the cochlea. In E. Zwicker and E. Terhardt (Eds.), *Psychophysical Models and Physiological Facts in Hearing*. Berlin: Springer-Verlag, 1974. P. 107.

23

Medical Management of the Hearing-Handicapped Child

Janet M. Stewart
Marion P. Downs

To the general primary care provider such as the family practitioner or pediatrician, a hearing-handicapped child has a moderate-to-profound hearing loss that had its onset at birth or during the first year of life. It is important to identify and manage these children properly, but their actual number is very small in private office or clinic. This same physician, however, will see many young children with mild hearing loss, frequently associated with chronic or recurrent serous otitis media. This hearing loss may be static or fluctuating. These children may have predisposing abnormalities such as a cleft palate or submucous cleft palate, but in most cases they are otherwise perfectly normal and healthy. There is increasing evidence that these children too are "hearing-handicapped." An up-to-date discussion of medical management of hearing-handicapped children therefore must have two sections: (1) the management of the child with a mild hearing loss, a situation in which the numbers are large and medicine has much to offer, and (2) the management of the child with a severe hearing loss, a less common problem but with the emphasis on identification, evaluation and habilitation.

EFFECTS OF MILD HEARING LOSS

Although there are other causes for a mild hearing loss, the most common one is otitis media. In the past this has been believed to be a temporary condition that clears with treatment and has no effect on language development. These assumptions appear to be wrong.

In 1972 Ling [31] compared achievement test results on two matched groups of school children: one group had hearing losses from 15 to 45 dB with histories of otitis media; the other group had no hearing loss or history of otitis media. Careful matching was made of the two groups for age, intelligence, environmental factors, and so on. The test results revealed that by 9 or 10 years of age the otitis media group was retarded 15 months in reading skills, 16 months in mechanical arithmetic, and 19 months in problem arithmetic. The degree of retardation correlated positively with the severity of the losses, but even the children with the mildest losses showed significant academic handicaps.

Quigley [37] further demonstrated the effect of very mild losses in a study of Illinois public school children with mild-to-moderate hearing impairments. He showed that children with hearing loss significantly less than 26 dB suffered measurably in their academic progress. Even children with hearing losses of 15 to 26 dB scored significantly lower than those with losses less than 15 dB in all the language-related subtests of the Stanford Achievement Tests.

But such static hearing losses are not the only culprits implicated in language retardation. Even mild, fluctuating hearing acuity can have marked effects on performance. Holm and Kunze [22] investigated the effects of the fluctuating hearing loss that is experienced in recurrent and chronic otitis media. They studied an experimental group of children aged $5\frac{1}{2}$ to 9 years who had no other medical problems except middle ear disease that had had its onset before age 2. The fluctuations in hearing levels of these children ranged from normal levels to greater than 25 dB. A matched control group of children with no history of otitis media was used for comparison. Each group was given a battery of tests including the Illinois Test of Psycholinguistic Abilities (ITPA), the Peabody Picture Vocabulary Test, the Templin-Darley Picture Articulation Screening Test, and the Mecham Verbal Language Development Scale. The results showed that the otitis media group was significantly deficient in all tests that required the receiving or processing of auditory stimuli or the production of a verbal response (with one minor exception). But in tests requiring visual skills the two groups showed no differences. In addition, all language skills were retarded in the otitis media group as compared with the control group. The authors expressed deep concern that physicians may consider such fluctuating hearing levels insignificant, particularly during early critical periods in the child's life. They cautioned physicians to be alert to the educational implications of the bouts of otitis media that occasion such losses.

The prevalence of these handicapping conditions may be inordinately higher than has been heretofore supposed, as suggested by some British studies. One, by Fry and Jones [18], evaluated what happens to children after an acute attack of otitis media that has been treated and is no longer symptomatic. Following the so-called cure of their acute otitis media episodes, 403 children were given audiometric evaluations at varying periods. Seventeen percent were found to have hearing losses of 20 dB or greater in two or more frequencies. In a matched control group only 4% were found with such levels. These authors consider that a 20 dB hearing level constitutes a handicapping degree of loss, and estimate that perhaps 25% of the child population is affected by acute otitis media. They are also concerned with physicians' indifference to the sequelae of otitis media in terms of mild hearing loss. Also in England, Lowe and co-workers [32] found in a similar study that 25% of the children had significant hearing loss 6 months after their attacks of otitis media. In 29% of the cases there was apparent failure to cure the disease. Fairly equivalent figures were reported by others in England [34] and in the United States [35].

The English studies reflect the concern that has been felt for milder hearing losses in Great Britain. A 20 dB level is considered a significant hearing loss, compared with 27 to 37 dB in the United States. However, it is becoming evident that even a lower point is more realistic, and that in addition the factors of age of onset, duration of loss, and frequency of reduced acuity between normal periods must all be taken into consideration. A case report from the files of the University of Colorado Medical Center is illustrative.

CASE REPORT: The patient is a 13-year-old white male who appeared first in the ENT clinic at age 6, having been referred by the school screening program for failing the hearing test. A long-term history of otitis media was elicited. Audiogram at admission showed bilateral conductive losses of 25 dB average, with slightly lowered bone conduction in the left ear for the high frequencies (Fig. 23-1). Otologic examination revealed serous otitis media, and myringotomies were performed with polyethylene tube insertions. Hearing levels following myringotomy were right-ear: 13 dB, left ear: 8 dB. A year and a half later the levels were right ear: 30 dB, left ear: 45 dB (Fig. 23-2). Note that the bone-

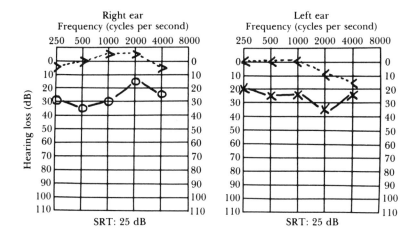

Figure 23-1. Audiogram showing bilateral conductive losses of 25 dB average, with slightly lowered bone conduction in left ear for high frequencies.

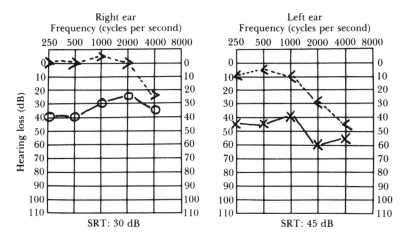

Figure 23-2. Audiogram 18 months after audiogram shown in Figure 23-1.

conduction level at 2000 Hz in the left ear had progressed to 30 dB from a previous 10 dB. Myringotomies were again performed, and the hearing levels improved to 10 dB and 16 dB. The sequence of reduced hearing, myringotomies, improved hearing, was repeated five more times during the following 7 years, with the hearing levels worse than 15 dB over half the time. The last audiogram taken showed the bone-conduction hearing had progressed further in the left ear and was beginning to progress in the right ear.

Language evaluations were made at this time (age 13). On the Raven Progressive Matrices he scored in the 90th percentile, indicating that he is superior in visual-related cognitive functioning. On the WISC test his performance IQ was 124, but his verbal IQ was only 77. This discrepancy between his functioning on visual and performance tasks and on that of verbal tasks demonstrates that he has been audiotorally deprived during critical learning periods, and that this potentially bright boy is now a language-handicapped child. In the classroom he was described as "retarded, unmotivated, and disinterested—a behavior problem."

In addition to the language retardation shown in this patient, another alarming fact is the indication of progression of the sensorineural component of the hearing loss. Progressive sensorineural hearing loss related to chronic otitis media has been previously described by English and colleagues [13] and by Paparella and Brady [36]. These authors suggest that the communication of infection through the round window may be responsible for the progression. Thus another sequela is added to the apparently mild symptoms of otitis media.

In the case cited, the child was given a hearing aid at the time of the last audiogram—13 years too late. The damages resulting in language retardation can no longer be repaired. It is probable that when he was first seen at age 6, irreversible deficits were already present. The difference between the verbal and the performance IQs is similar to what we have found in young deaf adults who have gone through special education classes throughout their school years [11]. It is also the same approximate IQ-point difference found by Dennis [8] and by Heber and Garver [21] in their respective studies on the effects of early experiential deprivation in the first years of life. Based on comparative tests of deprived and control populations, both these studies showed that in groups deprived of high-quality language input and other experiences during the first 2 or 3 years of life, differences of 30 to 50 IQ points will be found in their eventual performances as compared with the control groups.

Here we begin to understand the handicap of hearing impairment in terms of a test that is based on urban society's demands of its members. We also see that the handicap as measured is more age-dependent than it is degree-of-loss-dependent. For if both the deaf child and the child with mild hearing loss were able to receive high-quality language input before the age of 2, the differences between their potential abilities as measured by visual performance and that of their verbal skills would be markedly reduced.

In addition to the studies, a large number of reports continue to be published in the literature regarding the language sequelae of otitis media in early infancy.

Better controls are being introduced into the studies, and many disciplines are investigating the sequelae [4, 9, 25, 40, 42].

The reason that a slight hearing loss of 15 dB may be a handicap to a young child is obvious if one reflects on the nature of speech sounds. The voiced vowel and consonant sounds contain a great deal of speech energy. However, the unvoiced consonant sounds, like *s, f, t, p, k,* and *th,* contain less energy and are not heard as loudly as the voiced sounds. Many unvoiced consonants are not heard at all in normal conversation by the average listener, but their absence is not noted because once a word is learned, the listener can fill in mentally for the missed sound and will perceive the meaning. The child who has not learned the word cannot fill in; he must be able to hear all the sounds clearly if he is to learn the meaning of a word. Language learning can be seriously impeded if all the sounds are not heard clearly.

DEFINITION OF A HEARING HANDICAP

From the evidence previously cited we can begin to define more realistically where a hearing handicap begins. It is apparent that the revised criteria for a handicapping hearing loss should be as follows:

1. Hearing level of 15 dB or poorer
2. Indications of serous otitis media in a child less than age 2 more than half the time for 6 months
3. Fluctuating hearing levels from 0 to more than 15 dB, with levels worse than 15 dB more than half the time

When these criteria for a handicap are used, it becomes necessary to revise the epidemiologic figures of hearing losses. According to a National Academy of Sciences report [26], 30% of all children between 6 months and 3 years had evidence of middle ear disease declining to 15% by age 11. Seven percent of the 4- to 11-year-olds had hearing losses in the speech frequencies of 15 dB or greater. The age trend for hearing loss paralleled that for ear pathology, and although no hearing data were obtained for children less than 4 years, the study assumed that hearing loss must also be high in the young group. If we extrapo-

Table 23-1. Handicapping Effects of Hearing Loss

Average hearing 500–2000 Hz (ANSI)	Description	Condition	Sounds heard without amplification	Degree of handicap (if not treated in first year of life)	Probable needs
0–15 dB	Normal range	Serous otitis, perforation, monomeric membrane, tympanosclerosis	All speech sounds	None	None
15–25 dB	Slight hearing loss	Serous otitis, perforation, monomeric membrane, sensorineural loss, tympanosclerosis	Vowel sounds heard clearly; may miss unvoiced consonant sounds	Mild auditory dysfunction in language learning	Consideration of need for hearing aid; lipreading; auditory training; speech therapy; preferential seating
25–40 dB	Mild hearing loss	Serous otitis, perforation, tympanosclerosis, monomeric membrane, sensorineural loss	Hears only some louder-voiced speech sounds	Auditory learning dysfunction, mild language retardation, mild speech problems, inattention	Hearing aid, lipreading, auditory training, speech therapy
40–65 dB	Moderate hearing loss	Chronic otitis, middle ear anomaly, sensorineural loss	Misses most speech sounds at normal conversational level	Speech problems, language retardation, learning dysfunction, inattention	All the above, plus consideration of special classroom situation
65–95 dB	Severe hearing loss	Sensorineural or mixed loss from sensorineural loss plus middle ear disease	Hears no speech sounds of normal conversation	Severe speech problems, language retardation, learning dysfunction, inattention	All the above; plus probable assignment to special classes
More than 95 dB	Profound hearing loss	Sensorineural or mixed loss	Hears no speech or other sounds	Severe speech problems, language retardation, learning dysfunction, inattention	All the above; plus probable assignment to special classes

late from these figures we find that in the age 4 to 11 group, 47% of those with ear disease had significant hearing losses. This would mean that an equivalent number of the 6-month to 2-year-olds who had otitis media also had significant hearing losses, or almost 15% of the entire child population. Other studies tell us more about the occurrences: Feingold and associates [14] found that 62% of cases of acute middle ear infection occurred in children age 2 and less. In Alaskan natives, Beal [2] reported that 60% of all native children have at least one episode of acute middle ear infection in the first year of life. Some studies show peaks at ages 4 and 6, but all implicate a young age as the most likely period for otitis media.

If the prevalence of handicapping conditions is as high as 15%, we find that in addition to the known and well-measured hearing losses in the United States must be added a large number of children who will be handicapped by the presence of mild hearing loss or fluctuating ear disease and hearing loss.

Degree of hearing loss is not the only important variable when considering handicapping effects. Such factors as time of treatment, intellectual potential, and home environment may have profound effects on the amount of handicap that results from a given hearing loss. However, the degree of loss is the most accessible to measurement and does show a hierarchy of handicapping conditions. Table 23-1 attempts to summarize the effects that various hearing losses will have on children who are not given habilitation or treatment before age 2 years.

MANAGEMENT OF SEROUS OTITIS MEDIA

Medical

Medical treatment is the first line of defense for recurrent otitis media. Indeed, a recent report [19] strongly indicated that zealous medical treatment may forestall to some extent the recurrence of otitis media. However, many children treated with tympanotomy tubes may have already had recurrent otitis media or will continue to have recurrence despite replacements of tubes. For these children, even more vigor-

ous action may be necessary, particularly if early speech and language development is delayed. The questions then become how to determine whether speech and language delays are present, and what to do if they are found.

Educational

The first requisite step is screening and monitoring of all children for speech and language development as part of every regular health visit. As in the basic growth parameters of height, weight, and head circumference, unusual growth or lack of growth in speech and language indicates a need to explore the causes for change in the developmental pattern. Routine monitoring of speech and language development is the means of detecting unexpected changes. Change can also be positive, and this too, is important information in the educational management of a child.

In a child who has an ear infection or a history of recurrent otitis media, speech and language should be tested if more than 3 months have elapsed since the last screening. When the results of speech and language screening are part of a child's health record, comparisons can be made to determine whether language is beginning to drop below the child's previous developmental pattern.

It is important to administer speech and language screening at the beginning of medical intervention and at subsequent visits. During treatment, such evaluations will indicate whether the medical intervention is sufficient or more vigorous measures, such as a home stimulation program or referral to a speech and language pathologist, audiologist or both, are required.

Haskins and others [20] concluded that the most important aspects of early intervention programs are the need to refer the child to a language pathologist early enough and the need for language stimulation as soon as a problem is suspected or discovered.

For the child who shows a questionable speech or language delay, a home stimulation program should be implemented. Speech and language stimulation books should be used to select language stimulation activities appropriate for the child's language age level. These activities should be given to the parents to use at home. Speech and language screening should be repeated in 3 months. If in 3 months the child still has otitis media, the parents should continue to provide extra home stimulation, and the child should be screened again in 3 months. Screening can avoid an unnoticed decrement in speech and language development.

If the child shows a significant delay, or if after 6 months of language stimulation the otitis media is still present, he or she should be referred to a speech pathologist for consideration of more formalized speech and language therapy.

Whenever there is a significant language delay from recurrent serous otitis media, the use of a hearing aid should be considered, provided that the family situation is favorable.

Speech and language delays must not be approached with the belief that the child will outgrow them. Speech and language development are affected by every problem within the child's developmental system. Subtle organic, emotional, or developmental delays may be immediately apparent in speech and language skills, which are a very sensitive gauge of the child's overall development. Any fear that the referral will cause potential anxiety should be evaluated in terms of the danger of the problem being untreated until the later years, when intervention is less effective.

RESPONSIBILITY FOR DETECTION
Ideally, an infant is seen by a physician or by designee six to eight times during the first year of life for routine preventive care. This care includes assessment of physical growth parameters, development, diet, and other areas of parental concern. Included should be various methods of screening for hearing problems. Perhaps most important in this respect is a knowledge of the factors that make a child a high risk for hearing loss [3, 12].

Following is a list, *A* through *G,* of risk factors for hearing loss [23]:

*A*sphyxia, which may include infants with Apgar scores of 0 through 3, those who fail to exhibit spontaneous respirations by 10 minutes, and those with hypotonia persisting to two hours of age

*B*acterial meningitis, especially *Hemophilus influenzae*

*C*ongenital perinatal infections (e.g., TORCH syndrome [toxoplasmosis, rubella, cytomegalovirus, herpes simplex], syphilis)

*D*efects of the head or neck (e.g., craniofacial syndromal abnormalities, overt or submucous cleft palate, morphologic abnormalities of the pinna)

*E*levated bilirubin exceeding indications for exchange transfusion

*F*amily history of childhood hearing impairment

*G*ram birth weight less than 1500

Although this list can obviously be very extensive, these factors will account for a large percentage of children with a significant hearing loss. It has been shown that the application of a high-risk register in one center reduced the time required for diagnosis and amplification from 27 to 11 months [3]. Any child put into a high-risk category should be carefully tested for hearing loss, using office screening procedures with referral to an audiologist at the first sign of a questionable response.

At the time of each routine visit, the young child should be screened for a hearing loss. This can be done simply, accurately, and inexpensively, using a high-pitched squeeze toy and bells [10]. This screening must be done in such a way as to exclude all visual clues. The deaf child has exceptional visual alertness; indeed, this alertness itself may be an early clue to a hearing loss. It is also necessary to know the normal response to sound and its maturation [10, 12] to recognize properly and interpret an abnormality. A response that is developmentally delayed may indicate future intellectual deficit rather than a hearing loss. In addition to an actual screening test for hearing impairment, the physician should ask a series of questions at each visit [10]. These concern the infant's response to sound at home and his development of vocalization and speech. It is difficult to differentiate the babbling of a deaf infant from that of a normal hearing infant, but one investigator [24] has indicated that for the deaf child the quantity of noncrying vocalization during the first years of life may be considerably reduced. Again, essential to the interpretation of any questions about language is a thorough knowledge of normal language development [30].

Perhaps most important is to ask parents if they have any concern about their child's hearing. A positive answer to this question, with or without high-risk factors of positive physical findings, is a mandate for further evaluation. We must not forget that parents live with a child 24 hours a day and know his responses (or lack of them) better than any physician can in a short office visit.

REFERRAL

If the primary physician has any question about a child's ability to respond normally to sound, the first step is to refer the child to a pediatric audiologist. There is a misconception that a hearing loss cannot be diagnosed until age 2 or 3. This is *not* true. Although it may take more than one test to confirm or negate the suspicion, an experienced audiologist can estimate the degree of loss with considerable accuracy in even an infant. Once the loss has been confirmed, the second step is to refer the child to an otologist interested in hearing loss and experienced with young children. The purpose of this referral is to rule out any treatable otologic abnormalities that may be either causing or contributing to the hearing loss. This is particularly important if the loss is conductive or mixed.

In most cases, the loss is sensorineural and no medical or surgical treatment is available. The next step is amplification and appropriate speech and language training. Although hearing aid prescription and referral for therapy usually comes from the audiologist, it is vital that the primary physician continue his or her role at this point. The diagnosis of hearing loss, even if previously suspected, is a major emotional shock with widespread implications for the entire family [5, 43]. Understanding this impact, and its resulting feelings of anger, guilt, and denial is essential to assist the family in working through their feelings and channeling their energies into constructive work with their hearing-handicapped child.

The physician must also realize that hearing aids and speech therapy are expensive and beyond the means of many families. Public and private agencies can give financial assistance, and appropriate referrals should be made. The availability of speech and language therapy for the hearing-impaired child varies considerably from one geographic location to another. In one place, it may be just a question of selecting the best facility for the individual child, while in another, existing facilities must be adapted and modified to meet the needs of the child. In the latter instance, the physician should be prepared to use his or her knowledge of community resources to assist the family in finding appropriate therapy.

EVALUATION

The hearing loss has now been confirmed, amplification obtained, and therapy started. At this point, many questions are going through the minds of the parents. (1) What caused it? (2) Does this mean that there are other problems? (3) Will it happen again? (4) What does the future hold for our child? The primary physician must address each of these questions in turn.

What caused the hearing loss? In 50 to 75% of the cases it is possible to answer this question after a medical evaluation (which need be neither expensive nor elaborate). Since approximately 50% of all profound childhood deafness is genetic [16], attention is first turned to the family. A careful family history in pedigree form is taken, with specific questions about hearing loss and any of the other signs or symptoms seen in the more common deafness syndromes [27, 28]. This family evaluation may include audiograms and physical examinations of other family members. A detailed pregnancy history, including possible exposure to infectious diseases or ototoxic drugs, should be obtained. Birth records should be requested to determine birth weight, gestational age, Apgar scores, and the presence of neonatal problems such as jaundice, hypoxia, or meningitis. A physical examination of the affected child should include developmental and ophthalmologic evaluations.

Recommended laboratory tests will depend on the age of the child and the findings of the history and physical examination. In a young child (less than 12 to 24 months) viral titers and cultures may be helpful. A detailed discussion of the clinical evaluation of the deaf child and an appraisal of its value has been published by Ruben and Rozycki [38, 39].

With the exception of some of the more specialized laboratory tests, the medical evaluation can be done by the primary care physician. Laboratories at the university medical center, the state health department, and the Communicable Disease Center in Atlanta, Georgia, can provide assistance when necessary. In some medical centers, there is a congenital deafness clinic or team available to assist the physician in answering this or subsequent questions.

Does this mean that there are other problems? Whenever a child has been demonstrated to have one abnormality he is at an increased risk for having others. This is also true of the hearing-handicapped child. There is an increase in abnormalities in general [7, 15] and visual problems in particular [1, 29, 41]. A knowledge of the cause will guide the physician to suspicious areas: for example, choreoathetosis may be associated with hyperbilirubinemia; cataracts, congenital heart disease, mental retardation, or central learning disability may be associated with rubella; and renal anomalies may be associated with microtia. The physical examination of the child at the time of the evaluation should include those laboratory tests and x-ray studies necessary to investigate any suspected associated abnormalities.

Will our future children have a hearing loss? Rearing a deaf child is a considerable emotional and financial expense, and most families are extremely concerned about having a second child similarly affected. If this question is not specifically raised, the physician should initiate the discussion. Accurate genetic counseling depends on a specific diagnosis. In some cases (rubella, meningitis, hypoxia) the risk is minimal. Nevertheless, the recurrence risk should be discussed as there may be considerable confusion in the minds of the parents. The risk may be low (microtia, cleft lip or palate) or high (autosomal recessive, autosomal dominant, sex-linked). Numerous good articles discuss the genetics of deafness [6, 16, 17, 27, 28]. In many cases, however, the propositus is the first-born child with no associated abnormalities and no history that indicates a diagnosis. In these cases, an empiric 10% risk figure is given. If rubella can be effectively ruled out (negative titer at age 1), this figure should probably be increased to 15%.

What does the future hold for my hearing-impaired child? The answer to this question obviously depends on the presence or absence of associated abnormalities and on intelligence. Even in an otherwise normal deaf child, the question may be impossible to answer immediately. It requires periodic reassessment of the medical condition, audiologic status, emotional adjustment, and educational progress to allow an eventual prediction of the child's ultimate potential.

REEVALUATION

Once amplification has been obtained and therapy started, there is a tendency to assume that appropriate speech and language will automatically develop. At this stage, the management of the hearing-handicapped child is often left in the hands of the special-needs educator with periodic consultations as necessary. The importance of the continuing active participation of the primary care physician cannot be overemphasized. Periodic follow-up is necessary in the following five areas: (1) medical, (2) audiologic, (3) behavioral, (4) educational, and (5) genetic.

Medical

Yearly physical examinations are particularly important for the hearing-handicapped child. They should include careful otologic examinations to prevent associated ear disease and reinforce hearing conservation. In addition, the physical findings seen in some of the more important deafness syndromes may not be present at the time of the initial evaluation. The retinitis pigmentosa of Usher's syndrome may not appear until late in the first decade of life, and the goiter of Pendred's syndrome may not develop until adolescence. In Usher's syndrome, an early history of night blindness can often be elicited and an electroretinogram may then confirm the diagnosis.

Audiologic

Hearing should be checked at a minimum of 6-month intervals during early childhood and yearly thereafter. Genetic hearing loss and that caused by rubella may be progressive, and a more powerful hearing aid may be needed. At the time of the audiogram, the performance of the hearing aid should be checked. Many a hearing-handicapped child has worn a totally non-functioning aid for weeks with no one being the wiser!

Behavioral

A congenital hearing loss causes severe communication problems, and the first place that this becomes apparent is within the family unit itself. Because of delays in diagnosing the hearing loss, parents may have thought their hearing-impaired child stubborn or even retarded. This communication problem can form the basis for an abnormal parent-child relationship, and considerable management and behavioral problems may ensue. The frequency of behavior problems in hearing-handicapped school-aged children has been shown to be increased [33]. The physician must be aware of the possibility of behavior problems and either provide or assist families in finding appropriate conuseling when necessary.

Educational

It is beyond the scope of this chapter to discuss and compare the various educational approaches to the hearing-handicapped child. Among educators of the hearing-impaired there is considerable disagreement about the best method and, in cases of poor progress, an occasional tendency to blame the parent or the child rather than the educational approach. No single approach is ideal for all children. Medical, audiologic, and social factors should all be considered when an educational technique is selected and reevaluated. The deaf child needs an advocate, someone who is interested only in him and who has no vested interest in any technique. The physician is best suited for this role. He or she should be familiar with the educational approaches available and see that the child's progress in speech and language is periodically and impartially reassessed. He or she should

talk to parents and teachers about their concerns and facilitate a change in approach (if indicated) with a minimum of anger, reproach, disappointment, and guilt. He or she should be actively involved in his hearing-handicapped patient's educational planning until the best and definitive school setting has been found.

Genetic

Genetic counseling is not a one-time or static procedure. If retinitis pigmentosa or a goiter is discovered, an autosomal recessive syndrome has been diagnosed and the family should be recounseled with a 25% recurrence risk figure. With the birth of a sibling, it is the physician's responsibility to test the infant shortly after birth and to reassess hearing periodically. If a hearing loss is detected in the sibling, recurrence risk increases to as high as 25% and the family should be recounseled. Finally, the physician must remember genetic counseling for the hearing-impaired teenager as he or she passes through adolescence and approaches parenthood. The risk will depend on the hearing status and family history of the proposed mate. If a specific diagnosis has been made, a specific risk figure can be given; if not, empiric figures from the literature are used [6]. Genetic counseling clinics are available for this purpose.

TEAM MANAGEMENT

Congenital hearing loss is a severe disability with profound implications for communication and language development. It is best managed by a team of persons concerned with the child's education and care. Some medical centers have available a congenital hearing loss clinic or team consisting of a pediatrician, otologist, audiologist, speech pathologist, and social worker. In such cases, the child with a suspected hearing loss can be referred directly to this team for a full evaluation and long-range planning. The audiologist will confirm the hearing loss and determine its degree and type. The pediatrician will do the evaluation and counseling previously described. The otologist will search for treatable ear abnormalities and describe basic pathology. The social worker will assess the family unit, looking for financial and emotional strengths and weaknesses, and assist the family in obtaining the prescribed hearing aid and determine what resources are available for training in the home community. The speech pathologist will then determine the current level of language function as a baseline against which progress can be measured.

The final decision concerning a training program should consider information collected by *all* members of the team: medical, otologic, audiologic, and social. On the basis of this information, an appropriate referral can be made. This same team would then be involved in regular follow-up visits (every 6 to 12 months depending on age) with periodic reassessment of hearing, medical status, and language. The team would work closely with the community in molding a program appropriate for each child.

Team treatment is believed by many to be the ideal approach to the hearing-handicapped child. Each team member has a special interest in and is experienced in the child with a hearing loss. However, when team treatment is not available, can it be approximated? Otologists, audiologists, and speech pathologists are available in many places, if not directly in a small town, in an adjacent community. Each person can play a role but there must be one person who captains the team and who ensures good communication among professionals involved in the care of the child and between these professionals and the family. Because of his or her close contact with the entire family unit, the primary care physician may be the ideal person to do this. The ad hoc congenital hearing loss team can be assembled periodically to discuss the hearing-handicapped patient, assess his progress, and make future plans. The management of the hearing-handicapped child must go beyond the medical area and include an understanding of the behavioral, educational, financial, and genetic implications of childhood hearing loss.

REFERENCES

1. Alexander, J. C. C. Ocular abnormalities among congenitally deaf children. *Can. J. Ophthalmol.* 8:428, 1973.

2. Beal, D. D. Prevention of Otitis Media in the Alaska Native. In A. Glorig and K. S. Gerwin (Eds.), *Otitis Media.* Springfield, Ill.: Thomas, 1972.

3. Bergstrom, L., Hemenway, W. G., and Downs, M. P. A high risk registry to find congenital deafness. *Otolaryngol. Clin. North Am.* 4:369, 1971.

4. Brandes, P. J., and Ehinger, D. M. The effects of early middle ear pathology on auditory perception and academic achievement. *J. Speech Hear. Disord.* 46:301, 1981.

5. Broomfield, A. M. Guidance to parents of deaf children—A perspective. *Br. J. Discord. Commun.* 2:112, 1967.

6. Brown, K. S. The Genetics of Childhood Deafness. In F. McConnell and P. Ward (Eds.), *Deafness in Childhood.* Nashville: Vanderbilt University Press, 1967.

7. Danish, J. M., Tillson, J. K., and Levitan, M. Multiple anomalies in congenitally deaf children. *Eugenics Q.* 10:12, 1963.

8. Dennis, W. *Children of the Creche* (Century Psychology Series). New York: Prentice-Hall, 1973.

9. Dobie, R. A., and Berlin, C. I. Influence of Otitis Media on Hearing and Development. In "Otitis Media and Child Development," *Ann. Otol. Rhinol. Laryngol.* (Suppl. 60) 88:48–53, 1979.

10. Downs, M. P. Audiological evaluation of the congenitally deaf infant. *Otolaryngol. Clin. North Am.* 4:347, 1971.

11. Downs, M. P. The deafness management quotient. *Hear. Speech News* 42:8, 1974.

12. Downs, M. P., and Silver, H. K. The "A.B.C.D.'s" to H.E.A.R. *Clin. Pediatr.* 11: 563, 1972.

13. English, G. M., Northern, J. L., and Fria, T. J. Chronic otitis media as a cause of sensorineural hearing loss. *Arch. Otolaryngol.* 98:17, 1973.

14. Feingold, M., et al. Acute otitis media in children. *Am. J. Dis. Child.* 3:361, 1966.

15. Fishman, J. E., and Cristal, N. Sensorineural deafness: Familial incidence and additional defects—Study of a school for the deaf. *Am. J. Med. Sci.* 266:111, 1973.

16. Fraser, G. R. Profound childhood deafness. *J. Med. Genet.* 1:118, 1964.

17. Fraser, G. R. The genetics of congenital deafness. *Otolaryngol. Clin. North Am.* 4: 227, 1971.

18. Fry, J., Jones, R. E. M., and Kalton, G. The outcome of otitis media. *Br. J. Prev. Soc. Med.* 23:205, 1969.

19. Gebhart, D. E. Tympanostomy tubes in the otitis media prone child. *Laryngoscope* 91: 849, 1981.

20. Haskins, R., Finkelstein, N. W., and Stedman, D. J. Infant-stimulation programs and their effects. *Pediatr. Ann.* 7:123, 1978.

21. Heber, R., and Garver, H. An experiment in the prevention of cultural-familial mental retardation. Washington, D.C.: U.S. Department of Health, Education and Welfare, Office of Education, Educational Resources Information Center, ED 059762, PS 005367, 1970.

22. Holm, V. A., and Kunze, L. H. Effect of chronic otitis media on language and speech development. *Pediatrics* 43:833, 1969.

23. Joint Committee on Infant Hearing Position statement, 1982. *Pediatrics,* September 70(3):496, 1982.

24. Jones, M. C. Office aid to diagnosis of severe hearing impairment. *Clin. Pediatr.* 9:338, 1970.

25. Kessler, M. E., and Randolph, K. The effects of early middle ear disease on the auditory abilities of third grade children. *J. Acad. Rehab. Aud.* 12:6, 1979.

26. Kessner, D. M., Snow, C. K., and Singer, J. *Assessment of Medical Care in Children, Contracts in Health Status,* Vol. 3. Washington, D.C.: National Academy of Sciences, 1973.

27. Konigsmark, B. W. Hereditary deafness in man. *N. Engl. J. Med.* 281:713, 1969.

28. Konigsmark, B. W. Hereditary congenital severe deafness syndromes. *Ann. Otol. Rhinol. Laryngol.* 80:269, 1971.

29. Lawson, L. J., and Myklebust, H. R. Ophthalmological deficiencies in deaf children. *Except. Child.* 37:17, 1970.

30. Lillywhite, H. Doctor's manual of speech disorders. *J.A.M.A.* 167:850, 1958.

31. Ling, D. Rehabilitation of Cases with Deafness Secondary to Otitis Media. In A. Glorig and K. S. Gerwin (Eds.), *Otitis Media.* Springfield, Ill.: Thomas, 1972. Pp. 249–253.

32. Lowe, J. F., Bamforth, J. S., and Pracy, R. Acute otitis media: One year in a general practice. *Lancet* 2:1129, 1963.

33. Meadows, K. P., and Schlesinger, H. S. The prevalence of behavioral problems in a population of deaf school children. *Am. Ann. Deaf* 11:346, 1971.

34. Neil, J. F., et al. Deafness in acute otitis media. *Br. Med. J.* 1:75, 1964.

35. Olmsted, R. W., et al. The pattern of hearing following acute otitis media. *Pediatrics* 65:252, 1961.

36. Paparella, M. M., and Brady, D. R. Sensorineural hearing loss in chronic otitis media and mastoiditis. *Arch. Otolaryngol.* 74:108, 1970.

37. Quigley, S. P. Some effects of impairment upon school performance. (Prepared for the Division of Special Education Services, Office of the Superintendent of Public Instruction for the State of Illinois, 1970).

38. Rubin, R. J., and Rozycki, D. Diagnostic screening for the deaf child. *Arch. Otolaryngol.* 91:429, 1970.

39. Rubin, R. J., and Rozycki, D. Clinical aspects of genetic deafness. *Ann. Otol. Rhinol. Laryngol.* 80:255, 1971.

40. Sak, R. J., and Ruben, R. J. Effects of recurrent middle ear effusion in pre-school years on language and learning. *J. Dev. Behav. Pediatr.* 3:7, 1982.

41. Suchman, R. G. Visual impairment among deaf children. *Arch. Ophthalmol.* 77:18, 1967.

42. Teele, D. W., Klein, J. O., and Rosner, B. Epidemiology of Otitis Media in Children: The Greater Boston Project Proceedings of the Second International Symposium, Recent Advances in Otitis Media with Effusion. *Ann. Otol. Rhinol. Laryngol.* (Suppl. 68) 89:3, 5, 1980.

43. Vernon, M. C. Psychological aspects of the diagnosis of deafness in a child. *Eye Ear Nose Throat Mon.* 42:60, 1973.

24

Direct Stimulation of the Auditory Nerve

Derald E. Brackmann
William F. House

In recent years, great strides have been made in the rehabilitation of patients with hearing impairment. The development of surgery for otosclerosis (initially fenestration and then stapedectomy), and later of surgical techniques for chronic infection, has restored hearing to many. Restoring sensorineural loss has remained more of a problem. Developments in hearing aids have benefited persons with partial sensorineural loss. The major problem that remains is those patients with severe sensorineural hearing impairment who receive little or no benefit from hearing aids. Standard rehabilitation techniques, although helpful, have not solved the problem. Many patients born with profound sensorineural hearing impairment remain without speech and are severely handicapped. This chapter deals with a relatively new approach to patients with this severe problem, that is, direct electrical stimulation of the auditory nerve [19].

HISTORY OF ELECTRICAL STIMULATION OF HEARING

Knowledge that hearing could be produced by applying electrical currents to the ear is nearly as old as the knowledge of electricity itself. In 1790 Volta [34] inserted metal rods into each ear and connected them to a circuit that produced approximately 50 volts. On closing the circuit, he experienced a sensation that he described as a blow to the head followed by a sound like the boiling of viscid liquid. Perhaps because of Volta's unpleasant experience, there were only sporadic reports of similar experiments during the next 50 years.

In the latter half of the nineteenth century, interest in the electrical stimulation of hearing was revived. Textbooks were published that advocated the use of electrical stimulation to treat many hearing disorders. Politzer [26] was among the well-known otologists of the time to use this form of therapy. He treated a series of cases of tinnitus with electrical stimulation and reported improvement in some cases.

Gradenigo [11] was a strong advocate of electrical methods of diagnosis. He claimed

Sponsored by a grant from the House Ear Institute, an affiliate of the University of Southern California School of Medicine, Los Angeles.

that an acoustic sensation did not result from electrical stimulation of the normal ear, but only from stimulation of a diseased ear. During the late 1880s, most investigators attributed auditory sensations from electrical stimulation to the direct effect of the impulses on the auditory nerve. Near the turn of the century, electrical treatment became associated with quackery because it was advocated by many unscrupulous practitioners for many diseases for which it had absolutely no value. Reputable practitioners therefore completely abandoned its use.

In 1930, interest in electrical stimulation was revived by the discovery by Wever and Bray [37] of the electrical potential that arises in the cochlea as a result of acoustic stimulation. Their concept that the cochlea acted essentially as a transducer of acoustic to electrical energy recreated enthusiasm for the possibility of artificial hearing through direct stimulation of the acoustic nerve. At about this same time, several radio engineers discovered that tones could be produced by placing electrodes near the ear and stimulating it with a modulated alternating current. In 1937, Stevens termed this the electrophonic effect, and over the next several years, he, Flottorp, and Jones and Lurie [8, 15, 33] experimented with the production of hearing in this manner.

Electrophonic hearing results when an alternating electrical current in the audible frequency range is passed from an electrode to the skin surface. The electrode and the skin surface act as two plates of a condenser microphone, which results in a vibration that is transmitted to the cochlea by both air- and bone-conduction routes and produces auditory sensation. Electrophonic hearing requires a normal or near-normal cochlea. Frequencies may be heard from approximately 150 to 12,000 Hz. Patients report a maximum loudness of approximately 40 dB sensation level before pain threshold of the skin is reached.

Electrophonic hearing may be produced by placing electrodes in the external or middle ear as well as by having an electrode on the skin. In 1957, Djourno and Eyries [5] published the results of electrical stimulation of a totally deaf patient by a wire implanted into the cochlea. They reported that their subject perceived background sound and was greatly benefited in lipreading. With practice he was able to recognize a few words. This report ushered in the modern era of treatment of severe sensory hearing impairment by electrical stimulation.

PRINCIPLE OF DIRECT EIGHTH NERVE STIMULATION

There is a common misconception that a cochlear implant or stimulator is a type of hearing aid. In fact, a cochlear implant works on an entirely different principle from a hearing aid. A hearing aid increases the amplitude of the incoming acoustic stimulus to provide greater stimulation to the existing auditory mechanism. On the other hand, the cochlear implant attempts to replace a function of the cochlea that has been entirely lost.

The cochlea acts as a transducer of the mechanical energy of sound vibration to a form of energy capable of stimulating the eighth (auditory) nerve. The hair cells within the cochlea perform this function, and when they are absent, total hearing loss occurs. Cochlear stimulation attempts to replace the function of the lost hair cells in that it transforms the mechanical energy of sound to electrical energy, which directly excites or stimulates the remaining eighth nerve.

It is only those patients with loss of hair cells with remaining viable auditory neurons that can benefit from this device. It is therefore important to further define and differentiate types of hearing impairment that in the past have been grouped under the term *sensorineural hearing loss*.

Types of Sensorineural Hearing Impairment

In the past, four types of hearing impairment have been collectively termed sensorineural: (1) sensory, (2) neural, (3) brain stem, and (4) central. *Sensory* hearing loss occurs when the sensory elements of the cochlea (hair cells) are diseased and therefore incapable of stimulating the auditory nerve. An example of this is the hearing loss that occurs from ototoxic antibiotics. *Neural* hearing impairment occurs when the auditory nerve is diseased and incapable of conducting the impulses generated by the hair cells to the central nervous system. This type of loss is exemplified by acoustic neuromas. A *brain stem* loss occurs when brain stem structures are incapable of relaying the impulses from the auditory nerve to the cortex. Kernicterus is thought to produce this type of impairment. A *central* hearing loss occurs when the central nervous system is incapable of meaningfully interpreting the electrical impulses received from an intact peripheral mechanism. Central hearing loss is poorly defined, but cases have been documented in which the peripheral mechanism is intact but the patient is clinically deaf.

Even these four definitions are theoretical, and only extensive testing will determine to what degree the entities actually exist. Until recently we were totally dependent on histopathologic studies of temporal bones for knowledge in this area. Based on these studies, it is probable that most diseases that destroy the eighth nerve also destroy the hair cells; therefore, an isolated neural loss is rare and combined sensory and neural loss common. On the other hand, temporal bone studies have shown that with severe loss of sensory elements, some neurons frequently are present so that one can predict that a sensory loss will be the most commonly encountered. A brain stem loss is probably uncommon, and an isolated central deficit with a normal peripheral mechanism is rare.

Differentiation of Type of Sensorineural Hearing Loss. On a theoretical basis, it should be possible to determine the site of both inner ear and central deficits by measuring the electrical potentials generated from each site. Electrocochleography, brain stem audiometry, and cortical evoked response audiometry are used in an attempt to determine the site of the disorder.

It is possible to measure the cochlear microphonic from the hair cells, the eighth nerve action potential from the auditory nerve, the potentials generated in the brain stem, and finally the potentials from the auditory cortex. Theoretically, the first site from which a potential is not obtained would be the site of the defect, and the loss would be named accordingly. Theoretical conclusions are summarized in Table 24-1.

Table 24-1. Theoretical Types of Sensorineural Hearing Impairment

Physiologic finding	Type of loss
Cochlear microphonic absent	Sensory loss
Cochlear microphonic present Action potential absent	Neural loss
Cochlear microphonic present Action potential absent Brain stem response absent	Brain stem deficit
Cochlear microphonic present Eighth nerve action potential present Brain stem response present Evoked cortical response absent	Cortical defect

In practice, this theory is not workable because the production of each subsequent potential is dependent on the presence of an adequate potential preceding it. In other words, the cochlear microphonic is responsible for the action potential, the action potential is responsible for the brain stem potential, and so on. Thus, when the hair cells are nonfunctional, as they are in almost all cases of severe sensorineural loss, no potentials are produced in the eighth nerve or more centrally, even if these structures are intact. Therefore, when the cochlear microphonic is absent as a result of hair cell degeneration, recording of potentials will not determine if the central mechanisms are intact, and therefore will not separate sensory from neural hearing impairment. Although we believe that the study of electrical potentials of the inner ear is important for many other reasons, it is not possible to separate sensory from neural hearing impairment by this means when the impairment is severe.

Selection of Patients for Cochlear Implantation. Electrically stimulating the patient's inner ear through the same needle previously used for recording auditory potentials differentiates sensory from neural impairment [13]. A low-frequency (30–120 Hz), low-voltage (0.3–1.2 v) alternating current is applied. In effect, this current supplies an artificial cochlear microphonic to stimulate remaining neural elements. We are developing a technique to measure the brain stem and cortical responses thus evoked, but at the present time we simply ask the patient if he perceives an auditory sensation as a result of the electrical stimulation, an equivalent to pure-tone behavioral audiometry. Most patients have no difficulty differentiating auditory from tactile or other sensations. On the basis of whether the patients perceive an auditory sensation through the peripherally applied electrical stimulation, the impairment may be divided into sensory or neural.

If a patient perceives sound, we believe that this demonstrates that the auditory nerve and more central mechanism are intact, and we classify this as a sensory loss. On the other hand, if there is no response to electrical stimulation, we believe that this indicates a neural or more central impairment. We use this test to select patients for cochlear implant surgery. All patients thus selected have responded to the permanently implanted device to stimulate the auditory nerve directly.

FUNCTION OF THE NORMAL COCHLEA

The normal cochlea acts as a transducer in that it converts the mechanical energy of sound into a form capable of evoking an action potential in the eighth nerve. The mechanical vibration of the tympanic membrane and ossicles creates a fluid wave within the perilymph of the cochlea. The fluid wave causes a displacement of the basilar membrane, which results in a shearing action on the cilia of the hair cells. An alternating current–electrical potential that duplicates the frequency of the stimulus is produced [3].

The eighth nerve then discharges, but exactly what occurs to cause the eighth nerve action potential is not known. It is most likely that there is a chemical mediator that interacts between the hair cell and the eighth nerve and that the release of this mediator is related to the alternating current produced by the hair cells. The action potential produced in the eighth nerve is carried centrally through a series of synapses to arrive finally at the auditory cortex. The mechanism by which this impulse is interpreted into meaningful sound is unknown [10].

Two types of frequency information are encoded in the cochlea for transfer to the central nervous system. The first is volley information, sometimes called periodicity pitch. Each of the 30,000 auditory neurons is capable of repetitive firing up to approximately 500 or 600 cycles per second. Low-frequency stimuli may be perceived in this manner.

The second type of encoding of acoustic stimuli that occurs in the cochlea is by selective firing of specific neuron populations with each frequency. This is called place pitch. Bekesy demonstrated the traveling wave in the cochlea, pointing out that there is a specific site along the basilar membrane that produces a maximum displacement for each frequency [35]. Thus, a specific group of neurons is most sensitive to stimulation by a particular frequency. These neurons are said to have a characteristic frequency to which they best respond. High frequencies excite primarily the basal end of the cochlea, whereas low frequencies excite the whole cochlear partition to produce a maximum effect near the apex. At high intensities, many additional fibers are stimulated besides those of the characteristic frequency of the stimulus presented. Maximum stimulation, however, is still of those fibers with the characteristic frequency of the stimulus. High-frequency information is coded by the place principle, and this mechanism may also convey information of low frequency [17].

These impulses are conveyed centrally through the brain stem by several synapses. It is likely that the brain stem structures have functions in addition to a simple relay of impulses. Elective suppression of specific impulses may occur, but the exact role of this efferent system is not known. Also, we do not know how the central nervous system decodes this information. The normal cochlea is extremely complex, and whether it is possible to reproduce this miraculous structure artificially raises many serious questions.

Auditory Nerve Survival

The first question that has been raised is will the auditory nerve survive after the hair cells have deteriorated? If a cochlear implant is to be effective, some auditory neurons must remain viable after there has been total hair cell degeneration, but the exact number is not known. Histopathologic studies have shown that invariably there is loss of some ganglion cells in all cases in which there is severe loss of hair cells [18]. On the other hand, in almost all cases at least 5 to 10% of the ganglion cells and neurons remain, as experiments in animals and histopathologic study of human temporal bones have shown. Apparently the neurons are metabolically and physiologically independent of the hair cells, but they are somewhat dependent on the supporting cells of the organ of Corti. Therefore, any cochlear prosthesis must respect the integrity of the organ of Corti as much as possible.

This leads to the second question: will a cochlear implant destroy the remaining auditory neurons? Four types of damage can occur to the neural tissue: (1) mechanical, (2) chemical, (3) thermal, and (4) electrolytic.

Mechanical. Any electrode must be designed to produce the minimum amount of mechanical injury to the remaining cochlear structures and auditory nerve. The scala tympani seems to be the best site to place an electrode to produce the least amount of mechanical trauma. Placement of scala tympani electrodes in animals has shown little damage to the hair cells or neurons as demonstrated by no loss in the cochlear and neuronal potentials postoperatively [29]. On the other hand, an electrode in the scala vestibuli would likely injure Reissner's membrane, and this has been shown to be associated with neuronal degeneration.

The temporal bones of cats in which molded Silastic implants had been placed into the scala tympani have been studied [27]. It was found that although the cochlea was damaged as a result of the implant, there was little evidence of loss of spiral ganglion cells. Physiologic studies on the same cats showed that these cells were responsive to electrical stimulation several months after the implant. Patients who have been implanted with a similar Silastic molded scala tympani electrode have shown little change in stimulus parameters over the years. Similarly, patients implanted with a wire electrode in the scala tympani

have shown little change in their ability to be stimulated over a period of implantation of up to nine years.

Several of our patients have had one type of scala tympani electrode removed to be replaced by another type. In these cases there has been no change in the patients' response to electrical stimulation after the second operation. Based on these cases, it appears that implantation with currently used scala tympani electrodes will not compromise the use of more advanced electrode types when they are developed.

Electrodes placed directly into the auditory nerve through the modiolus have been shown to be well tolerated in cats and, in one case of long-term implantation, in a human being [28, 30]. All this evidence, therefore, points to the likelihood that the auditory nerve will survive the mechanical effect of long-term electrode implantation.

Chemical. The second type of damage that can occur as a result of electrode placement is chemical, which can be minimized by the selection of chemically inert materials. After testing many different types of metals, it is generally concluded that platinum, iridium, and titanium are all suitable electrode materials. These materials are all highly resistant to corrosion and to alkalis. Teflon, Silastic, and various types of varnishes are available for insulation. Of these, Teflon is the least likely to develop insulation leaks. All are well tolerated by tissue, as shown in animal experiments and clinical use.

Thermal. Thermal damage may also occur as a result of electrical stimulation of neural tissue. Fortunately, the current levels necessary to stimulate the auditory nerve are so low that thermal damage is not likely. The heat dissipation capabilities of the tissue environment exceed the heat that is produced by current adequate for stimulation. Studies [36] have shown that modiolar electrodes in the eighth nerve have the lowest levels of current necessary for eighth nerve stimulation. Although scala tympani electrodes require a higher current level, it is still in the microampere range (less than 200 μA), well below the level found to cause damage by heat.

Electrolytic. The fourth type of injury that can result from electrical stimulation is electrolytic damage. The use of alternating current is much less likely to produce electrophoresis than is a direct current. It is generally agreed, therefore, that the stimulus should be alternating current. Fortunately, the low currents necessary for stimulation also reduce the hazard of electrolysis. From previous experience, it is unlikely that charged ions such as chlorine will accumulate in sufficient quantity to be injurious. Electrolysis may also cause loss of electrode surface. Again, from the experience gathered to date, it appears that electrodes small enough to be introduced into the scala tympani or the modiolus will have sufficient surface area so that they will have a long life with the small amount of electrolysis that occurs.

Thus, it appears that the auditory nerve will survive implantation of either modiolar or scala tympani electrodes and that both the nerve and the electrode will withstand long-term continuous alternating current stimulation. These findings have been most encouraging.

INFORMATION TRANSFER BY ELECTRICAL STIMULATION
How much information can be transferred by electrical stimulation of the auditory nerve? To what degree can the function of a normal organ of Corti be duplicated? These are important but difficult questions that are not yet answered. One thing is certain: it will be impossible to reproduce exactly the normal cochlear function that discretely innervates approximately 30,000 auditory neurons. The question then becomes whether sufficient information can be passed to make a device useful and whether speech discrimination, which would be the ultimate goal of such a device, is possible.

The normal cochlea encodes pitch by two mechanisms, volley and place pitch. It has been established, both through animal experimentation and with patients implanted to date, that volley information can be produced with electrodes in the eighth nerve, modiolus, and scala tympani. Pitch discrimination is good up to approx-

imately 800 Hz with stimulation through a single electrode. A good deal of information can be passed through a single channel that produces this periodicity pitch. Background information is provided, and a rhythm is imparted to speech, which greatly improves the patient's ability to read lips. It has become apparent, however, that a single channel producing only periodicity pitch will not provide information sufficient for any but limited speech discrimination. Multiple-channel stimulation will be necessary to reach this goal. It does appear that this will be possible.

Our first three patients each had a five-wire electrode placed into the scala tympani. This electrode was hard-wired to an external button embedded in the mastoid bone. Extensive testing of these patients showed the possibility of place pitch discrimination, taking advantage of the spatial distribution of the auditory neurons in the cochlea. These patients repeatedly reported that pitch increased as electrodes were stimulated progressively closer to the basal end of the cochlea. This discrimination of place pitch held true for several different frequencies tested from 25 to 800 Hz. These patients were also able to reliably discriminate periodicity pitch on each electrode, namely, the pitch increased as the pulse repetition rate increased. Thus, these patients reported increasing pitch as the frequency of the stimulus was increased progressively during the stimulation of electrodes from the apical to the basal end. It therefore appears that an auditory prosthesis that takes advantage of both periodicity and place pitch can be constructed.

A problem that has become apparent through both animal experimentation and treatment of human beings is that the dynamic range of electrical stimulation is reduced from the dynamic range of the normal cochlea. During acoustic stimulation, discharge rates of single auditory neurons increase over a range of 20 to 40 dB. On the other hand, the discharge rate of single auditory neurons for electrical stimuli increases over a range of only 4 dB [16]. Thus the dynamic range for electrical stimulation is only one fifth to one tenth of the normal range of acoustic stimulation. The large range of intensities to which the patient is exposed must be compressed to a range that will be acceptable through electrical stimulation, which can be done with compression circuits.

SUMMARY OF CLINICAL EXPERIENCE AND PRESENT STATUS OF DIRECT EIGHTH NERVE STIMULATION

Simmons and associates [31] performed important early studies on electrical stimulation. In 1964 they reported an experiment in which bipolar stimulation of the eighth nerve was performed during a posterior craniotomy under local anesthesia. Electrodes were spaced approximately 4.5 mm apart on the eighth nerve. Bipolar square-wave stimulation was used. This patient was able to distinguish rate differences easily between 20 to 900 pulses per second. Above that level the rate difference detection diminished considerably.

In 1966 Simmons [28] reported the results of a study in which he implanted small electrodes into the auditory nerve through the modiolus. The electrodes were well tolerated for several months, during which time the patient was studied intensively. Simmons found that electrical pulses through such electrodes could be used to excite relatively discrete groups of nerve fibers. There was a dynamic range of approximately 15 to 25 dB from threshold to a loudness level to which the patient objected. At threshold levels excitation of two discrete groups of fibers did not summate or otherwise interact. At higher intensities, the fibers did interact, either at the cochlea or more central level. At times simultaneous stimulation in two electrodes produced sensations that retained their perceptual identity; at other times they fused to form a different third sound. Subjective pitch sensation was influenced by electrode selection, stimulus repetition rate, and current intensity. From this study Simmons concluded that both periodicity and place pitch were possible with modiolar electrodes. Speech and speech-modulated waveforms were recognized by Simmon's patient, primarily on the basis of their irregular envelopes and amplitudes. The patient did not learn, however, to identify words or phrases. The electrode was re-

moved after completion of the study. More recently Simmons and associates [32] have conducted further studies with a multiple-channel modiolar implant.

In 1971 Michelson [22, 23] reported on four patients who had been implanted with a bipolar electrode system in the scala tympani. (Subsequently a fifth patient has been implanted with a bipolar electrode with wires embedded in a Silastic mold of the basal portion of the cochlea.) The electrodes terminate in a small amplitude modulation radio receiver placed beneath the skin of the mastoid. This radio receiver is driven by an external antenna placed over the receiver. Externally applied sound thereby generates an audio-electric field within the electrodes in the cochlea.

Merzenich and his associates [20] have since studied these patients intensively. They have found that the patients respond to sinusoidal electrical stimulation across the frequency range of approximately 25 Hz to more than 10,000 Hz. With increasing frequency of stimulation, the subjective sensation changes from a low tone to a higher one. Pitch changes as a function of stimulus frequency from approximately 50 to 500 Hz. At levels of more than 500 to 600 Hz, the pitch changes little with increasing frequency. Merzenich [21] and Michelson [24] confirmed the finding of a narrowed dynamic range to electrical stimulation in their cases. As a result of their experiments, they concluded that the useful range of discriminative hearing is limited to frequencies of less than 400 to 600 Hz. The resulting discrimination is due to encoding of the time order of discharge of auditory neurons analogous to periodicity pitch. There is no place pitch encoding with the single-channel electrode.

Michelson and Schindler [24] recently reported a patient who achieved significant speech discrimination with a multiple-channel electrode connected in series with a single-channel stimulator. Merzenich and colleagues [21] continue research with the aim of developing a true multiple-channel device. In addition to work in the United States, several centers in other countries are also active in cochlear implant programs. In France, Pialoux and his associates [25] have gained considerable experi-

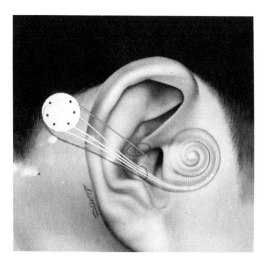

Figure 24-1. Placement of electrodes in the scala tympani and scala vestibuli. Note five active electrodes in the scala tympani and the single ground, or inactive, electrode in the scala vestibuli. (From J. Urban, Proceedings of the First International Conference on Electrical Stimulation of the Acoustic Nerve as a Treatment for Profound Sensorineural Deafness in Man. San Francisco, 1974.)

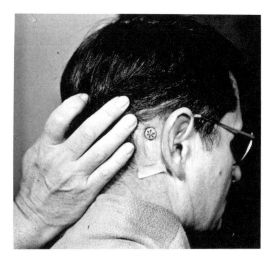

Figure 24-2. The electrode button in place with the protective cap removed. (From J. Urban, Proceedings of the First International Conference on Electrical Stimulation of the Acoustic Nerve as a Treatment for Profound Sensorineural Deafness in Man. San Francisco, 1974.)

ence with cochlear implants. Burian and his associates [1] in Austria report success in achieving significant speech discrimination in one patient. In England, a group [9] has investigated the feasibility of extracochlear stimulation with success. Clark and his group [2] in Australia continue to develop a multiple-channel device.

In Los Angeles, House and Urban [14] initiated work on eighth nerve stimulation at the House Ear Institute in the early 1960s. The first three patients were implanted with a five-contact electrode placed through the round window into the scala tympani (Fig. 24-1).

This electrode was connected to a five-place button embedded in the bone of the mastoid cortex (Fig. 24-2). One of these buttons was rejected in the immediate postoperative period. The other two patients were studied extensively. These patients were able to discriminate both periodicity and place pitch with this electrode array. These results are surprising because it was speculated that the impedance of the perilymphatic fluid would be so low as not to allow discrete stimulation of multiple electrodes. Repeated tests have shown,

however, that stimulation of discrete populations of nerve fibers can be accomplished with this electrode array.

It was the initial concept of House and Urban [14] to produce a multichannel stimulator that would take advantage of both place and periodicity pitch. A stimulator was constructed in which a complex incoming signal could be divided in bandwidths. The higher frequency bandwidths were then fed into the electrode near the basal turn, and the lower bandwidths were progressively connected to electrodes nearer the apex. It was also possible to count down or divide the incoming frequencies by factors of 1 through 22. A time delay could also be created between the electrodes to simulate the lag that occurs with the traveling wave in the normal cochlea. Work with this device was aimed toward establishing the specifications for an external stimulating device that would most nearly reproduce the function of the normal cochlea. Before this objective was achieved, however, shunting problems occurred between the electrodes and the external button, which prevented further investigation. Because these two patients gained so much from single-channel stimulation, efforts were focused on the development of a portable single-channel device.

A device has been developed consisting of a single active electrode placed into the scala tympani via a mastoid-facial recess approach. The ground wire is placed into the attic area. These leads connect to an induction coil, which is embedded in the bone of the mastoid cortex. The external unit produces a 16,000 Hz carrier wave. Incoming acoustic stimuli are converted to a signal that produces a 90% amplitude modulation of the carrier wave. The use of an amplitude-modulated carrier wave for stimulation was arrived at empirically. The first patient was allowed to select the stimulus mode from which he derived the most benefit. Through trial and error he selected these stimulus characteristics. The first patient has worn this device continuously since May 1972. The other patients have been fitted with similar devices. Technically, our patients perceive periodicity pitch at frequencies to approximately 800 Hz.

Although significant speech discrimination has not been achieved, our patients derive considerable benefit from the implants. Our patients have led us to appreciate other aspects of hearing in addition to speech discrimination [4]. Implant users indicate that they are able to identify differences among music, environmental sounds, and speech. Multiple sounds occurring simultaneously are differentiated. They also report improved perception of sounds at a distance. Many sounds are also perceived at a comfortable listening level.

Relative to their auditory memory, patients commonly use words like *mechanical, tinny, metallic, distorted,* and *muffled* to describe the sounds. A frequent description is of an "untuned" or "off-station" radio where differences between speech and music can be heard, but where understanding is not possible. The cochlear implant seems to enhance appreciation and enjoyment of music for many patients.

Patients consistently report that the cochlear implant provides useful auditory information. That they consider this information beneficial is demonstrated by the fact that the large majority use their implant all day, every day. Interviews with patients and their spouses or relatives indicate that the implant and rehabilitation program have improved the quality of their lives. Implant users report that they feel less concerned about their safety, less isolated, and less upset about their hearing loss. They state that they feel more comfortable in social situations and find communication less difficult and less frustrating. Reports from patients also indicate that they feel that their relationships with their families are more satisfying and that they feel that they are less of a burden to their families. In addition, relatives report that the cochlear implant program has improved their own quality of life.

Patients describe few problems with the implant. The most common problem seems to be alignment of the external coil relative to the internal coil. When the coils are not aligned, the signal strength is weakened and the eyeglass-mounted external coil must be repositioned. Interference from two-way, or citizens band, radios also has been reported.

In general, observations and patient reports [12] indicate that the single-electrode cochlear implant system offers substantial auditory and "quality of life" benefits to persons for whom little else has been available or successful.

FUTURE OF DIRECT EIGHTH NERVE STIMULATION

The experience gained from single-channel stimulation makes it apparent that such a device will not provide information sufficient for speech discrimination, which is the goal of research in this field. Only with multiple-channel stimulation can we hope for enough bits of information to enable understanding of speech. It has been estimated that 8 to 12 channels each stimulating a different population of nerve fibers may provide sufficient information for this understanding. An appealing (but perhaps naive) hope is that placing electrodes within the scala tympani in the area of the fibers whose characteristic frequencies cover the speech range may result in the sensation of these speech frequencies.

From the results of our study of patients with multiple electrodes, we know that electrical stimulation will provide some place information. Pitch-matching experiments have been extremely difficult, however, so that we do not know the range of pitches that are elicited. Animal experimentation has shown that nerve fibers respond entirely differently to electrical than to acoustic stimulation [16]. Therefore, it is unlikely that information artificially produced will so easily duplicate the normally functioning cochlea.

No matter how sophisticated a cochlear prosthesis may be, it will likely supply a different type of information than is normal to the central nervous system. What is hoped is that a prosthesis will supply sufficient bits of information so that the brain will be able to decode this information and speech discrimination will result. It is interesting to speculate that perhaps the patient with congenital hearing loss without an auditory memory might learn this new code with more facility than a patient with an auditory memory, who must in effect unlearn one language before learning another.

With the larger electrodes in use, it is difficult to reach the apical portion of the cochlea where the speech frequencies are normally perceived (17–28 mm from the round window). It has been proposed that a finer, more flexible electrode could be made by techniques of coating thin, flexible films with conductive metals. It may be, however, that electrical stimulation of fibers whose characteristic frequency to acoustic stimulation is in the speech frequencies will not respond in this manner to electric stimulation. In this case, placement of electrodes into the apex may not be necessary. Perhaps as much information can be produced by stimulating 8 to 12 discrete groups of fibers near the basal end of the cochlea.

In any event, the basic concept is that speech signals will then be divided into 8 to 12 bandwidths. Each bandwidth will stimulate a separate electrode. It is hoped that electrodes placed in the area of the cochlea whose fibers are of characteristic frequency of the speech range will be stimulated. It is not known if this will be the case. It may be that only periodicity pitch to the range of 800 Hz can be produced, and the speech frequencies will have to be reduced from 500 to 2000 Hz to 50 to 800 Hz.

Another problem for the future will be the coupling of the external device to the internal cochlear or modiolar electrode. Because of the risk of infection, any device that protrudes through the skin may not be satisfactory for long-term stimulation. For single-channel stimulation, induction coils have worked very well. One can use the same induction coil principle for multiple-electrode stimulation by using external and internal buffers with high speed serial memories [6]. Other suggestions for coupling are with the use of light-emitting diodes and ultrasonic transmission. Although further discussion of this problem is beyond the scope of this text, the engineering aspects of direct eighth nerve stimulation are within the scope of current technology. The problem that remains is to outline the specifications necessary for the unit, which is not an easy task.

REFERENCES

1. Burian, K., Hockmair-Desoyer, I. J., and Hockmair, E. S. Cochlear implants: Further clinical results. *Acta Otolaryngol.* 91:629, 1981.
2. Clark, G. M., and Tong, Y.-C. A multiple-channel cochlear implant. *Arch. Otolaryngol.* 108:214, 1982.
3. Davis, H. Transmission and transduction in the cochlea. *Laryngoscope* 68:359, 1958.
4. Davis, H., and Silverman, S. R. *Hearing and Deafness.* New York: Holt, Rinehart & Winston, 1970.
5. Djourno, A., and Eyries, C. Prothese auditoire par excitation electrique a distance due nerf sensoriel a l'aide d'un bobinage inclus a demeure. *Presse Med.* 35:14, 1957.
6. Dobelle, W. H., et al. Data processing—LSI will help to bring sight to the blind. *Electronics,* January 24, 1974.
7. Eddington, D. K. Multiple-Channel Intracochlear Stimulation. In D. E. Brackmann (Ed.), *Neurological Surgery of the Ear and Skull Base.* New York: Raven, 1982.
8. Flottorp, G. Effect of different types of electrodes in electrophonic hearing. *J. Acoust. Soc. Am.* 25:236, 1953.
9. Fourcin, A. J., et al. External electrical stimulation of the cochlea: Clinical psychophysical, speech, perceptual, and histologic findings. *Br. J. Audiol.* 13:85, 1979.
10. Galambos, R. Neural mechanisms in audition. *Laryngoscope* 68:388, 1958.
11. Gradenigo, G. Die erkrankungen des nervus acousticus. *Arch. Ohrenh.* 27:105, 1888.
12. House, W. F., and Berliner, K. I. (Eds.).

Cochlear implants: Progress and perspectives. *Ann. Otol. Rhinol. Laryngol.* (Suppl. 91):1, 1982.

13. House, W. F., and Brackmann, D. E. Electrical promontory testing in differential diagnosis of the sensorineural hearing impairment. *Laryngoscope* 84:2163, 1974.

14. House, W. F., and Urban, J. Long-term results of electrode implantation and electric stimulation of the cochlea in man. *Ann. Otol. Rhinol. Laryngol.* 82:504–510, 1973.

15. Jones, R. C., Stevens, S. S., and Lurie, M. H. Three mechanisms of hearing by electrical stimulation. *J. Acoust. Soc. Am.* 12: 281, 1940.

16. Kiang, N. Y. S., and Moxon, E. C. Physiological considerations in artificial stimulation of the inner ear. *Ann. Otol. Rhinol. Laryngol.* 81:714, 1972.

17. Kiang, N. Y. S., and Moxon, E. C. Tails of tuning curves of auditory nerve fibers. *J. Acoust. Soc. Am.* 55:620, 1974.

18. Lawrence, M., and Johnsson, L. G. The role of the organ of Corti in auditory nerve stimulation. *Ann. Otol. Rhinol. Laryngol.* 82:464, 1973.

19. Merzenich, M. M., Schindler, R., and Sooy, F. Proceedings of the First International Conference on Electrical Stimulation of the Acoustic Nerve as a Treatment for Profound Sensorineural Deafness in Man. San Francisco, 1974.

20. Merzenich, M. M., et al. Neural encoding of sound sensation evoked by electrical stimulation of the acoustic nerve. *Ann. Otol. Rhinol. Laryngol.* 82:486, 1973.

21. Merzenich, M. M., et al. Cochlear implant prostheses: Strategies and progress. *Ann. Biomed. Eng.* 8:361, 1980.

22. Michelson, R. P. Electrical stimulation of the human cochlea. *Arch. Otolaryngol.* 93: 317, 1971.

23. Michelson, R. P. The results of electrical stimulation of the cochlea in human sensory deafness. *Ann. Otol. Rhinol. Laryngol.* 50: 914, 1971.

24. Michelson, R. P., and Schindler, R. A. Multi-channel cochlear implant: Preliminary results in man. *Laryngoscope* 91:38, 1981.

25. Pialoux, P., et al. Indications and results of the multichannel cochlear implant. *Acta Otolaryngol.* 87:185, 1979.

26. Politzer, A. *Diseases of the Ear.* Philadelphia: Henry Lea's Son & Co., 1883.

27. Schindler, R. A., and Merzenich, M. M. Chronic intracochlear electrode implantation. Cochlear pathology and acoustic nerve survival. *Ann. Otol. Rhinol. Laryngol.* 83: 202, 1974.

28. Simmons, F. B. Electrical stimulation of the auditory nerve in man. *Arch. Otolaryngol.* 84:24, 1966.

29. Simmons, F. B. Permanent intracochlear electrodes in cats, tissue tolerance and cochlear microphonics. *Laryngoscope* 77:171, 1967.

30. Simmons, F. B., and Glattke, T. J. Comparison of electrical and acoustical stimulation of the cat ear. *Ann. Otol. Rhinol. Laryngol.* 81:731, 1972.

31. Simmons, R. B., et al. Electrical stimulation of acoustical nerve and inferior colliculus. *Arch Otolaryngol.* 79:559, 1964.

32. Simmons, F. B., et al. A functioning multichannel auditory nerve stimulator. *Acta Otolaryngol.* 87:170, 1979.

33. Stevens, S. S., and Jones, R. C. The mechanism of hearing by electrical stimulation. *J. Acoust. Soc. Am.* 10:261, 1939.

34. Volta, A. On the electricity excited by more contact of conducting substances of different kinds. *Trans. R. Soc. Phil.* 90:403, 1800.

35. von Bekesy, G. V. *Experiments in Hearing.* New York: McGraw-Hill, 1960.

36. Walloch, R. A., and Cowden, D. A. Placement of electrodes for the excitation of the eighth nerve. *Arch. Otolaryngol.* 100:19, 1974.

37. Wever, E. G., and Bray, C. W. The nature of the acoustic response: The relation between sound frequency and frequency of impulses in the auditory nerve. *J. Exp. Psychol.* 13:373, 1930.

25

Tinnitus

Jack A. Vernon

Tinnitus is a symptom that is associated with nearly every known hearing disorder. It is an unresolved problem and a collection of paradoxes. Tinnitus has plagued humankind since the beginning of history and yet, to date, no cure has been found. The United States Health Survey of 1962–1963 estimates that 36 million American adults have tinnitus in one of its forms and 7.2 million have severe tinnitus. Patients afflicted with tinnitus do not, as a rule, make it a common topic of conversation because they fear that others would think they were "a little crazy." As a general rule, tinnitus patients suffer in silence.

Tinnitus has been likened to external sound with qualities of pitch and loudness, yet tinnitus does not follow rules that apply to hearing or to the physics of sound. Tinnitus patients often report that their tinnitus is worse at bedtime, but this likely is due to the quietness and the subsequent lack of interference from ambient sounds.

It is paradoxic that the loudness of severe tinnitus is actually at very low sensation level. Tinnitus is not always accompanied by audiometric loss, and in fact it occurs in approximately 10% of normal hearing patients [39]. The masking of tinnitus represents another paradox because it does not obey any of the laws that we associate with psychoacoustic masking. For example, "noiselike" tinnitus is easily masked by a pure-tone stimulus. It has been commonly believed that in ordinary masking there is a greater spread of effect toward the higher frequencies than toward the lower ones. Recently, Zwicker and Jaroszewski [46] emphasized that the spread of masking is level dependent and that the upward spread was limited to the more intense levels.

CLASSIFICATION OF TINNITUS

Various schemes of classifying tinnitus have been attempted [16, 17, 24, 30, 31] with limited success. Part of the problem is that it is not easy to determine the pitch of tinnitus, and traditionally most classification schemes rely on pitch. For example, noise-induced tinnitus is usually a ringing high-pitched tone. Most likely, the tinnitus is not a pure tone, but rather a very narrow band of noise that possesses a great deal of tonality. An interesting aspect of noise-induced tinnitus is the fact that all people who have noise-induced tinnitus have, in addition, noise-induced hearing loss. But all who have noise-induced hearing loss, even severe hearing loss, do not have tinnitus. It has been suggested that deliberate induction of temporary tinnitus by brief noise exposure may provide a basis for predicting patients who are highly susceptible to noise damage [38]. If successful, such a screening procedure would have obvious utility in assigning people into industrial noise conditions where sound levels cannot be controled.

Another broad classification of tinnitus compares Meniere's disease with otosclerosis. The tinnitus associated with Meniere's disease is usually in the middle-pitch region and more of a noise than a tone [41], often described by patients as a "roaring sound." The tinnitus associated with otosclerosis is usually a low-pitched, roaring noise. In both otosclerosis and Meniere's disease, symptomatic relief of the medical condition usually removes the tinnitus. The tinnitus of middle ear infections is often a pulsatile roaring noise. These different kinds of tinnitus represent an attempt to classify tinnitus according to etiology.

Subjective Tinnitus

Subjective tinnitus is the experience of hearing auditory sensation in the absence of sound. The fact that subjective tinnitus has no known objective indicator is one of the reasons tinnitus has received so little investigative attention. There are many limitations to the study of an entity that exists only as a subjective experience in the mind. In the absence of an objective indicator, all measures of tinnitus lack validity. The reliability of each test can be determined by measuring the consistency of response with test-retest situations.

Objective Tinnitus

Objective tinnitus can be heard by others, yet is not always heard by the patient. One common form of objective tinnitus is pulsatile tinnitus generated by the vascular system. The perceived pulses are in synchrony with the patient's pulse and can be heard by others, although a stethoscope or some form of amplification may be required. Another form of objective tinnitus is palatal myoclonus, a spasm of the soft palate.

Objective tinnitus may also be a continuous pure tone that is emitted from the patient's ear. Etiology of such an occurrence is unknown, but the resulting tinnitus is usually high pitched. This kind of objective tinnitus, known as spontaneous acoustic "echoes," is the most puzzling of the various types of objective tinnitus [25].

Spontaneous echoes have been recorded from the ears of both human beings and animals. When the patient hears the echo with the same ear that is emitting the sound, the pitch heard by others does not match the pitch heard by the patient [44, 45]. Spontaneous echoes appear at lower frequencies and interact with external sounds in a manner much different than does tinnitus. Spontaneous echoes can be reduced by proper application of an external sound. Kemp [26] has concluded that the echo coming from the ear as a result of either stimulated emissions or spontaneous emissions is due to mechanical action within the cochlea. Furthermore, he states that spontaneous echoes are most often found in normal hearing ears. Kemp indicates that spontaneous echoes are changed (often increased) by manipulation of the static pressure in the external ear canal. It is also true that severe tinnitus, in some cases, can be altered by increasing or decreasing the static pressure in the ear canal. In almost every case in which a change occurs, it is, however, a reduction of the tinnitus. That tinnitus can be reduced by alteration of the static pressure in the ear canal has been a puzzle but, in such cases, it is highly suggestive that the tinnitus is related to some sort of a mechanovibratory disturbance. The relationship between spontaneous echoes and tinnitus is far from clear. With the evidence at hand, however, the most reasonable conclusion is that severe tinnitus is not produced by spontaneous echoes.

Spontaneous Tinnitus

Spontaneous tinnitus is almost always a thin, weak, high-pitched tone that lasts for a very brief time. The typical course of the development of spontaneous tinnitus is as follows: first, the person notices a sensation of pressure in one ear; next, they notice that hearing on that side is impaired, followed rapidly by the rise of a weak, thin, high-pitched tone. This tone maintains itself for a few seconds and then gradually fades out. It is often difficult to determine exactly when it disappears, but when one is no longer aware of the tone it is also the case that the sensation of pressure has ceased and hearing on that side has returned to its usual level.

PAST RELIEF PROCEDURES FOR TINNITUS

The fact that there is today no cure for tinnitus is a telling commentary on our lack of understanding of this problem. For the most part it is difficult to evaluate past procedures for relief because they usually represent case history reports. In our clinic, we have seen many patients who insist, adamantly, that they have found the cure for tinnitus. They may advocate a rigidly controlled diet that usually contains some special item, such as the seeds of apples or scrapings from inside of the apple peel, vitamin C, B_{12}, or E, or cod liver oil. Such reports are not based on objective evidence. Spontaneous remission of tinnitus may occur, and if tinnitus disappears when the patient is trying out some self-generated prescription for relief, the procedure being tried is likely to get the credit.

Nicotinic Acid

The medication prescribed most frequently for tinnitus is nicotinic acid. The rationale for using nicotinic acid in an attempt to relieve tinnitus is the belief that tinnitus can be produced by a "vascular accident." However, there is no direct evidence that tinnitus can be produced by vascular accident. Most likely, the vascular accident theme was a convenient explanation offered to patients who were concerned as to the cause of their tinnitus.

It is difficult to understand, however, how nicotinic acid, a peripheral vasodilator, could influence the auditory system in any direct manner. If the organ of Corti and its hair cells are suspected as the cul-

prits causing tinnitus, then nicotinic acid could almost surely exert no influence. The organ of Corti is not in the peripheral vascular supply but is fed by the vas spirale, vessels that contain no muscles and therefore cannot dilate or contract.

The claim for nicotinic acid is supported by Flottorp and Willie [10]. The study suffers by not identifying the kinds of tinnitus experienced by the patients serving as subjects, nor was either a placebo or a blind procedure used. The need for an orally administered medication to relieve tinnitus is primary, but nicotinic acid is not the answer [6, 21].

Injections of Local Anesthetics

Studies involving injected local anesthetics have received recent attention by Melding and associates [29] and Melding and Goodey [28], although the technique was originated as early as 1937 by Lewy [27]. It is surprising that a local anesthetic such as lidocaine, when injected intravenously, can produce brief, temporary relief of tinnitus. The mechanism that can produce such relief and not produce either more general effects or neurologic symptoms is unknown.

The use of lidocaine for relief of tinnitus has recently undergone a rigorous test by Israel and colleagues [22], who used a placebo, double-blind cross-over paradigm. They found that 19 of 26 patients (73%) obtained temporary relief of their tinnitus when lidocaine was administered. No change in their tinnitus occurred when saline was used.

Goodey [13] uses the results of intravenous injections of lidocaine in a clinical setting as a screening procedure with which to recommend subsequent treatment. If the lidocaine produces either prolonged relief or no response, the patient is then evaluated for possible use of tinnitus maskers, hearing aids, or both. When there is a good response to lidocaine, the patient is then placed on a trial period using anticonvulsant medication such as carbamazepine. Goodey and associates [14] studied 59 patients who were screened according to this procedure. They found that 58% of the patients responded to both lidocaine and masking, 12% responded to neither, 19% responded to lidocaine alone, and

11% to masking alone. Patients who responded to both masking and lidocaine usually had noise-induced hearing losses. Patients who responded to neither masking nor lidocaine tended to have essentially normal hearing and tinnitus of unknown etiology.

CURRENT PROCEDURES TO RELIEVE TINNITUS

Different treatment methods are currently available to tinnitus patients. The classes of relief procedures are masking, biofeedback, electrical stimulation, and drug therapy. Because so little is known about tinnitus it is usually not possible to prejudge whether these relief procedures will be successful. Only through actual trial can their effectiveness be determined.

Masking

The first reference to relieving tinnitus by masking was made by Jones and Knudsen in 1928 [23]. They developed a noise generator using a transformer and a loudspeaker that were activated by ordinary 60 Hz household electricity. The unit was placed on the bedside table and exerted its sound influence on the tinnitus patient during sleep. Jones and Knudsen had hoped to cure tinnitus in this manner by "burning out" the offending portion of the ear. Most likely, their sound generator produced sound composed of frequencies well below those corresponding to the pitch of most tinnitus. That is, the majority of patients suffering from severe tinnitus hear a high-pitched tone within the 4000 to 12,000 Hz region. It seems reasonable to assume that the tinnitus patients seen by Jones and Knudsen also had high-frequency tinnitus and thus, their masking unit did not have much of a chance to effect masking.

It was the high-pitched character of tinnitus that hampered our early attempts to mask tinnitus in our laboratory at the University of Oregon Medical Center [43]. The initial tinnitus masker produced a band of noise that peaked at approximately 1500 Hz and provided little energy above approximately 3000 Hz. Thus, we were unable to generate sounds of sufficiently high frequency, and what little

masking noise we could generate, the patient was unable to appreciate because of hearing losses. Fortunately, 12% of tinnitus patients can be masked by any sounds, and in such cases, it is not necessary to match the pitch of the masking noise to the tinnitus to effect proper masking.

There are three ways of masking tinnitus: (1) hearing aids, (2) tinnitus maskers that can provide low-, medium-, and high-frequency bands of noise, and (3) the tinnitus instrument, which is the combination of a hearing aid and a tinnitus masker.

Hearing Aids. Another form of masking previously used as relief for tinnitus was the hearing aid [32, 33]. The primary concern was with the tinnitus that accompanies otosclerosis. Theoretically, the hearing aid would amplify environmental noise and thereby mask the patient's tinnitus. This technique is of value today when the patient's tinnitus is sufficiently low pitched as to be reached by the sound reproduced through hearing aids. However, when surgical treatment of otosclerosis restores the hearing loss the associated tinnitus usually disappears. Thus, the idea of using hearing aid amplification to mask tinnitus fell into disuse with the advent of surgery.

The modern-day role of the hearing aid in the relief of tinnitus is a significant one, although it is effective in slightly less than 10% of the cases. When it works, it provides a double advantage; the tinnitus is relieved and the patient's hearing is improved. The tinnitus only disappears while the hearing aids are in use.

The Tinnitus Masker. It is assumed when the hearing aid (or aids) is effective in relieving tinnitus it is due to a form of masking. That is, the environmental sounds have been amplified so that the patient can now hear them and they, in turn, can serve to mask the tinnitus. In addition, some masking may come from the broadband background noise present in the electronics of the hearing aid. In patients with normal hearing, the availability of normal environmental noise is obviously not sufficient to mask tinnitus. For this purpose, the tinnitus masker was developed.

The tinnitus masker went through sev-

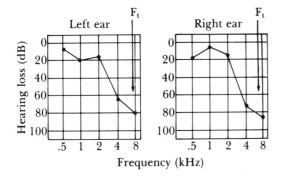

Figure 25-1. *Typical case of noise-induced hearing loss and noise-induced tinnitus. Tinnitus frequency (F$_t$) is determined by the pitch matching procedure explained in the text (see p. 298). The loudness of the tinnitus is not represented by the length of the arrow, which only denotes the frequency best corresponding to the pitch of the tinnitus.*

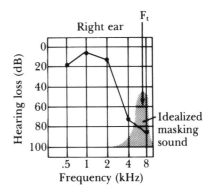

Figure 25-2. *The idealized masking noise for patient represented in Figure 25-1. Unfortunately, the kind of noise represented by the stippled area does not exist in a wearable tinnitus masking unit. A system such as this would prevent stimulation in unwanted frequency areas.*

eral stages of development in which the major effort was to produce bands of noise centered at different frequencies. There were low-, medium-, and high-frequency maskers and several breeds of high- and higher-frequency maskers, as well as a power masker.

The audiogram in Figure 25-1 is from a farmer who spent more than 20 years driving loud farm machinery. The hearing in both of his ears has been damaged, but the right ear has the more severe tinnitus.

The important point for this patient and many others like him is the relationship between the hearing loss and the frequency of the tinnitus. The frequency corresponding to the pitch of the tinnitus (F$_t$) is 7800 Hz. At 7800 Hz the hearing in the tinnitus-affected ear is depressed by approximately 70 to 75 dB, and more importantly, that hearing loss at 7800 Hz is characterized by a steep slope. The problem for tinnitus masking is to produce a band of noise, at or around 7800 Hz, that is sufficiently narrow as not to produce excessive stimulation at lower frequencies where the hearing is much better. The ideal schematized representation of this condition is shown in Figure 25-2.

Unfortunately, the idealized conditions as depicted in Figure 25-2 do not exist. It is not possible to make filters with steep skirts and package them in small hearing aid cases. Moreover, an ability to contract

and expand the width of the noise band would be most desirable and, of course, constant variable tuning of the center frequency would be essential. With such an arrangement, masking could be maximized and idealized for the patient by a precise custom fitting.

The situation that occurs with most patients is represented in Figure 25-3. Note that the band of masking noise spills over to greatly affect the hearing below those frequencies needed for masking of the tinnitus, and that portion of the masking sound is perceived as loud. In many cases, this arrangement is unsatisfactory, causing the patient to find the masking sound to be as objectionable as the tinnitus itself. After all, masking is merely substituting a more acceptable external sound for the internal one.

Using available equipment, it is possible to alter the frequency spectrum of the masking sound by manipulating the tubing used to fit the unit to the ear. Variables such as tube size, insertion depth, and length of tube can be manipulated to achieve better agreement between the patient's tinnitus and the masking sound. As a general rule a nonoccluding ear mold is required for patients with high-frequency hearing losses.

The Tinnitus Instrument. The dilemma of having hearing loss at the frequency posi-

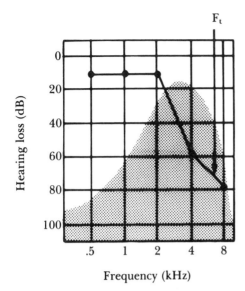

F_t

Hearing loss (dB)

Frequency (kHz)

Figure 25-3. A realistic representation of the masking available for the patient in Figure 25-1. That the masking sound, as indicated by the stippled area, unnecessarily stimulates many frequencies below the F_t can, and often does, render the masking sound unacceptable to the patient, even when it completely covers up the tinnitus.

tion where masking is needed for relief of tinnitus presents special problems. The solution came from a dentist with long-term exposure to a high-speed dental drill. He had a bilateral high-frequency hearing loss with severe bilateral tinnitus. Hearing aids could help his hearing, but they provided no relief for his tinnitus. High-frequency tinnitus maskers were not powerful enough to mask his tinnitus. He tied the hearing aid and the tinnitus masker together with a rubber band, fitted the branches of a Y-tube into each unit, and inserted the stem of the Y-tube into his ear. By judicious adjustment of the volume of each unit, he was able to completely relieve the tinnitus in his ear. With engineering improvements this combined unit is now known as a *tinnitus instrument*. In our tinnitus clinic, we recommend the tinnitus instrument to approximately 75% of all patients who receive instrument recommendations.

If masking alone does not work, how can the tinnitus instrument be successful? It appears that the hearing aid part of the unit improves the ability to hear high frequencies and the masker enriches the sound environment needed to cover up (or mask) the tinnitus.

There is another interesting puzzle concerning the tinnitus instrument. In routine masking with a tinnitus masker, the masking sound must cover up the tinnitus to produce an acceptable substitution for the tinnitus. That is, as the intensity of the masking sound is increased, the intensity of the tinnitus *does not* decrease. One does not end up with a reduced level of tinnitus that is acceptable to the patient. But in some cases with a tinnitus instrument, the patient will report that the tinnitus instrument is incapable of complete masking of the tinnitus but the remaining perceptible tinnitus is greatly reduced in loudness and thus acceptable.

Some Results with a Masking Program. For any new relief procedure, those concerned will always ask what is the percentage of success? That is not a simple question. A file of 598 patients who attended the Tinnitus Clinic at the Oregon Health Sciences University were surveyed [34], with the following results.

The 178 patients in the "no recommendation" category represented many different conditions. The tinnitus presented by some of these people simply could not be masked, no matter what kind of sound was used.

Of the 362 patients receiving a specific recommendation for either tinnitus maskers or tinnitus instruments, a random selection of 130 patients were contacted by telephone. Each patient was queried as to (1) whether they went to the dispenser and conducted a trial period, (2) whether they purchased the recommended unit, and (3) whether they obtained relief of tinnitus with the recommended unit after 1 to 2 years of using the unit.

Of the 130 patients contacted, tinnitus maskers were recommended for 33 patients (25%) and tinnitus instruments were recommended for 97 patients (75%). Of the 33 patients to whom maskers were recommended, 29 (88%) conducted the trial period. Of these, 21 (72%) purchased the units at the end of the trial period. All masking units were placed on trial for 1

Table 25-1. 1980 Survey of 598 Patients
Evaluated at Tinnitus Clinic

Recommendation	Number of patients	Percent of patients
None	178	30
Tinnitus masker	106	18
Tinnitus instrument	256	43
Hearing aid	58	9
N = 598		100%

Table 25-2. Random Telephone Survey of 130
Tinnitus Masker and Tinnitus Instrument
Users

	Tinnitus masker	Tinnitus instrument
Number recommended	33	97
Number who conducted trial period	29	81
Number who purchased unit	21	51
Number who obtained relief of tinnitus	18	45

month before purchase of the unit. Note that 28% of the patients did not purchase the recommended tinnitus masker.

Of the 97 patients to whom tinnitus instruments were recommended, 81 (84%) conducted the trial period. Of these, 51 (63%) purchased the unit. Note that 30 patients (37%) did not purchase the tinnitus instrument. The results are summarized in Tables 25-1 and 25-2.

Of the patients conducting the trial period, we have a total of 38 patients who did not purchase the recommended unit. We asked these patients about their decision since relief (we thought) had been demonstrated; 21 of them (55%) indicated they could not afford the purchase price. Twelve of the patients (32%) found the masking sound to be ineffective. The remainder of the nonpurchasing group offered a variety of reasons for their actions, such as "tinnitus has become mild," "vanity," "apparatus too much bother," and "wanted a cure, not a chronic relief procedure." Of the 21 patients (86%) who purchased maskers, more than 1 year later 18 were still obtaining relief from tinni-

tus. Of the 51 patients who purchased tinnitus instruments, more than 1 year later 45 (88%) were still obtaining relief by use of the unit.

Biofeedback
Regardless of the interpretation of our results, it is clear that although some patients could be relieved of tinnitus, others could not. Could relief have been possible by some improved, or more precise, form of masking? Also, what other relief procedures can be recommended to those for whom masking is inappropriate? Biofeedback, as practiced by House [18], is recommended to such patients. It is her contention that tinnitus can generate high levels of stress and that such patients need to learn coping procedures to handle the stress. House and colleagues [19] report the immediate results of 41 patients receiving biofeedback training, 33 (80%) reported some degree of improvement, whereas 8 felt there had been no change in their tinnitus.

Suppression of Tinnitus by
Electrical Stimulation
Electrical stimulation seems to have been used at one time or another for almost every known malady affecting the human being. Thus, it is not surprising to find that Field [9] in 1893 reported the suppression of tinnitus during electrical stimulation of the ear. At the present time, Cazals [3] and Aran and Cazals [1] are engaged in the exploration of electrical stimulation as a relief procedure for tinnitus.

Aran's method is to deliver constant current square wave pulses between the ear and the ear lobe or mastoid. Electrodes are placed on the round window membrane or on the promontory and on the ear lobe or mastoid. The train of electrical pulses can be either only positive or only negative currents or alternating currents. The intensity of the current can be precisely controlled from 1 to 30 mA.

Aran has examined 106 patients who were profoundly deaf and who were candidates for a cochlear implant. Approximately 84 of these patients complained of tinnitus, and electrical stimulation was applied to see if tinnitus could be relieved. Several interesting findings have resulted.

1. Only positive currents (current flowing from promontory or round window electrode to the mastoid or ear lobe electrode) were capable of suppressing tinnitus. Negative currents were capable of producing an auditory experience that was perceived in addition to the tinnitus.
2. The intensity of current necessary for suppressing tinnitus varies considerably with each patient.
3. When a round window electrode was used, 60% of the patients experienced total suppression of the tinnitus. Use of a promontory electrode suppressed tinnitus in 43% of the patients, and only 25% of those experienced total suppression.
4. The suppression only lasts the duration of the electrical stimulation.
5. Alternating currents did not suppress tinnitus.
6. Electrical suppression is ineffective when the tinnitus appears to be the result of a central lesion. Also, it does not work in a contralateral arrangement, which means that bilateral tinnitus requires electrode arrangements for each ear to effect suppression of the tinnitus. One significant aspect is that properly applied electrical stimulation was able to suppress tinnitus in totally deaf patients.

The major problem with electrical suppression of tinnitus is tissue damage. Direct current is known to be capable of producing tissue damage. Alternating currents are much less likely to produce damage but, unfortunately, they do not suppress tinnitus [16]. It would appear that where there is no net transfer of electrons, the tinnitus is not suppressed. It is also the case that a net transfer of electrons is not always sufficient to suppress tinnitus, being effective in about 60% of Aran's patients.

House [20] reports that patients receiving cochlear implants that deliver electrical stimulation presumably to the remaining primary afferent fibers of the eighth nerve often experience relief of tinnitus. This kind of suppression does not appear to be a case of masking, because the relief usually does not appear until after the implant has been in use for a matter of weeks. Also, the cochlear implant uses an alternating current so that presumably there should be no net transfer of electrons. Thus, the cochlear implant may present a special case of tinnitus suppression using electrical stimulation. These findings strongly suggest the need for continued investigation of electrical stimulation for tinnitus suppression.

Drug Therapy for Tinnitus

Brown and associates [2] list over 100 drugs as producing tinnitus, of which about one half also produce hearing loss. Some of these drugs have been used as treatment for tinnitus. Understandably, many patients with severe tinnitus also experience mental depression. It is common to treat depression with tricyclic antidepressants, all of which list tinnitus as a side effect. Often, the treatment of depression increases the tinnitus, which in turn increases the depression.

One of the stronger claims of relief for tinnitus using drugs has come from Emmett and Shea [4, 5]. These investigators have treated patients with tocainide, which is an oral analogue of lidocaine. Their data provide encouragement for drug treatment of tinnitus. Prior to the use of tocainide, Shea and Emmett [35] reported an 82% incidence of relief of tinnitus using carbamazepine in a study of 27 patients. The present state of drug treatment for tinnitus is far from satisfactory, but there is little doubt that more effective agents will be found.

DESCRIPTION OF TINNITUS

We believe that a minimum of four different kinds of measures are necessary to properly describe tinnitus. They are (1) its pitch, (2) its loudness, (3) its maskability, and (4) the production of residual inhibition [46].

Pitch

It would seem a simple matter to present a variety of tones to the tinnitus patient, allowing him to select the one most similar to his tinnitus. Most patients confuse pitch and loudness, thus the first requirement for the comparison sound is that it be at the *same loudness as the tinnitus.* Seldom is it the case that a patient cannot reliably match the loudness of their tinnitus; even patients with complex tinnitus composed of several sounds at differing loudness levels can perform reliable loudness estimates. In most cases of severe tinnitus the tone is high pitched: as reported in a previous study [39], we found in approximately 80% of the patients with tinnitus, the pitch was between 2000 and 12,000 Hz.

If a random sample of audiometric tones is presented one at a time to the patient, he will usually be able to select a tone most like his tinnitus. The reliability of this procedure, however, is not good. Octave confusion occurs when the patient selects one tone matching the pitch of his tinnitus and that tone is usually one octave below the best match. Therefore, a test for octave confusion must be performed each time a patient selects a tone as a pitch match for his tinnitus.

Loudness
It was Fowler [11, 12] who first found that the sensation level (SL) that duplicated the loudness of the tinnitus was surprisingly low, usually on the order of 5 to 10 dB SL. Fowler's work was primarily done with the comparison tone at the tinnitus frequency, or perhaps an octave below it, since he did not test for octave confusion. We find two groups of patients according to loudness matching frequency independent and highly frequency specific. For the frequency independent, the same, and very low, sensation levels will be selected to match the tinnitus loudness, regardless of the frequency of the comparison tone. For the frequency specific, frequencies that are dissimilar to the tinnitus frequency effect a loudness match with the tinnitus. For this group, for example, a comparison tone at 500 Hz may require an SL of 50 to 55 dB to match the loudness of the tinnitus, which is at 8000 Hz. As the frequency of the comparison tones approaches the frequency of the tinnitus, the SL of the loudness match systematically reduces so that, in the previous example, it may be only 5 dB SL at 8000 Hz. Frequencies above the tinnitus frequency also tend to require a low SL to effect the loudness

match. With patients in this group the loudness match may tend to lead one into the identification of the tinnitus frequency [37].

Maskability
It is obvious that if a masking procedure is used as a relief for tinnitus, the maskability of the tinnitus should be quantified. Additionally, however, statements as to the maskability of tinnitus most certainly contribute to the description and understanding of tinnitus. Moreover, the information on maskability may eventually help select the treatment procedures as well as indicate underlying mechanisms.

The maskability of tinnitus has been investigated by Feldman [7], who used pulsed tones as the masking stimulus. We have investigated the maskability of tonal tinnitus using continuous tones [42].

In one study, we used the audiometric frequencies as masking tones measuring the minimal amount of sound required to just mask the tinnitus; this we call the minimum masking level (MML). Three groups of masking curves resulted.

Group I. All tones used were capable of masking the tinnitus at approximately the same sensation level, which was only 4 or 5 dB SL. Of the 32 patients studied, 12% fit into group I.

Group II. The amount of masking required for MML progressively increased as the frequency of the masking tone fell below that of the tinnitus, 52% of the patients fit into group II.

Group III. Masking was found to be independent of frequency as in group I, except that the amount of masking required was high, being in excess of 20 dB SL; 22% of the cases fit the group III pattern.

For 8% of the patients, no masking was possible regardless of intensity or frequency of the masking tone. It is of interest that these "unmaskable" patients were often those where the tinnitus was suspected to have been caused by head injury. The remaining 6% of the patients did not clearly or reliably fit any of the categories.

In our tinnitus clinic, we used the determination of maskability to help predict the outcome of masking as a relief procedure. We use a narrow band of noise centered at the tinnitus frequency as the masking sound and with it, measure the MML for the affected ear. If the MML is 5 dB or less, we predict that masking will work well. If MML is between 5 and 15 dB SL, we have doubts about a masking program, and if MML is 20 dB SL or more, then it is almost certain that masking as a relief procedure is inappropriate.

Production of Residual Inhibition
Residual inhibition is the temporary suppression or temporary cessation of tinnitus after removal of the masking sound. Residual inhibition, though not called by that name, was discovered by Spaulding in 1903 [36].

We have developed a standardized test of residual inhibition, using conditions that for the most part were arbitrarily chosen. For the masking sound, we use a tone at the tinnitus frequency and, additionally, a narrow band of noise centered at the tinnitus frequency. The masking sound is presented to the ipsilateral ear at MML plus 10 dB for 60 seconds. On cessation of the masking sound, the patient is required to estimate the magnitude of the residual inhibition using a visual analogue device that can be set at any position from 0 to 100%. In addition, the time required for recovery to the normal level of tinnitus is determined. As a general rule, this test can produce complete residual inhibition (tinnitus = 0%) lasting for about 25 to 30 seconds and partial residual inhibition of 15 to 20 seconds. There are many different patterns of residual inhibition, and we are only now beginning to understand some of the patterns.

Recently, we tested residual inhibition in 15 patients. The amount and duration of residual inhibition was measured after masking at MML plus 10 dB for 60 seconds, where many different frequencies were used as the masking tone [8]. Previously, we had thought that the instigation of residual inhibition was highly frequency specific, that is, we expected residual inhibition to result only when tones near the tinnitus frequency were used as maskers. As it turned out, however, such was

not the case. In a group of 12 patients, all with tonal tinnitus, 9 of them displayed residual inhibition at all the frequencies used as masking tones. For masking tones, we used the audiometric frequencies, plus the tinnitus frequency, and one-half octave below the tinnitus frequency. Only three patients displayed a decrease in residual inhibition as the frequency of the masking tone moved progressively away from the tinnitus frequency. Eight patients had greater than 80% residual inhibition at *all* test frequencies. There were five patients who displayed maximum residual inhibition at the tinnitus frequency and five whose maximum was at minus one-half octave. There were four patients who displayed such prolonged residual inhibition that it was necessary to discontinue testing until another day. From these data, we conclude that whatever specificity obtains for residual inhibition it is not necessarily a matter of frequency of the masking tone.

These findings, though far from conclusive, cause us to make the following generalizations about residual inhibition [40]:

1. It is clear that tinnitus can be temporarily turned off or repressed by proper manipulation of external sounds.
2. Most sounds that mask tinnitus also produce residual inhibition.
3. Residual inhibition tends to accumulate over time.
4. Residual inhibition is primarily ipsilateral. Contralateral residual inhibition does occur rarely.
5. Patients using hearing aids as effective maskers for their tinnitus do *not* experience residual inhibition after use of the hearing aid.
6. Residual inhibition can be used in some cases to dissect the tinnitus. For example, complex tinnitus composed of a tone and a noise can have the noise remain and the tone in residual inhibition by tonal masking, or the tone may remain and the noise in residual inhibition by noise masking.
7. When tinnitus is bilateral and one ear is placed in residual inhibition, the tinnitus in the other ear is often judged as

having increased in loudness. At this point, we do not know whether this is a contrast phenomenon or if the tinnitus actually increases.

8. In the case of tonal tinnitus, residual inhibition is better produced by tonal masking than by noise masking for most patients.

9. In our clinic, 78% of the patients demonstrate some form of residual inhibition; 35% display complete residual inhibition, and 43% display only partial residual inhibition.

REFERENCES

1. Aran, J.-M., and Cazals, Y. Electrical suppression of tinnitus. In D. Evered and G. Lawrenson (Eds.), *Tinnitus* (CIBA Symposium 85). London: Pitman Books, 1981.

2. Brown, D. R., et al. Ototoxic Drugs and Noise. In D. Evered and G. Lawrenson (Eds.), *Tinnitus* (CIBA Symposium 85). London: Pitman Books, 1981.

3. Cazals, Y., Negrevergne, M., and Aran, J.-M. Electrical stimulation of the cochlea in man: Hearing induction and tinnitus suppression. *J. Am. Audiol. Soc.* 3:209, 1978.

4. Emmett, J. R. Drugs in the Treatment of Tinnitus (discussion). In D. Evered and G. Lawrenson (Eds.), *Tinnitus* (CIBA Symposium 85). London: Pitman Books, 1981.

5. Emmett, J. R., and Shea, J. J. Treatment of tinnitus with tocainide hydrochloride. *Otolaryngol. Head Neck Surg.* 88:442, 1980.

6. Engler, C. W. Treatment of tinnitus. *J.A.M.A.* 163:615, 1956.

7. Feldmann, H. Homolateral and contralateral masking of tinnitus by noise-bands and pure tones. *Audiology* 10:138, 1971.

8. Fenwick, J. A., and Vernon, J. A. Frequency specificity for the production of residual inhibition in tonal tinnitus. In press, 1984.

9. Field, G. P. *A Manual of Diseases of the Ear.* London: Balliere, Tendall and Cox, 1893.

10. Flottorp, G., and Willie, C. Nicotinic acid treatment of tinnitus: A clinical-audiological examination. *Acta Otolaryngol.* [Suppl.] 118:85, 1955.

11. Fowler, E. P. The illusion of loudness of tinnitus—Its etiology and treatment. *Ann. Otol. Rhinol. Laryngol.* 52:275, 1942.

12. Fowler, E. P. Control of head noises: Their illusions of loudness and timbre. *Arch. Otolaryngol.* 37:391, 1943.

13. Goodey, R. J. Drugs in the Treatment of Tinnitus. In D. Evered and G. Lawrenson (Eds.), *Tinnitus* (CIBA Symposium 85). London: Pitman Books, 1981.

14. Goodey, R. J., Hutchinson, R., and Coddington, K. Masking, drugs and tinnitus. *N. Z. Med. J.*, 93:32, 1981.

15. Goodhill, V. A tinnitus identification test. *Ann. Otol. Rhinol. Laryngol.* 61:778, 1952.

16. Graham, J. M., and Hazell, J. W. P. Electrical stimulation of the human cochlea using a transtympanic electrode. *Br. J. Audiol.* 11:59, 1977.

17. Graham, J. T., and Newby, H. A. Acoustical characteristics of tinnitus: Analysis. *Arch. Otolaryngol.* 75:162, 1962.

18. House, J. W., Miller, L., and House, P. R. Severe tinnitus: Treatment with biofeedback training. *Trans. Am. Acad. Ophthal. Otolaryngol.* 84:697, 1977.

19. House, P. R. Personality of the Tinnitus Patient. In D. Evered and G. Lawrenson (Eds.), *Tinnitus* (CIBA Symposium Vol. 85). London: Pitman Books, 1981.

20. House, W. F. Cochlear implants. *Ann. Otol. Rhinol. Laryngol.* (Suppl.) 185:127, 1976.

21. Isono, H., et al. Some experience in the use of nicotinic acid in the treatment of tinnitus. *Otolaryngology* (Tokyo) 29:855, 1957.

22. Israel, J. M., et al. Lidocaine in the treatment of tinnitus aurium: A double-blind study. *Arch. Otolaryngol.* 108:471, 1982.

23. Jones, I. H., and Knudsen, V. O. Certain aspects of tinnitus, particularly treatment. *Laryngoscope* 38:597, 1928.

24. Kafka, M. M. Tinnitus aurium: Etiology, differential diagnosis, treatment and review of 25 cases. *Laryngoscope* 44:515, 1934.

25. Kemp, D. T. Stimulated acoustic emissions from within the human auditory system. *J. Acoust. Soc. Am.* 64:1386, 1978.

26. Kemp, D. T. Physiologically Active Cochlear Mechanisms—One Source of Tinnitus. In D. Evered and G. Lawrenson (Eds.), *Tinnitus* (CIBA Symposium Vol. 85). London: Pitman Books, 1981.

27. Lewy, R. Treatment of tinnitus aurium by the intravenous use of local anesthetic agents. *Arch. Otolaryngol.* 25:178, 1937.

28. Melding, P. S., and Goodey, R. J. The treatment of tinnitus with anticonvulsants. *J. Laryngol. Otol.* 93:111, 1979.

29. Melding, P. S., Goodey, R. J., and Thorne, P. R. The use of intravenous lignocaine in the diagnosis and treatment of tinnitus. *J. Laryngol. Otol.* 92:115, 1978.

30. Nodar, R., and Graham, J. T. An investigation of frequency characteristics of tinnitus associated with Meniere's disease. *Arch. Otolaryngol.* 82:28, 1965.

31. Reed, G. F. An audiometric study of two

hundred cases of subjective tinnitus. *Arch. Otolaryngol.* 71:94, 1960.

32. Saltzman, M. Tinnitus aurium in otosclerosis. *Arch. Otolaryngol.* 50:440, 1949.

33. Saltzman, M., and Ersner, M. S. A hearing aid for the relief of tinnitus aurium. *Laryngoscope* 57:358, 1947.

34. Schleuning, A. J., Johnson, R. M., and Vernon, J. A. Evaluation of a tinnitus masking program: A follow-up study of 598 patients. *Ear Hear.* 1:71, 1980.

35. Shea, J. J., and Emmett, J. R. The Medical Treatment of Tinnitus. In M. M. Paparella and W. L. Meyerhoff (Eds.), *Sensorineural Hearing Loss, Vertigo and Tinnitus.* Baltimore: Williams & Wilkins, 1981.

36. Spaulding, A. J. Tinnitus with a plea for its more accurate musical notation. *Arch. Otolaryngol.* 32:263, 1903.

37. Vernon, J. A. The loudness(?) of tinnitus. *Hear. Speech Action* 44:17, 1976.

38. Vernon, J. A. The other hearing problem produced by excessive noise exposure. *Natl. Safety Conf. Trans.* 21:21, 1977.

39. Vernon, J. A. Information from UOHSC tinnitus clinic. *ATA Newsletter* 3:14, 1978.

40. Vernon, J. A. Some Observations on Residual Inhibition. In M. M. Paparella and W. L. Meyerhoff (Eds.), *Sensorineural Hearing Loss, Vertigo and Tinnitus.* Baltimore: Williams & Wilkins, 1981.

41. Vernon, J. A., Johnson, R. M., and Schleuning, A. J. The characteristics and natural history of tinnitus in Meniere's disease. *Otolaryngol. Clin. North Am.* 13:611, 1980.

42. Vernon, J. A., and Meikle, M. B. Tinnitus Masking: Unresolved Problems. In D. Evered and G. Lawrenson (Eds.), *Tinnitus* (CIBA Symposium Vol. 85). London: Pitman Books, 1981.

43. Vernon, J. A., and Schleuning, A. J. Tinnitus: Treatment and management. *Laryngoscope* 88:413, 1978.

44. Wilson, J. P., and Sutton, G. J. Acoustic Correlates of Tonal Tinnitus. In D. Evered and G. Lawrenson (Eds.), *Tinnitus* (CIBA Symposium Vol. 85). London: Pitman Books, 1981.

45. Zurek, P. M. Spontaneous narrow-band acoustic signals emitted by human ears. *J. Acoust. Soc. Am.* 69:514, 1981.

46. Zwicker, E., and Jaroszewski, A. Inverse frequency dependence of simultaneous tone-on-tone masking patterns at low levels. *J. Acoust. Soc. Am.* 71:1508, 1982.

Appendix

Programmed Instruction in the Decibel

Charles I. Berlin

To study the decibel, you must first review something about the logarithm. Logarithms are simply exponents, and you know what an exponent is; in the expression $10^2 = 100$, the 2 is an exponent.

exponent

(1) In the expression $10^2 = 100$, the 2 is an _____.

exponent

(2) We have said that a logarithm is an _____.

logarithm

(3) Therefore, the number 2 in the expression $10^2 = 100$ is both an exponent and a _____.

The exponent or logarithm above the number 10 tells us how many times to use the ten in multiplication. Thus, 10^2 means the same as 10×10 or 100.

multiplication

(4) The expression 10^3 means use the number 10 three times in _____.

ten, multiplication

(5) The expression 10^4 means use the number _____ four times in _____.

6

(6) The expression $10^{—}$ means use the number 10 six times in multiplication.

10, 10, 10

(7) The expression 10^3 means the same as _____ × _____ × _____, or 1,000.

$10 \times 10 \times 10 \times 10 \times 10$ or 100,000

(8) The expression 10^5 means the same as _____.

(9) In the expression 10^5 the number 10 is called the base, while the number 5 is the

This is a revised and expanded version of "Programmed Learning on the Decibel," which originally appeared in the *Maryland Journal of Speech and Hearing* 11(1):5, 1963.

The decibel work was supported by NINDB Research Career Development Award 5K3-NB 19,488, and by the Information Center for Hearing, Speech, and Disorders of Human Communication, a part of the Neurological Information Network of the National Institute of Neurological Diseases and Blindness, supported under contract No. PH 43-65-23.

logarithm
multiplication

exponent or _____, which tells you how many times to use the base in _____.

(10) In the expression 4^3 and 10^3 the exponents are the same (the number three) but the bases are _____ and 10 respectively.

4

(11) If 10^3 means $10 \times 10 \times 10$, then 4^3 must mean _____ $\times$ _____ $\times$ _____.

4, 4, 4

(12) In the expression 10^6, we mean use the number _____ (how many) _____ times in multiplication.

10   6

(13) Thus, $10^6 =$ (whole number) _____.

1,000,000

(14) And $10^4 =$ (whole number) _____.

10,000

(15) The number 1,000 can be expressed as 10^-.

3

(16) The logarithm in the expression 10^4 is the number _____, while the base is the number _____.

4
10

(17) $10^2 =$ _____.

100

(18) The logarithm of 100 is _____.

2

(19) $10^3 = 1,000$, which can be expressed as the log of 1,000 is _____.

3

(20) The log of 10,000 is _____.

4

You may have noticed that when the base is 10, the exponent tells you how many zeroes appear after the number 1. Thus, 10^2 is the number 1 followed by two zeroes, or 100. The expression 10^4 is the number 1 followed by four zeroes or 10,000.

In dealing with decibels, the base we will be concerned with will always be 10. When we ask, "What is the logarithm of 100," for example, we mean, "What is the logarithm *to the base 10?"*___

(21) 10^9 is the number 1 followed by _____ zeroes, or the whole number _____.

9
1,000,000,000

(22) It follows then that $10^1 =$ _____ and $10^0 = 1$.*

10

* Items 21 and 22 show techniques for helping you remember that the log of 1 is 0. Mathematically, *any number* with an exponent of zero will equal one. Here's why: When you multiply numbers such

It is very important to the concept of the decibel to remember that the *logarithm of 1 is zero.*

1	0
0	

(23) $10^0 =$ _____ . $10^{—} = 1$. The log of 1 is _____ .

logarithm

(24) The _____ of 1 is zero.

3	
3	

(25) The log of 1,000 is _____ . This is the same as $10^{—} = 1,000$.

2	
2	

(26) The log of 100 is _____ . This is the same as $10^{—} = 100$.

1	
1	

(27) The log of 10 is _____ . This is the same as $10^{—} = 10$.

0	
0	

(28) The log of 1 is _____ . This is the same as $10^{—} = 1$.

1

(29) The log of _____ is zero.

We must also review a bit about ratios. If we divide a number by itself, as in 198/198, we get a ratio of 1. If we divide 3,456 by 3,456, we still get a ratio of 1. If we divide 0.05 by 0.05, we still get a ratio of 1.

1

(30) If we divide 0.0002 by 0.0002, we get a ratio of _____ .

1

(31) Regardless of the magnitude of the number, any number divided by itself equals _____ .

10	1

(32) $0.002/0.0002 =$ _____ or $10^{—}$.

100	2

(33) $0.02/0.0002 =$ or $10^{—}$.

10,000	4

(34) $2/0.0002 =$ _____ or $10^{—}$.

1	0

(35) $0.0002/0.0002 =$ _____ or $10^{—}$.

---

as $10^4 \times 10^4$, you add the exponents and get 10^8. This is expressed as:

$$10^4 \times 10^4 = 10^{4+4} \text{ or } 10^8$$

When you divide such numbers, you *subtract* exponents, like this:

$$10^4/10^3 = 10^{4-3} \text{ or } 10^1$$

Now suppose we divide a number by itself like this: $10^8/10^8$. Regardless of the magnitude of the numbers, the answer is *always* 1. But we said when we divide numbers we subtract the exponents, so $10^8/10^8 = 10^{8-8}$ or 10^0; but, since to get 10^0 we have divided 10 by itself and arrived at 1, clearly 10^0 equals 1 just as readily as $10^8/10^8 = 1$.

THE DECIBEL IN MEASUREMENTS FROM A POWER REFERENCE

Study the following equation:

Number of decibels $= 10 \times \log (W_O/W_R)$
$W_O =$ watts per cm² (power) output, and
$W_R =$ watts per cm² (power) reference.

output

(36) $W_O =$ watts per cm² power _____,
and $W_R =$ watts per cm² power reference.

(37) $W_O =$ watts per cm² power output,
whereas $W_R =$ watts per cm² power _____.

reference

watts per cm² power output

(38) $W_O =$ _____.

watts per cm² power reference

(39) $W_R =$ _____.

To solve the equation, first find the numerical value of W_O/W_R. This is a ratio.

(40) If $W_O = 100$ and $W_R = 0.1$, then the
1,000   ratio = _____.

(41) If $W_O = 1,000$ and $W_R = 1,000$, then
1   the ratio = _____.

If your mathematics is sufficiently advanced to permit you to answer Item 42, you may then skip to Item 54.

(42) If $W_O = 10^{-12}$ and $W_R = 10^{-16}$, then
10^4 the ratio of W_O/W_R is 10,000 or _____.

If you could not answer Item 42, you must read the next section before you can go on; otherwise, go to Item 54.

The numbers such as the 3 in 10^3, called logarithms or exponents, tell you how many times to use the base 10 as a factor in multiplication. The exponents with a *minus* sign before them, such as the -3 in 10^{-3} tell you how many times to use the base *in division*, like this:

If $10^3 = 10 \times 10 \times 10$, then $10^{-3} = 1/10 \times 10 \times 10$ or $1 / 1,000$ or 0.001.

(43) If 10^4 means $10 \times 10 \times 10 \times 10$, then
$1/10 \times 10 \times 10 \times 10$ or 0.0001 or 10^{-4} means _____.
    1/10,000

These exponents are basic to what is called scientific notation, a language that will be clarified in a later program. If 10^4 means 10,000, then 10^{-4} means $1/10,000$.

Now you recall from the footnote on page 307 that when you multiply numbers such as $10^4 \times 10^8$, you *add* the exponents like this: 10^{4+8}, or 10^{12}. If you were to divide 10^8 by 10^3, as in this expression: $10^8 / 10^3$, you *subtract the exponent like this:* 10^{8-3}, or 10^5.

Try these:

(44) $10^7 \times 10^3 = $ _____ .

10^{10}

If you got that correct, you successfully multiplied 10 million by 1,000 to get an answer of 10 billion or 10,000,000,000, which is more simply expressed as 10^{10}.

10^8

(45) $10^6 \times 10^2 = $ _____ .

10^5

(46) $10^8 / 10^3 = $ _____ .

Now the next is a critical item:

10^{-3}

(47) $10^8 / 10^{11} = $ _____ .

That was a difficult frame. It teaches that the subtraction of the exponents requires that the lower figure (the denominator) be subtracted from the upper figure (the numerator) *regardless of which number is larger*

10^{-2}

(48) $10^3 / 10^5 = $ _____ .

10^{-13}

(49) $10^4 / 10^{17} = $ _____ .

10^{-1}

(50) $10^{-8} / 10^{-7} = $ _____ .

10^1

(51) $10^{-4} / 10^{-5} = $ _____ .

If you correctly answered Item 51, you knew that when you subtract numbers that are preceded by a minus sign, you essentially do this: $(-4) - (-5) = (-4) + 5$ or 1.

10^4

(52) $10^{-5} / 10^{-9} = $ _____ .

10^4

(53) $10^{-12} / 10^{-16} = $ _____ .

If you answered this item correctly, you have learned Item 42, which stopped you before. You may recall the item said: If $W_O = 10^{-12}$ and $W_R = 10^{-16}$, then the ratio is 10^4 or 10,000.

If you did not answer Item 53 correctly, go back to Item 43 and begin again.

If you missed Item 53 a second time, stop working on the program and see your mentor. Be sure this mathematical hurdle is cleared before you try to go any farther.

You recall we said that $W_O / W_R = 10^{-12}$ watt per $cm^2 / 10^{-16}$ watt per cm^2, or 10,000.

10

40

130

1

0

0

0

equal

1
0
0   0

(54) Then we multiply the log of 10,000 by _____ as in $10 \times \log 10{,}000$.

Remember that when we use numbers such at 10^4 or 10^2, the exponents are the logarithms; but if we used the numbers 10,000 or 100, we would have to find their logarithms before we could multiply them by 10.

(55) Thus, when $W_O = 10^{-12}$ and $W_R = 10^{-16}$, the decibel output with regard to the reference is $10 \times \log (W_O / W_R)$ or _____ decibels.

(56) If W_O is 10^{-3} and the reference is 10^{-16} watt per cm², then the decibel output with regard to the reference is _____ decibels.

Physicists and engineers have settled on an Intensity Level Reference of 10^{-16} watt per cm². We will use a reference of 10^{-16} watt per cm² when we talk about references from which to make Intensity Level (IL) measurements.

(57) If $W_O = 10^{-16}$ and W_R also $= 10^{-16}$, then the ratio of W_O over W_R is _____.

We have now come to one of the most critical parts of this program.

(58) When $W_O = W_R$ as in the case of $W_O = 10^{-16}$ and $W_R = 10^{-16}$, the ratio of the reference to the output is 1; but the logarithm of 1 is *zero*, therefore, the decibel output with regard to the reference is _____ dB.

(59) If the ratio between W_O and W_R equals 1, and we know that the logarithm of one equals _____, then the decibel output with regard to the reference is also _____ dB.

Thus, 0 dB does *not mean* silence, or absence of sound or absence of power, nor does it mean very faint sound or power. *It simply means that the power output of the system is exactly* _____ to the reference from which the decibel measurement is started.

(60) When $W_O = W_R$, the ratio is _____, the logarithm of 1 is _____, and $10 \times$ _____ = _____ dB.

(61) For example, if we chose as our reference point (or W_R) the value 100 watts

power
output
1

0

0

per cm², and W_O or (2 words) _____ _____ is also 100 watts per cm², the ratio of W_O/W_R would still equal _____, the logarithm of that ratio would still be _____, and the resultant decibel output *with regard to this new and different reference would still be* _____ dB.

Thus, either 10^{-16} watt per cm² or 100 watts per cm² can equal 0 dB, if they are chosen as references from which to make other measurements. It is quite permissible to choose any reference point from which to make a dB measurement. In fact, strictly speaking, every decibel measurement is a *decibel difference from 0 or decibel difference with regard to the reference from which the measurement was made.*

reference

(62) The word *decibel* alone implies no fixed dimension of its own because the _____ from which it is measured can be any value the experimenter chooses.

It is critical, therefore, to know the references from which various decibel measurements are made. The most common reference for measuring acoustic intensity differences, when the variable is *power,* is 10^{-16} watt per cm². Decibels described by the equation $10 \times \log W_O/W_R$ are expressed as dB IL or *decibels Intensity Level.*

$10 \times \log W_O/W_R$

70

(63) If you must calculate the number of decibels a 10^{-9} watt per cm² power will generate, the equation to use is: _____, and the dB re 10^{-16} watt per cm² is _____.

10^{-16}

(64) The most common and most likely reference point from which this measurement will be made is _____ watt per cm².

(65) However, if the reference were 10^{-12} watt per cm², a 10^{-9} watt per cm² signal will be only _____ dB.

30

(66) All that is required of the reporter in describing his decibel is that he *always specify the* _____.

reference

(67) When you see the phrase dB IL or dB intensity level, it usually means that the reference was _____ watt per cm².

10^{-16}

Henceforth, let us assume a reference of 10^{-16} watt per cm² equals zero dB IL.

120

10

20

30

60

base

10

(68) If the power output is 10^{-4} watt per cm², dB = _____.

(69) When $W_O = 10^{-15}$, dB = _____.

(70) When $W_O = 10^{-14}$, dB = _____.

(71) When $W_O = 10^{-13}$, dB = _____.

(72) When $W_O = 10^{-10}$, dB = _____.

Notice that as the power is *multiplied by 10*, the dB output simply increases *additively by units of 10*. Thus, the power required to move from 0 dB to 60 dB is *not sixty units* greater than 10^{-16} watt per cm², but 10^6 or 1,000,000 times greater than 10^{-16} watt per cm². For your own use, construct a table like this:

Power Measurements
dB = $10 \times \log W_O/W_R$, where
$W_R = 10^{-16}$ watt per cm²

Watts per cm² (W$_O$) output	(W$_O$/W$_R$) Ratio	Log	dB
10^{-16}	1	0	0
10^{-15}	10	1	10
10^{-14}	100	2	20
10^{-13}	1,000	3	30
10^{-12}	—	—	—

THE DECIBEL IN MEASUREMENTS FROM A PRESSURE REFERENCE

In acoustics we make pressure measurements more often than power measurements so we should know how to convert powers to pressures. Scientists have known for many years that powers (watts) and pressures (dynes) have a special relationship. *Sound pressure* ratios are usually proportional to the square root of corresponding power ratios, or *power : pressure²*.

(73) The exponent is a number that tells you how many times to use the _____ in multiplication.

(74) If we start with: dB (power) = _____ $\times \log W_O/W_R$, and we say that to make power figures proportional to pressure, we must square the pressures:

$$dB = 10 \times \log \frac{(P_O)^2 \text{ (now a pressure output)}}{(P_R)^2 \text{ (now a pressure reference)}}$$

When we square a number we multiply its

logarithm by 2, and we can rewrite the equation in this way:

$$dB \text{ (pressure)} = 10 \times 2 \times \log \frac{\text{pressure output}}{\text{pressure reference}}$$

Therefore

20

(75) $dB = \underline{\hspace{2cm}} \times \log \dfrac{P_O \text{ (pressure output)}}{P_R \text{ (pressure reference)}}$

Now we have obtained the equation for the decibel when the reference is in terms of sound pressures, instead of powers.

log

(76) No. $dB = 20 \times \underline{\hspace{2cm}} P_O/P_R$ where $P_O = $ pressure output and $R_R = $ pressure reference.

20

(77) No. dB (from a pressure reference) = $\underline{\hspace{2cm}} \times \log P_O/P_R$.

reference

(78) In this equation $P_O = $ pressure output from a phone or speaker, while $P_R = $ pressure $\underline{\hspace{2cm}}$.

output

(79) $P_R = $ pressure reference, while $P_O = $ pressure $\underline{\hspace{2cm}}$.

pressure
pressure reference

(80) $P_O = \underline{\hspace{2cm}}$ output, while $P_R = $ (2 words) $\underline{\hspace{2cm}}$ $\underline{\hspace{2cm}}$.

(81) To solve the equation $dB = 20 \times \log P_O/P_R$, we must first find the numerical value of the ratio expressed by P_O divided by $\underline{\hspace{2cm}}$.

P_R

logarithm

(82) Then we find the $\underline{\hspace{2cm}}$ of that value.

ratio

(83) Note that *first* we must find the numerical value of the $\underline{\hspace{2cm}}$ expressed by P_O/P_R.

logarithm

(84) *Then* we find the $\underline{\hspace{2cm}}$ of that value.

multiply

(85) The next step is to $\underline{\hspace{2cm}}$ the logarithm by 20.

P_R
0

(86) If the ratio between P_O and P_R is 1, that is, where $P_O = \underline{\hspace{2cm}}$, we obtain a logarithm of $\underline{\hspace{2cm}}$.

0

(87) If the logarithm then is 0, the entire equation yields a value of $\underline{\hspace{2cm}}$ dB for the pressure reference.

(88) Note again that *0 does not mean silence, or absence of sound, or the faintest level at which a sound can be heard, or any modification of such verbal conve-*

equal

P_0

2
40

3
20

log   6

2

L

0.0002 dyne per cm²

S

SPL

0.0002 dyne per cm²

watt

20
0.0002 dyne per cm²

niences; 0 dB simply means that the output of our speaker or phone is exactly _____ to the reference pressure we have chosen.

(89) Should we change the ratio of _____ over P_R to a ratio of 100, then, because the log of 100 is _____, we would get 20×2 = _____ dB.

(90) Suppose the output pressure then became 1,000 times as great as the reference pressure; the logarithm of 1,000 is _____ and thus we have _____ $\times 3 = 60$ dB.

(91) Suppose the output pressure is set at 1,000,000 times the reference pressure; the _____ of 1,000,000 is _____ and the resultant decibel value is 120 dB.

For various practical and historical reasons, acoustic scientists most often use 0.0002 dyne per cm² as a reference from which to measure sound pressure levels.

(92) Sound pressure level measurements in decibels are often based on 0.000 _____ dyne per cm².

(93) Sound pressure level is logically abbreviated SP _____.

(94) Thus, if you read a research paper in which the signals were given at 65 dB SPL, it means that the reference pressure was _____.

(95) A signal presented at 40 dB _____ PL has as its reference 0.0002 dyne per cm².

(96) Thus, the abbreviation (3 letters) _____ _____ _____ means specifically *s*ound *p*ressure *l*evel, and tells you that the reference from which the dB was specified was _____.

(97) Remember that 60 dB SPL has as its reference 0.0002 dyne per cm², while 60 dB IL has as its reference 10^{-16} _____ per cm².

You have already constructed a table for power ratios and decibel measurements using the equation $10 \times \log W_0/W_R$. Now do the same thing for pressure ratios using 0.0002 dyne per cm² as a reference. We will start for you:

Pressure Measurements
(98) dB = _____ $\times \log P_0/P_R$ where P_R = (numbers) _____.

Dyne per cm^2 output (P_O)	Pressure ratio (P_O/P_R)	Log	dB
0.0002	1	0	0
0.002	10	1	20
0.02	100	2	40
0.2	1,000	3	60

and so forth. You may add figures up to 140 dB. When you compare the table for power measurements (p. 312) with the table for pressure measurements, *note* that power and pressure are in a constant ratio to one another. When power is increased by a factor of 100, there is a 20 dB increase; however, a 100 times increase in power only generates a 10 times increase in pressure since *power : pressure²*. Increasing pressure by 10 *still* generates the 20 dB difference, just as a 100 times increase in power generates the same 20 dB difference because of the relationship of power to pressure.

Now let us review.

Decibels are ratios expressed as logarithmic numbers, so we must understand the logarithm to understand the decibel.

3

(99) The log of 1,000 is _____.

3

(100) This means that to obtain a numerical value of 1,000 you use the base (which is the number 10) _____ times in multiplication.

1

(101) The log of 10 is _____.

1,000

(102) The log of _____ is 3.

100

(103) The log of _____ is 2.

10

(104) The log of _____ is 1.

1

(105) The log of _____ is 0.

no. dB = 10 × log W$_O$/W$_R$

(106) When we use a *power reference,* our equation for determining the number of decibels reads _____.

no. dB = 20 × log P$_O$/P$_R$

(107) When we use a *pressure reference* for determining decibels, our equation reads _____.

(108) When P$_O$/P$_R$ is 1 (that is, when the output pressure is the same as the reference pressure), we have a log value of

0

_____.

reference

(109) Therefore, 0 dB is obtained when the pressure (or power) output equals the pressure (or power) _____.

10^{-16}

0.0002 dyne

(110) In the measurement of acoustic powers, the reference point used is _____ watt per cm².

(111) In measuring sound pressure levels, the P_R chosen is _____ per cm².

THE DECIBEL AND ITS USE IN CLINICAL AUDIOMETRY

The decibel, as you have learned, is always measured from an arbitrary reference. Occasionally in the literature you will see as reference points dB re: 1 microbar or 1 dyne per cm², or dB re: 1 volt or 1 millivolt. These are all different from 0.0002 dyne per cm² or 10^{-16} watt per cm², and must be so interpreted.

We shall now learn about still another kind of decibel reference.

10^{-16} watt per cm²

0.0002 dyne per cm²

(112) When you see dB IL, you know the reference was _____.

(113) When you see dB SPL, you know that the reference was _____.

You will now learn what the dB *Hearing Level* or HL uses as its reference.

Hearing
Level

(114) dB means decibel _____ _____.

The decibel hearing level uses as its reference the sensitivity of the normal human ear at various frequencies. As you know, the human ear needs more sound pressure to hear a 250 Hz tone than it needs to hear a 1000 Hz tone.

0.0002

(115) The following table shows the sound pressure re: _____ dyne per cm² necessary to reach the normal human ear's threshold (according to ASA 1951 standard).

Frequency and Sound Pressure Combinations, Considered to Be the Standard for Normal Hearing According to the 1951 ASA Standard (in a Standard Coupler)

Frequency (Hz)	dB SPL (0.0002 dyne per cm²)
125	54.5
250	39.6
500	24.3
1000	16.7
2000	17.0
4000	15.1
8000	20.9

54.5

1,000

39.6

15.1

more

22.9

17.0

SPL or re: 0.0002 dyne per cm²

102

109.3

(116) This table tells you that the normal listener needs _____ dB SPL to report hearing a 125 Hz tone.

(117) But this normal listener needs only 16.7 dB SPL to report hearing a _____ Hz tone.

(118) The table says that _____ dB is required to reach our hypothetical normal listener's threshold at 250 Hz, but only _____ dB SPL is needed to hear 4000 Hz.

(119) Thus, you need (more or less?) _____ sound pressure to make a 250 Hz tone audible than is needed to make a 1000 Hz tone audible.

(120) Obviously, you need more sound pressure to make the 250 Hz tone audible; in fact, you need _____ dB more pressure than is needed to make the 1000 Hz tone audible.

If you believed that 0 dB HL (that is, 0 dB setting on the audiometer) meant that at all frequency settings the audiometer generated the same sound pressure, you can see now why you were mistaken. The previous table shows that different sound pressures are needed at each frequency to reach human threshold. The figures on this table are the pressure references for 0 dB HL. *Thus, each figure given on the table equals 0 dB HL* at the specified frequency. If you increase the dB HL output by 10 dB, each pressure output increases by 10 dB.

(121) If you had a clinical audiometer in front of you that was calibrated to the ASA 1951 standard, and it was set to 2000 Hz, 0 dB HL, you would be generating _____ dB SPL.

(122) Now leaving the frequency at 2000 Hz, if you turned the HL dial to 40 dB you would be generating 57 dB _____.

(123) With the frequency selector still at 2000 Hz, turn the HL dial to 85 dB. You are now generating _____ dB SPL.

(124) Now leave the HL dial at 85 dB and change the frequency to 500 Hz. You are now generating _____ dB SPL.

(125) With the settings of 500 Hz and 85 dB HL and 2000 Hz and 85 dB HL, both

normal

10^{-16} watt per cm²

0.0002 dyne per cm²

normal

frequency

20

SL

SL

30

−40 dB

10^{-16} watt per cm²

0.0002 dyne per cm²

normal

signals are the same level above normal human hearing. Thus, the reference for calculating dB HL is _____ human hearing.

(126) You have now learned three notations that tell about the reference from which decibels are often calculated: dB IL means that the reference was _____.

(127) dB SPL means that the reference was _____.

(128) dB HL means that the reference was the sound pressure necessary for a _____ human listener just to perceive tones of various frequencies. The sound pressure reference for 0 dB HL *varies with* _____.

Now you will learn about one more set of letters that often follow the term dB.

(129) If a person has a 40 dB *hearing* level, and you present a tone to him at 60 dB HL, he is getting a tone _____ dB above his threshold, or 20 dB *Sensation Level* (SL).

(130) Thus, if a man has a 25 dB HL and is receiving a 40 dB HL tone, he is receiving a 15 dB (abbreviate) _____ tone.

(131) If a man has normal hearing, that is, 0 dB HL at all frequencies, all tones at 20 dB HL also are at 20 dB _____ to him.

(132) But if he has −10 dB HL hearing, then the same 20 dB HL tones are at _____ dB SL to him. If he had a 60 dB HL, the 20 dB HL tone would be at _____ SL.

So you see that there is also a decibel, the reference for which is the person's own hearing. This is the decibel *sensation level,* or dB SL.

(133) Now we have four modifying abbreviations that follow the letters "dB," which must be reviewed:

dB IL means that the reference was _____.

dB SPL means that the reference was _____.

dB HL means that the reference was the sound pressure necessary for a _____ human listener to hear tones of various

frequency

person's

frequencies. This reference changes with the _____ of the tone.

dB SL means that the reference was the _____ own threshold.

A NOTE ON LOUDNESS VS INTENSITY

Notice that you have also clarified the difference between intensity and loudness. A 125 Hz tone of 25 dB SPL has notable intensity re: 0.0002 dyne per cm², but no loudness to the average normal listener. On the other hand, a 1000 Hz tone of 25 dB SPL would have both intensity and loudness to a normal listener. *However, do not speak of the decibel as an index of loudness.* Loudness grows in quite a different way from sound pressure; other means of measuring loudness (magnitude estimation, sones, phons, noys, etc.) are needed, and the decibel is not appropriate.

ACKNOWLEDGMENTS

The author's appreciation goes to his students and colleagues who helped with previous versions, especially to Dr. Dixon Ward, who deleted critical errors and made clarifications. Thanks also go to Drs. Richard Riedman, Jack Katz, S. Thomas Elder, John Black, Victor Garwood, Joseph Chaiklin, William G. Hardy, Moise Goldstein, Henry Mark, and to Jack Cullen and Robert Daly. Special thanks are due to Lois Lunin and Drs. John Bordley and Francis Catlin and the staff of the information center for their kind assistance and encouragement in developing the decibel program. Editorial and production matters related to the decibel program were handled by Dr. Carl Thompson, who deserves special appreciation for his diligence. He and Gae Decker were responsible for this format and improved readability.

Index

Index